D0202573

Basic Pharmacology and Clinical Drug Use in Dentistry

For Churchill Livingstone

Commissioning Editor Mike Parkinson
Project Controller Nancy Arnott
Copy Editor Julie Gorman
Sales Promotion Executive Duncan Jones

Basic Pharmacology and Clinical Drug Use in Dentistry

R. A. Cawson MD(Lond) BDS FDS RCPS (Glasg) FRCPath
Emeritus Professor of Oral Medicine and Pathology in the University of London, Guy's Campus, United Medical & Dental Schools, London, UK;
Visiting Professor, Baylor University Medical Center and Dental College, Dallas, Texas, USA

R. G. Spector MD PhD FRCP FRCPath
Emeritus Professor of Applied Pharmacology, Guy's Campus, United Medical & Dental Schools, London, UK

Ann M. Skelly MDS (Lond) FDS RCPS (Glasg)
Senior Lecturer/Consultant in Dental Sedation, Guy's Campus, United Medical & Dental Schools, London, UK

SIXTH EDITION

CHURCHILL LIVINGSTONE
EDINBURGH HONG KONG LONDON MADRID MELBOURNE NEW YORK AND TOKYO 1995

CHURCHILL LIVINGSTONE
Medical Division of Longman Group Limited

Distributed in the United States of America by Churchill Livingstone Inc., 650 Avenue of the Americas, New York, N.Y. 10011, and by associated companies, branches and representatives throughout the world.

First edition 1975
Second edition 1978
Third edition 1982
Fourth edition 1985
Fifth edition 1987
Sixth edition 1995

ISBN 0 443 05107 0

British Library Cataloguing in Publication Data
A catalogue record for this book is available from the British Library.

Library of Congress Cataloging in Publication Data
A catalog record for this book is available from the Library of Congress.

Produced by Longman Singapore Publishers (Pte) Ltd.
Printed in Singapore

The publisher's policy is to use **paper manufactured from sustainable forests**

Contents

Preface

The teaching of pharmacology and therapeutics to dental students is a subject which often provokes strong feelings among those who are involved with it, and even more among those who are not. Traditionally, many have regarded pharmacology as largely irrelevant to dentistry, even though most dentists are administering potent drugs – especially local anaesthetics – many times every working day. Dental teachers also tend to forget that they practise their craft in an unusually sheltered environment. When anything goes wrong – if, for instance, the patient is tactless enough to have a heart attack – experts are called in and the matter is dealt with. Students perhaps do not always appreciate that, once qualified and in practice, they are quite on their own and considerably more vulnerable to the slings and arrows of outrageous fortune.

This problem has been emphasised by the 1990 Report of the Expert Working Party on General Anaesthesia, Sedation and Resuscitation in Dentistry. Among other matters, the Report advised that since a patient can unexpectedly collapse at any time, dentists must be aware of any current medication taken by the patient and be fully competent in resuscitation techniques. To this end the Working Party listed no fewer than 15 drugs and 2 infusion solutions, 'which should be available in *every* dental practice'. Coroners and lawyers supporting medicolegal claims pay considerable attention to such recommendations. It follows, therefore, that dentists must take them seriously and understand how drugs should be used. This is particularly important, because some drugs, if not given appropriately, can be dangerous and potentially lethal.

Thus, there is growing pressure on the dental profession to acquire some knowledge of drugs and how they should be used. Quite apart from their duty to protect their patients, dentists would be wise to arm themselves as best they can against possible medicolegal complications.

In view also of the greater emphasis on basic science, this book has been organised to meet both the needs of dental teaching and of providing an adequate background for drug use in general practice. The first section is therefore devoted to the scientific aspects of pharmacology and how drugs act on the various body systems. At the same time the relevance of this information to dental practice is made clear. The second section deals with drugs of special importance in dentistry. The information provided should also be more than adequate for those seeking higher qualifications.

Since a brave attempt has been made to keep the text as short as possible, no suggestions have been made as to further reading. Pharmacology is so rapidly advancing a subject that the British National Formulary has to be revised every 6 months and it is more appropriate that teachers should keep their students advised about up-to-date further reading.

Change has been forced upon us too and the advances in pharmacology and its teaching have made yet another edition of this book necessary.

London, 1995

R.A.C.
R.G.S.
A.M.S

Acknowledgements

I am most grateful to Mr Sidney Luck for his unstinting help in finding the relevant literature, to Mr Peter Erridge *MBE* DGPDS RCS, Director of the Special Needs Department, for his expert advice on cross-infection control and to Mrs Anne Prasad FRPharmS for her invaluable comments on management of emergencies. I also take this opportunity to express again my gratitude for the great kindness shown to me by Professor Lord Ian McColl, Director of Surgery at Guy's Hospital, for allowing me to work in his distinguished department.

R.A.C.

Publisher's note

Some illustrations have been reproduced from:

Sacks S, Spector R 1993 Aids to pharmacology, 3rd edn.
Rees J, Ritter J, Spector R 1993 Aids to clinical pharmacology and therapeutics, 3rd edn.

Both books are published by Churchill Livingstone, Edinburgh.

SECTION 1

Basic pharmacology

1. Drugs: an introduction

Pharmacology is the study of drugs. Pharmacologists investigate the actions of drugs in vitro, on animals and less frequently on humans. Indeed a pharmacologist may spend a lifetime studying the effect of drugs on isolated guinea-pig intestine and never see a drug given to a human being. Clearly, however, it is important to have some idea of how drugs can affect diseases or be affected by human variables such as age, genetic abnormalities, other concomittantly administered drugs or the disease itself.

Therapeutics (sometimes called clinical pharmacology) is the study of the effect of drugs on patients and their diseases.

A drug is any substance used for the prevention, treatment or diagnosis of disease, or to modify a physiological process. Obviously enough, penicillin given for an infection is a drug, but occasionally the categorisation of some substances is more difficult to decide. A soap used for the usual hygienic or cosmetic reasons is obviously not a drug, but a soap could be a drug if used to treat a skin disease such as acne vulgaris. More difficult still is the status of vitamins: these are foods, present in a normal diet; but if it cannot be absorbed from food, as in pernicious anaemia, vitamin B_{12} has to be administered as a drug.

Originally, all drugs were crude plant, animal or mineral substances, but currently used drugs are highly purified or even entirely synthetic products built up from relatively simple chemical precursors. Aspirin and ephedrine, for example, were originally plant derivatives, but are now synthesised de novo. Nevertheless, many drugs are still extracted from plants, microorganisms or tissues; examples are digoxin, antibiotics and many hormones.

For many patients the term 'drug' conveys unjustifiable overtones of addiction and it is usually better to use the term 'medicine' under such circumstances.

DRUG ACTION

Drug receptors

A remarkable property of many drugs is that they can act at phenomenally low concentrations. Frequently drugs are so highly diluted by body fluids that only a few molecules are available to act on each cell. Even so the drug's effect can be profound and widespread. These considerations suggest that there are highly sensitive sites in each cell on which the drug acts. These sites are *drug receptors*, which are specific for different drugs. If the specific receptor is present and a drug binds to it, the receptor becomes changed and stimulates the cell as a whole to produce an observable result. By contrast, cells which lack receptors for a particular drug will not respond to it.

Even minor alterations in the structure of a drug can produce large changes in its effects. Its actions may be enhanced, or abolished, or its selectivity changed with the result that its action is enhanced on one organ but diminished on another. An example is the modification of isoprenaline to produce salbutamol. Isoprenaline relaxes bronchial smooth muscle but also stimulates the rate of heartbeat. Salbutamol, by contrast, relaxes bronchial muscle but has little effect on heart rate. This suggests that isoprenaline receptors in the bronchi are different from those in the heart – the bronchial receptors can also be stimulated by salbutamol, whilst those in the heart pacemaker are little affected.

The formulae in Figure 1.1 illustrate the fact that an apparently trivial structural change results in a major difference in effect.

ISOPRENALINE

SALBUTAMOL

Fig. 1.1 Although the structure of isoprenaline is closely similar to that of salbutamol, the latter has a major bronchodilator action with only a relatively slight effect on the heart as a consequence of the difference in the receptors in those sites.

Competitive inhibition and receptor blocking drugs

Some drugs (receptor blockers) can bind to specific receptors but do not necessarily stimulate the cell. As a consequence, if such a drug and a related stimulatory agent, which both bind to the same receptor, are given at the same time, they compete for that receptor. The higher the concentration of the competitor, the more completely it binds to the receptor and blocks the action of the other drug.

Antihistamines are commonly used drugs which make use of this principle of *competitive inhibition* to block some of the actions of histamine in minor allergic diseases. Histamine, however, stimulates two different types of receptor, namely H_1 and H_2. Stimulation of H_1 receptors causes increased capillary permeability and relaxation of smooth muscle in some organs. An H_1 antihistamine such as chlorpheniramine blocks these actions of histamine by binding to the receptors on capillary endothelium and smooth muscle, and by so doing may lessen the effects of minor allergies.

The H_2 actions of histamine, by contrast, are on receptors on gastric parietal cells to stimulate gastric acid secretion. To prevent this effect a quite different type of antihistamine, an H_2-receptor blocker such as cimetidine, has to be used and is effective in the treatment of peptic ulcer (Ch. 12).

Because of this mode of action antihistamines are *receptor blockers*, but other drugs can be used to antagonise the actions of histamine (to continue with the same example) by quite different means, as discussed in later chapters.

Receptor function

The structures and functions of receptors are many and varied. One important type is a protein connected to an ionic channel in a cell membrane (Fig. 1.2). When a drug or natural chemical transmitter binds to a specific recognition site on

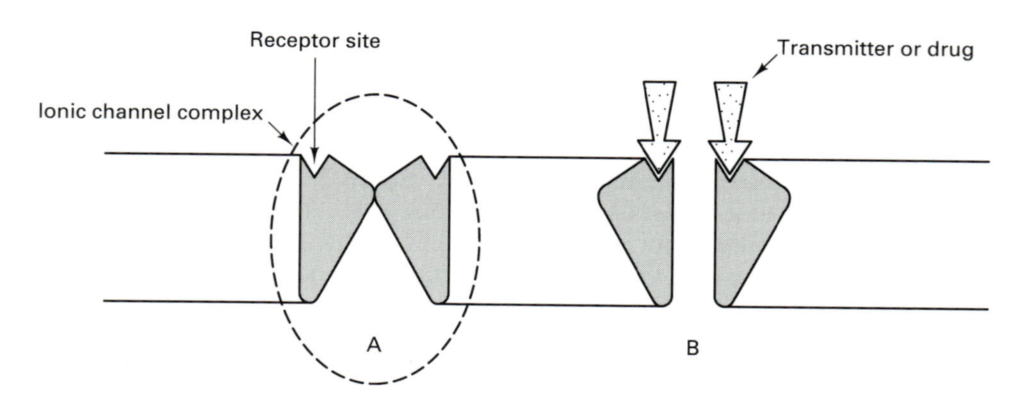

Cawson & Spector 986/01-02

Fig. 1.2 **A** An ionic channel in the resting (closed) state. **B** A natural transmitter or drug, attaching to a receptor site, changes the permeability of the ion channel to permit movement of ions which affect the excitability of the cell.

the protein, the permeability of the ionic channel is changed. This enhances or depresses the excitability of the cell. For example, the nicotinic actions of acetylcholine are mediated by enhancing the permeability of the cell to Na^+ and K^+. This causes depolarisation and excitation of the target cell. By contrast, the inhibitor neurotransmitter, γ-aminobutyric acid (GABA) increases the permeability of nerve cell membranes to chloride ions; this results in lowered excitability (Ch. 3).

Another group of membrane receptors acts by setting off secondary chemical reactions. Binding to the receptor changes the activity of an enzyme such as adenyl cyclase or phospholipase, which in turn can change the concentration of intracellular chemicals such as cyclic AMP, inositol pyrophosphates and diacylglycerol. Such chemicals modulate many cell functions, including ionic movements, energy generation and protein activity. Receptors which act in this way include the muscarinic receptor for acetylcholine and the adrenergic receptors.

The steroid hormones bind to intracellular receptors which regulate the transcription of specific genes via mRNA production (Ch. 10).

Transmitters

The biological function of cell receptors is to respond to chemical signals (transmitters), which include neurotransmitters and hormones. When a transmitter reaches its specific receptor, it initiates a series of steps which end with a detectable response by the cell. The response may be secretion, movement or a change in electrical excitability, according to the nature of the cell. Drugs that act like transmitters to initiate a sequence which leads to a response by a cell are termed *agonists*. By contrast, drugs may only bind to receptors without causing any further change. The result is that the specific transmitter or agonist drug cannot bind to the receptor and the cell cannot respond to it. This type of receptor-blocking drug is termed an *antagonist*.

The response to rising doses of an agonist can be plotted graphically. Such graphs usually show a threshold below which no response can be detected, and a maximum response (such as death, for example) beyond which further increases in dose cause no greater response (Fig. 1.3).

When some receptors are blocked by antagonist molecules, the responses to a particular dose of the agonist are of course diminished, because the agonist cannot reach all its receptors. Nevertheless, with many types of antagonist, raising the doses of the agonist can overcome the block and induce a maximum response. The higher the concentration of antagonist, the higher the dose of the agonist has to be raised to reach the threshold and maximum responses (Fig. 1.4). This pattern of blockade is termed *competitive antagonism*.

Species specificity

A final example of some of the many diverse properties of drugs is that of species specificity. Bacterial chemotherapy is an application of this phenomenon. The essential requirement of antibacterial drugs is that they destroy bacterial cells within patients without harming patients themselves. One mechanism by which this is attained is by inhibiting or destroying a bacterial cell component, which is not present in the host's cells. Penicillin and the cephalosporins, for example, prevent the synthesis of an adequate bacterial cell wall. Animal cells possess no cell wall and are therefore completely unharmed.

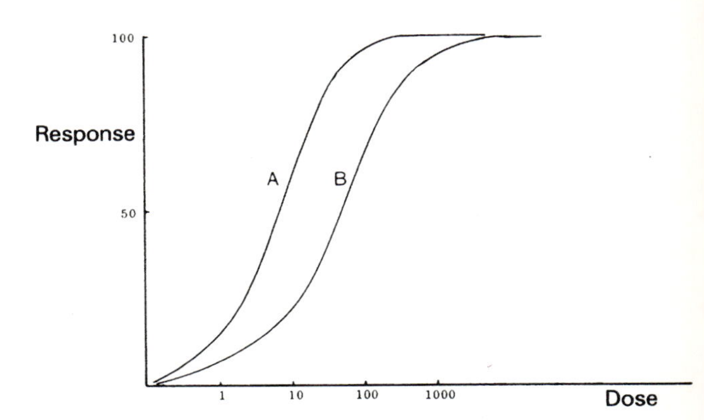

Fig. 1.3 Dose–response curve (semi-logarithmic plot). Drugs A and B. (Reproduced with permission from *Aids to Pharmacology*.)

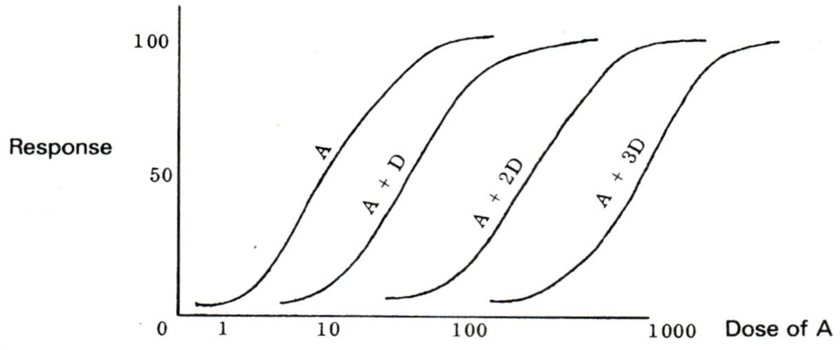

Fig. 1.4 The dose–response curve of agonist A in the presence of increasing concentrations of agonist D. (Reproduced with permission from *Aids to Pharmacology*.)

PHARMACOKINETICS

The way in which drugs are handled in the body is of great clinical importance. The study of the time-course of the absorption, distribution, metabolism and excretion of drugs is the definition of pharmacokinetics. In other words, pharmacokinetics is what the body does to drugs.

Although pharmacokinetics may sound a discouraging term, dental surgeons (like Molière's M. Jourdain, who was surprised to learn that he was speaking prose) are unconsciously using their knowledge of pharmacokinetics in the everyday practice of their speciality.

To give a simple example, nitrous oxide is widely used for dental sedation because, as a gas, it is almost instantaneously absorbed through the lungs into the bloodstream and then acts on receptors in the brain with great rapidity. This drug is very little metabolised, but is quickly excreted from the lungs. When administration stops, the patient wakes. These are some of the great advantages of nitrous oxide.

By contrast, diazepam (also used for dental sedation), has to be given by injection to achieve a reliably rapid effect. It affects brain receptors almost as rapidly as nitrous oxide, but remains active for very much longer because it has to be metabolised in the liver, and is recirculated via the bile. Metabolites of the drug are also active, so that patients require at least an hour to awake, take very much longer to recover completely, and have to be managed accordingly. Even in a normal person it may be several days before all traces of diazepam metabolites are finally excreted. Further, if the patient has liver disease, recovery may be even more delayed or the dose may have to be reduced.

Local anaesthetics, used many times every day in dental surgery, are an example of the way in which the pharmacokinetics of a drug can be modified. To render lignocaine ionisable and soluble for injection it is given as its hydrochloride. To achieve a high tissue concentration the local anaesthetic is injected in close proximity to the nerve, where it penetrates the axonal membrane to block sensory transmission. However, lignocaine is also rapidly absorbed into the blood, carried to the liver and quickly metabolised by amidases. The half-life of lignocaine, once it has entered the circulation, is therefore brief, although neural transmission recovers rather more slowly. To prolong analgesia therefore, local ischaemia is induced by adding a vasoconstrictor (adrenaline) to the solution. Lignocaine is thus held captive in the area and, unaffected by liver enzymes, maintains its activity often for 2 h or longer.

Pharmacokinetics thus includes all those processes covered by the acronym ADME – Absorption, Distribution, Metabolism and Excretion.

Absorption of drugs

The most important mechanism for drug absorption at cellular level is passive diffusion. This is not dependent on metabolic energy but determined merely by a concentration gradient and the ability of the drug to pass through the cell membrane. Since cell membranes contain a large amount of lipid, lipid-soluble uncharged forms of the drug are generally able to pass through. Many drugs contain acidic or basic parts in their molecules and these may exist in ionised (charged) or unionised (uncharged) forms. The unionised forms are more fat soluble and these more readily pass through cell membranes. Thus, basic drugs are best absorbed in an alkaline environment and acidic drugs in an acidic environment. Non-polar and lipid substances are usually well absorbed.

Drug administration

The most rapid and certain method of introducing a drug into the body is by injection, but oral administration is simpler, safer, cheaper and less unpleasant. Possible routes of administration are as follows:

1. Oral
2. Parenteral (injections)
   a. subcutaneous and submucosal
   b. intramuscular
   c. intravenous
3. Inhalational
   a. gases and vapours
   b. aerosols and powder inhalers
4. Transcutaneous and transmucosal.

Absorption from the alimentary tract

Oral administration is preferred by patients, but limited by the fact that some drugs, such as benzyl penicillin and insulin, are inactivated by gastric acid or destroyed by digestive enzymes. Absorption into the bloodstream is also relatively slow and sufficiently high plasma levels may not be achieved. In addition, the drug passes via the portal veins to the liver where it may be metabolised to a greater or lesser degree. This process, termed *first-pass metabolism*, affects nitrates used for the treatment of anginal pain. The usual way in which they are given is therefore as a sublingual tablet for transmucosal absorption into veins, avoiding the portal circulation.

A few drugs (such as aspirin and alcohol) are partly absorbed through the stomach wall, but most drugs given by mouth are absorbed in the upper part of the small intestine.

Drugs which are irritant to the stomach can be made tolerable by giving them a coating which only dissolves in the intestine (enteric coating).

Pro-drugs. First-pass metabolism can be a serious limitation on some drugs given by mouth, but advantage has been taken of this phenomenon to produce a variety of pro-drugs. These are drugs which are metabolised by the liver to release the active component into the systemic circulation. *Pivampicillin* for example releases the antibiotic, *ampicillin*; it is more effectively absorbed than the latter and causes less gastric upset. *Benorylate* releases *paracetamol* and *aspirin*, and lessens any gastric irritant action of the latter.

Bioavailability. Bioavailability is, in simple terms, the extent to which the drug is taken into the body and can act on the target tissues. The many variables which affect bioavailability include:

1. The drug's physical properties, which affect its absorption
2. Gastrointestinal factors affecting absorption
3. The degree of hepatic metabolism
4. The physical properties of the drug once absorbed.

The bioavailability of a drug is measured by the plasma levels achieved by the active component. However, an essential requirement of drugs which are to act on the brain is their ability to penetrate the blood–brain barrier – for this purpose, centrally acting drugs need to be lipid soluble.

Injection of drugs

Subcutaneous injection of a drug is simple but allows only a small volume to be given and absorption is relatively slow. These factors may, however, be advantages in the case of a potent drug such as adrenaline.

Submucosal injection is a common route for local anaesthetics as it allows them to act precisely where required.

Intramuscular injection is a common route for giving drugs when a more rapid effect is needed or if, as in the case of benzyl penicillin for example, the drug is destroyed in the gastrointestinal tract.

However, intramuscular injection can cause pain by pulling muscle fibres apart, and this may limit the volume of drug that can be administered by this route. Some drugs such as erythromycin are so irritant that they are not given in this way.

Intravenous injection allows a drug to act almost immediately and reach a high plasma concentration. Large volumes of drug can be given in this way, but there are disadvantages such as:

1. Skill is required to insert the needle into a vein; a haematoma may be produced if the vein wall is torn
2. Infection may be carried into the bloodstream (a major hazard for addicts)
3. The sudden entry of the drug into the blood can cause toxic or particularly severe allergic reactions (the antibiotic, *vancomycin* for example is so toxic that it is administered intravenously in dilute solution over 100 min – this is termed *intravenous infusion*)
4. Some drugs or their solvents (notably propylene glycol used to dissolve diazepam) are irritant to vessel walls and can cause thrombophlebitis.

Pulmonary absorption

Anaesthetic gases and vapours, liquid aerosols and solid particles are given and absorbed via the lungs. Absorption into the circulation is mainly from the alveoli and alveolar ducts. In the adult human lung the area of these respiratory surfaces is $60\,m^2$, which is equivalent to the area of the deck of a large motor cruiser.

An important advantage of delivering bronchodilator aerosols such as salbutamol directly into the respiratory tract by this route is that they are sprayed into the lungs to provide a high local concentration. The blood levels are relatively low and this lessens the danger of systemic toxic effects.

The absorption of anaesthetic gases is governed by their solubility, their rate of entry into the tissues and the rates of pulmonary blood flow and respiration. The longer the time for which a patient is exposed to an inhaled anaesthetic, the greater the amount of anaesthetic agent that enters the tissues from the plasma. The plasma/tissue difference in concentration therefore falls during exposure to the anaesthetic.

Having entered the body, the main route of excretion of volatile anaesthetics is from the lungs. Some of the drug remains for several hours in adipose tissue and other cells, but this is usually a relatively small proportion.

Liquid aerosols and solid particles can be inhaled as far as the bronchioles if the droplet or particle size is less than 2 μm. Particles of 10 μm reach the small bronchi. Thus the smaller the particle size, the greater the surface area reached for absorption.

Drug absorption through the oral mucosa

Drugs applied to the oral mucosa are mostly used for a purely local effect, but some are absorbed to a significant degree and can have a systemic effect, particularly if they are held under the tongue where there are large superficial veins. Since such drugs are absorbed directly into blood vessels, they avoid the portal circulation and hepatic (first-pass) metabolism.

Drugs which can be given sublingually are *nitrates*, which are used for angina pectoris (Ch. 5), and the opioid analgesic *buprenorphine*. Morphine can also be given in this way to avoid injections, and special adhesive preparations have been made to hold the drug in place in the mouth while it is being absorbed. However, injection remains the most effective route for administration of morphine.

Drug absorption through the skin

Drugs are applied directly to the skin particularly to treat skin diseases. Apart from the local physical properties of the application – which may in themselves be beneficial – local application gives a high tissue concentration to the affected part and, usually, little is absorbed into the circulation to give a significant concentration elsewhere. Even for local effectiveness some of the drug must be absorbed and this takes place through the stratum corneum. Absorption is most rapid where the stratum corneum is thinnest and further enhanced by warming the skin and increasing its hydration. Plastic occlusive dressings over steroid creams (for instance) greatly enhance and prolong their action, and also increase systemic absorption.

Glyceryl trinitrate, used for the treatment of angina pectoris, can be absorbed from an application to the skin in the form of a cream.

Protein binding

Once a drug has been absorbed it travels throughout the body in the plasma. Although some of the drug is simply dissolved in the plasma, some is bound to plasma protein. The protein-bound form is generally inactive, and it is the free form which is pharmacologically active. Many drugs are partly bound to the albumin component of the plasma proteins. These include the coumarin anticoagulants, indomethacin, aspirin, barbiturates, digitalis and tetracyclines.

One consequence of drugs being protein bound is prolongation of their effect. Drugs which are mainly bound to plasma proteins have a prolonged action because only the free, unbound form of the drug is attacked by drug-metabolising enzymes and excreted in the urine.

For any particular concentration of a drug in the blood, only a proportion (corresponding to the unbound form) is pharmacologically active (Fig. 1.5). One type of harmful drug interaction can result from this situation. *Warfarin*, for example, is a drug used to prevent extension of thrombi because of its anticoagulant action. It is partly protein bound in the plasma. If another drug (such as *chloral*) is given, it displaces

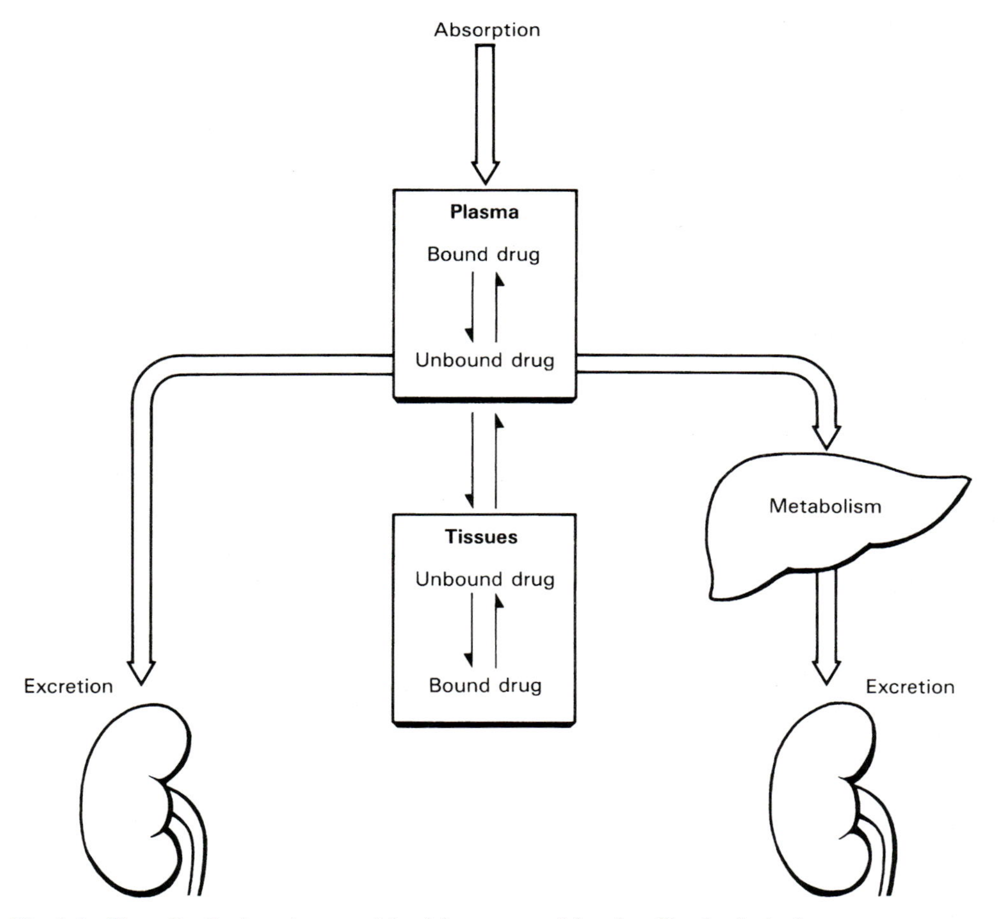

Fig. 1.5 Drug distribution: the essentials of the process of drug handling by the body.

warfarin from its binding sites on the albumin molecule. A higher proportion of warfarin is then free to act. The pharmacological effect of the warfarin is therefore enhanced and this can result in haemorrhage.

Metabolism and fate of drugs in the body

The effect produced by a drug does not persist indefinitely, but sooner or later ceases. The fall in plasma concentration of the drug often parallels the decline in the effect of the drug. The graph of plasma concentration against time generally follows a logarithmic pattern and therefore the rate of descent of the curve can be expressed as a half-life ($t^1/_2$) in the same way as other processes, such as radioactive decay, which diminish in a logarithmic pattern. This is due partly to metabolic destruction of the drug and partly to excretion. The relative importance of these two mechanisms varies from drug to drug.

The liver is the principal organ involved in drug metabolism, but others (such as kidney and intestine) are also involved to a lesser extent. Within the cell, the most important organelle carrying out metabolic transformations of drugs is the smooth endoplasmic reticulum. This constitutes the so-called 'microsomal fraction' of the cell.

Drugs may be metabolised by two types of mechanism:

1. Conversion
2. Synthesis.

Metabolic conversion

The structure of drugs may be modified in the body by simple chemical reactions. Important examples are oxidation and hydrolysis.

Many drugs, such as morphine and most of the barbiturates, are inactivated by oxidation by microsomal (drug-metabolising) enzymes in the liver. In severe liver disease (such as advanced cirrhosis) or in patients who have been given monoamine oxidase inhibitor drugs (for depression) these oxidising systems do not function adequately. Thus, if morphine or a barbiturate is given to such patients, it will cause profound and prolonged sedation with deep depression of respiration.

Suxamethonium is a muscle relaxant drug which acts on the motor end-plate. It has a very short action (usually less than 5 min) because it is rapidly hydrolysed by plasma pseudocholinesterase (Ch. 2). This drug is therefore used when brief muscular relaxation is wanted. However, about 1 in 4000 of the population lack plasma pseudocholinesterase. These people appear perfectly normal until given suxamethonium. This causes muscular (including respiratory) paralysis for many hours. During this time, life has to be maintained by applying positive-pressure artificial respiration until the effects of the suxamethonium have ceased.

Metabolic synthesis

Synthesis in the present context means conjugation of the drug with another chemical grouping or molecule. This may confer greater polarity and water solubility, less pharmacological activity and greater ease of excretion.

One form of conjugation of drugs is with glucuronic acid. Glucuronic acid is derived from glucose, and combines with some drugs in the liver. Glucuronidation is carried out by the smooth endoplasmic reticulum of the hepatic parenchymal cells. Aspirin and chloramphenicol are examples of two drugs handled in this way. In newborn infants – particularly those born prematurely – the drug-conjugating mechanisms may be incompletely developed and fail to function for several days after delivery. If such a child is given chloramphenicol during the early days of life, very little of the drug is converted to chloramphenicol glucuronide (inactive) and most remains in the non-conjugated active form. Thus, unusually high blood levels of the free antibiotic are reached and cause toxic effects, in particular circulatory collapse.

Factors which modify drug metabolism

These include the following categories:

1. Genetic
2. Physiological

3. Disease
4. Environmental influences.

Genetic constitution. This is a fairly common cause of variation in drug metabolism. As mentioned earlier, plasma pseudocholinesterase which greatly prolongs the action of suxamethonium, is inherited as a non-sex-linked (autosomal) recessive trait.

About a third of Europeans have inherited the ability to inactivate some drugs rapidly by acetylation. Thus they quickly inactivate such drugs as the antituberculous agent isoniazid, the antihypertensive hydralazine and the antidepressant phenelzine.

Genetic factors may also alter responsiveness to drugs and their ability to cause toxic effects. Thus some patients are genetically resistant to anticoagulants of the coumarin type such as warfarin. Warfarin is also widely used as a rat poison because the large amounts they consume in poisoned bait cause fatal internal haemorrhage. However, large populations of rats and mice have also developed resistance to warfarin as a result of genetic selection.

An example of enhanced vulnerability to a particular toxic effect is the inherited deficiency of the red cell enzyme glucose-6-phosphate dehydrogenase. Such patients may develop acute haemolytic anaemia when given certain antimalarial drugs (such as primaquine and pamaquine), antibacterial drugs (such as nitrofurantoin and sulphonamides) or, in some cases, aspirin.

Physiological factors. *Age* is one such variable. In the newborn, as mentioned earlier, excessively high levels of drugs such as chloramphenicol may result from immaturity of the microsomal drug-conjugating system. In old age, toxic effects from digoxin (a cardiac glycoside) and streptomycin (an antibiotic) are common, partly as a result of diminished renal function and impaired excretion.

Disease. Severe malnutrition may prolong the action of some drugs (in particular the hypnotics and anxiolytics) due to poor hepatic function. Liver disease, including cirrhosis and obstructive jaundice, may also slow down removal of drugs which are conjugated and then excreted into the bile.

Environmental influences. Previous exposure to drugs is an example. The barbiturates are powerful inducers of drug-metabolising enzymes. Even a few doses of a barbiturate increase the ability of the liver to metabolise a wide range of drugs. Thus if a patient is taking a barbiturate regularly and at the same time requires treatment with the anticoagulant warfarin, the latter has to be given in a higher than usual dose to produce the same anticoagulant effect. This is because the metabolism of warfarin by the liver has been accelerated. A well-recognised danger of this situation is that if patients suddenly stop taking barbiturates, but continue to take the same dose of warfarin, they may suffer serious haemorrhage. This is because withdrawal of the barbiturate allows the drug-metabolising enzymes in the liver quickly to fall to their previous (non-induced) level of activity. The warfarin is not then broken down so rapidly and attains much higher blood levels. Similarly, in women barbiturates may cause the contraceptive pill to become ineffective unless the dose of the oestrogen component is raised.

By contrast, monoamine oxidase inhibitor drugs, such as phenelzine, used for treatment of depression, inhibit oxidising enzymes in the liver. If morphine, which is normally oxidised in the liver, is given at the same time as phenelzine, it will have an enhanced effect and may precipitate coma.

Drug excretion

Drugs may leave the body unchanged or in a metabolically altered form. The most important organ of excretion is the kidney. Most renal excretion is via the glomerular filtrate. Arterial blood flows into the afferent arterioles of the glomeruli of the kidney and some of the plasma is filtered through the glomerular membrane and enters the lumen of the renal tubules. Some of the solutes in the filtered plasma (including electrolytes, metabolites and drugs) are to a variable extent reabsorbed via the tubular epithelium into the plasma. The remainder enters the collecting ducts to be excreted in the urine. An important consequence is that the less the tubular reabsorption of a drug, the more rapidly will it appear in the urine. To some extent this can be varied with individual drugs, particularly if they are acids or bases.

Acids and bases exist in uncharged (undissociated) and charged (ionised) forms. In acid solutions, acids are mainly undissociated while bases are mainly ionised. In alkaline conditions the situation is reversed – acids are mainly ionised and bases non-ionised.

It is a general rule that drugs can enter cells if they are uncharged, but cannot pass through even the outer cell membrane if they carry a charge. These phenomena are used in the treatment of some forms of drug overdose. Aspirin is a weak acid. When an overdose has been taken, excretion can be greatly accelerated by making the urine alkaline – usually by infusion of sodium bicarbonate. The alkalinity of the urine encourages dissociation of the aspirin (Fig. 1.6).

The ion thus formed carries a charge and, therefore, cannot be reabsorbed by the tubular epithelial cells. The aspirin which has entered the lumen of the renal tubule has then only one way out and this is via the collecting ducts into the urine.

Conversely, amphetamine, which is basic, can be excreted more rapidly by raising the acidity of the urine.

Many drugs retain their charge virtually unchanged throughout the entire pH range possible in body fluids. Streptomycin, for example, remains strongly positively charged at all physiological pH values, and the entire amount of streptomycin is filtered via the glomeruli and is excreted in the urine with almost no renal tubular epithelial reabsorption.

Occasionally, renal excretion of a drug exceeds that entering the tubule via the glomerulus. This is due to active secretion of the drug by the renal tubular epithelial cells. These cells take up and concentrate the drug from the plasma and secrete

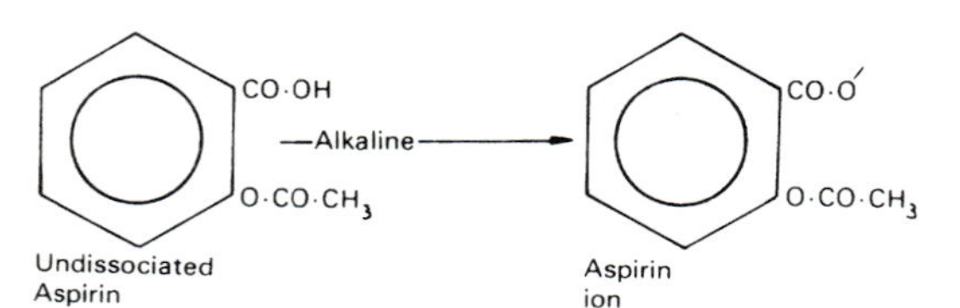

Fig. 1.6 Alkalinisation of the urine causes aspirin to dissociate and accelerates its excretion after an overdose.

it directly into the tubular lumen. For this reason penicillin has an extremely high excretion rate.

It is possible to block this secretion mechanism with another drug – probenecid. When probenecid is given with penicillin, the blood levels of penicillin are higher and its action more prolonged.

Some drugs, such as the volatile anaesthetics, leave the body partly via the lungs and are exhaled unchanged. This is a great advantage as it allows rapid control of the level of anaesthesia.

Many substances are excreted in the bile. Drugs which appear in the bile are mainly conjugated as glucuronides or sulphates, for example. These then enter the gut and leave the body in the faeces – although some may be de-conjugated by intestinal organisms and reabsorbed into the circulation (Fig. 1.7). This phenomenon of enterohepatic recirculation contributes considerably to resedation after wakening when diazepam is given for dental sedation (Ch. 18).

Some drugs, such as the aminoglycoside antibiotics, many of which are nephrotoxic, may inhibit their own excretion.

Drug elimination

The time course of the appearance and disappearance of a drug in the blood after a single dose can be plotted (Fig. 1.8).

The right-hand part of the curve shows a falling concentration of the drug. Its early part is known as the *redistribution phase* because, initially, the drug moves from the blood to other compartments in the body. The elimination phase corresponds to a falling drug concentration due to excretion or metabolism or both. Both these phases show an exponential form of decay and each can be described mathematically by a half-life ($t_{\frac{1}{2}}$). This is the time taken for a blood concentration of a drug to be halved. The elimination half-life is often used to give an idea of for how long a drug acts. For example, the long-acting sedative diazepam has a $t_{\frac{1}{2}}$ of 20–50 h while the similar but short-acting drug midazolam has a $t_{\frac{1}{2}}$ of 2 h.

Some drugs are not eliminated in this pattern (exponential or *first-order decay*) but have a linear (*zero-order*) pattern (Fig. 1.9). For example,

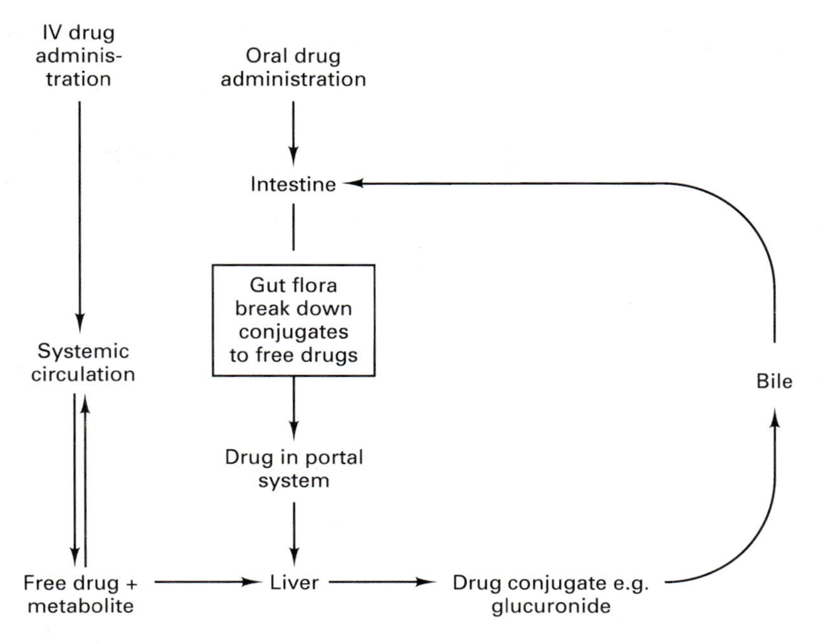

Fig. 1.7 Enterohepatic recirculation. Drugs undergoing this process include diazepam, oestrogens and thyroxine.
IV, intravenous.

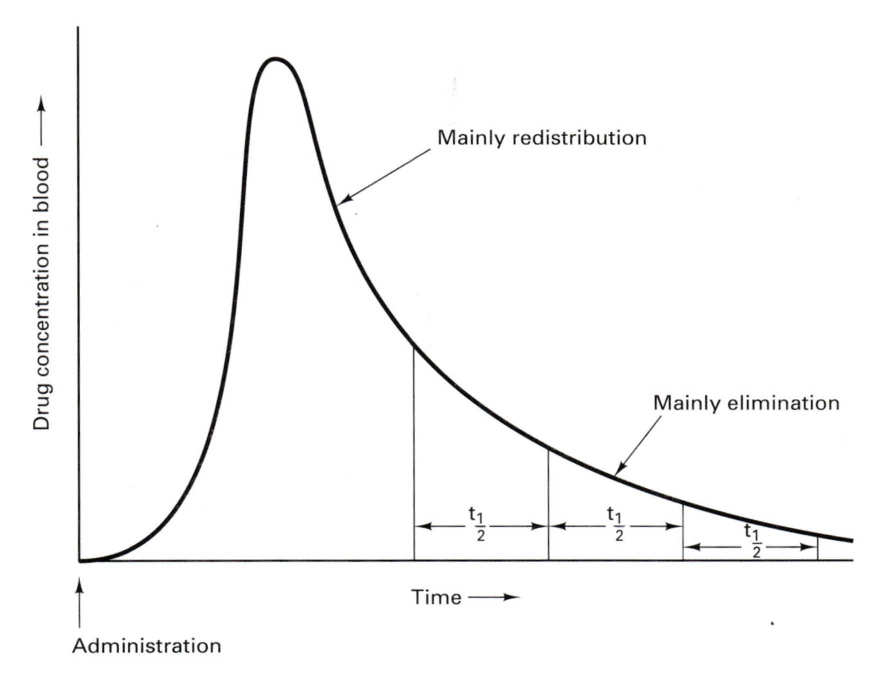

Fig. 1.8 First-order elimination: time course of concentration of drug in the blood following a single administration ($t_{1/2}$ is the elimination half-life). The right-hand part of the curve shows a falling concentration. The early part of this is known as the redistribution phase, because initially the drug moves from the blood to other compartments in the body. The elimination phase corresponds to a fall in drug concentration due to excretion or metabolism, or both.

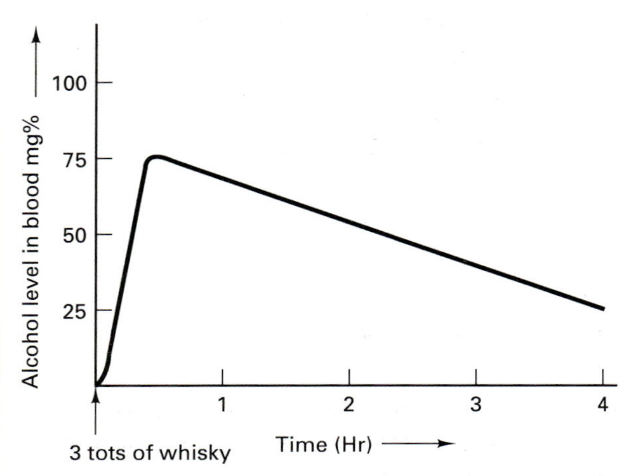

Fig. 1.9 Zero-order elimination: time course of alcohol in the blood following a single drink of three tots of whisky (about 80 ml, which contains 35.9 g of alcohol).

alcohol elimination does not have a single half-life, but the same amount is eliminated in unit time, namely 8 g of alcohol per hour (the amount in a single gin or half a pint of bitter).

The main aspects of drug handling by the body are summarised in Box 1.1.

Box 1.1 Essentials of drug handling by the body

1. Drugs may be given orally, by injection, by inhalation or by local application to the skin or mucous membranes. The route chosen depends on such factors as the chemical properties of the drug, the rapidity with which a response is required and whether local or systemic effects are required
2. The most important mechanism for drug absorption at cellular level is passive diffusion and is largely determined by a concentration gradient. In general, lipid-soluble, uncharged forms of a drug most readily pass through the lipid-rich cell membrane
3. Drugs can act in minute concentrations by binding to specific receptors on cells which may respond in a variety of ways according to their nature and that of the drug
4. Concomittantly administered drugs can compete for receptors. As a result the action of one drug may be blocked by another
5. Drugs which are eliminated mainly by metabolism are usually inactivated in the liver, although other organs may be involved
6. The principal organ of drug excretion is the kidney

2. The nervous system
I. The neuromuscular junction and the autonomic nervous system

Most activities of the body are under the control of the nervous system. In simple terms, with only minor exceptions, there are:

1. *The voluntary nervous system* – this mediates conscious control of muscular activity
2. *The involuntary (autonomic) nervous system* – this controls in an automatic fashion the function of such structures as the heart and blood vessels, intestines and glands.

The arrangement of nerve connections in the efferent (outflow) fibres differs in the voluntary from that in autonomic nervous systems. The neuronal outflow from the spinal cord illustrates these differences (Fig. 2.1).

THE VOLUNTARY NERVOUS SYSTEM AND THE NEUROMUSCULAR JUNCTION

The pharmacological basis of muscular contraction and the activation of the neuromuscular junction by chemical agents is of considerable practical importance, particularly in general

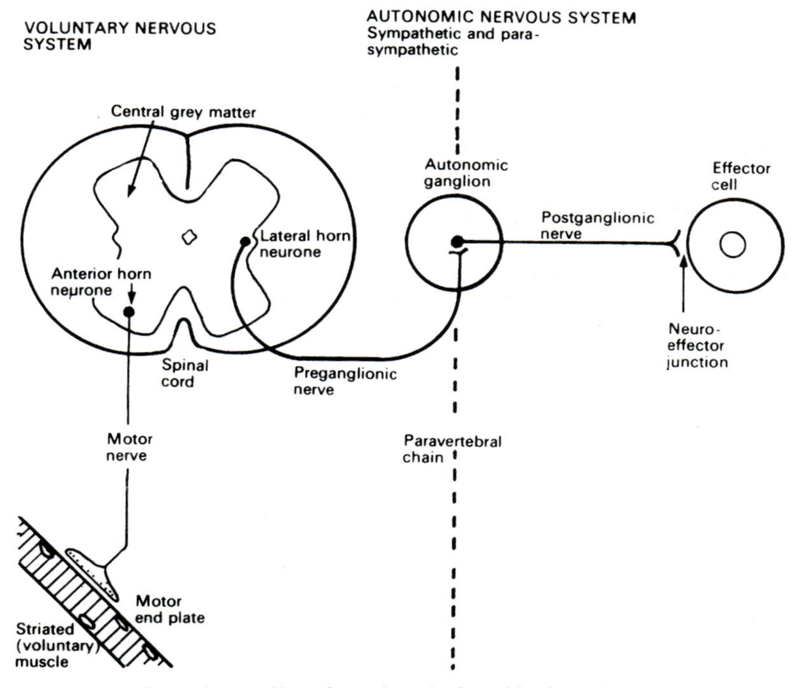

Fig. 2.1 Outflow of nerve fibres from the spinal cord in the voluntary and autonomic nervous systems.

anaesthesia. For many kinds of operation it is essential to have muscular relaxation. This can be achieved during light anaesthesia by using drugs (muscle relaxants) which block the chemical processes involved in muscle contraction.

Mechanisms

The efferent nerve fibres in the voluntary nervous system are the axons of the motor nerve call bodies in the anterior grey horn. These bundles of axons are the motor nerves. They travel without interruption to carry nerve impulses from the central nervous system to striated muscles whenever a voluntary movement is initiated.

On the surface of the muscle the axon splits up into several fine nerve branches. These do not touch the muscle fibres, but are separated from them by a minute gap of about 20 nm. The region of the termination of the motor nerve on the surface of the muscle fibre is the *motor end-plate.*

Electrical excitation spreads down the motor nerve, into its terminal branches, and induces electrical excitation in the muscle fibres. This is followed by contraction of the muscle. There is no electrical continuity between the motor end-plate and muscle, but the terminal filaments of motor nerves contain vesicles of acetylcholine. When an action potential passes down to the end of the nerve fibre, these vesicles empty into the gap between the nerve ending and the surface of the muscle fibre. Acetylcholine then diffuses across the gap and binds to receptors on the surface of the muscle (Fig. 2.2). This allows an influx of sodium ions, causing a wave of electrical excitation to pass along the muscle fibre. This is followed by contraction.

In electrical terms, an excitable cell such as a nerve or muscle, in a resting (non-stimulated) state, is not conducting waves of electrical activity. Under these conditions there is a negative charge within the cell relative to the outside. This is the

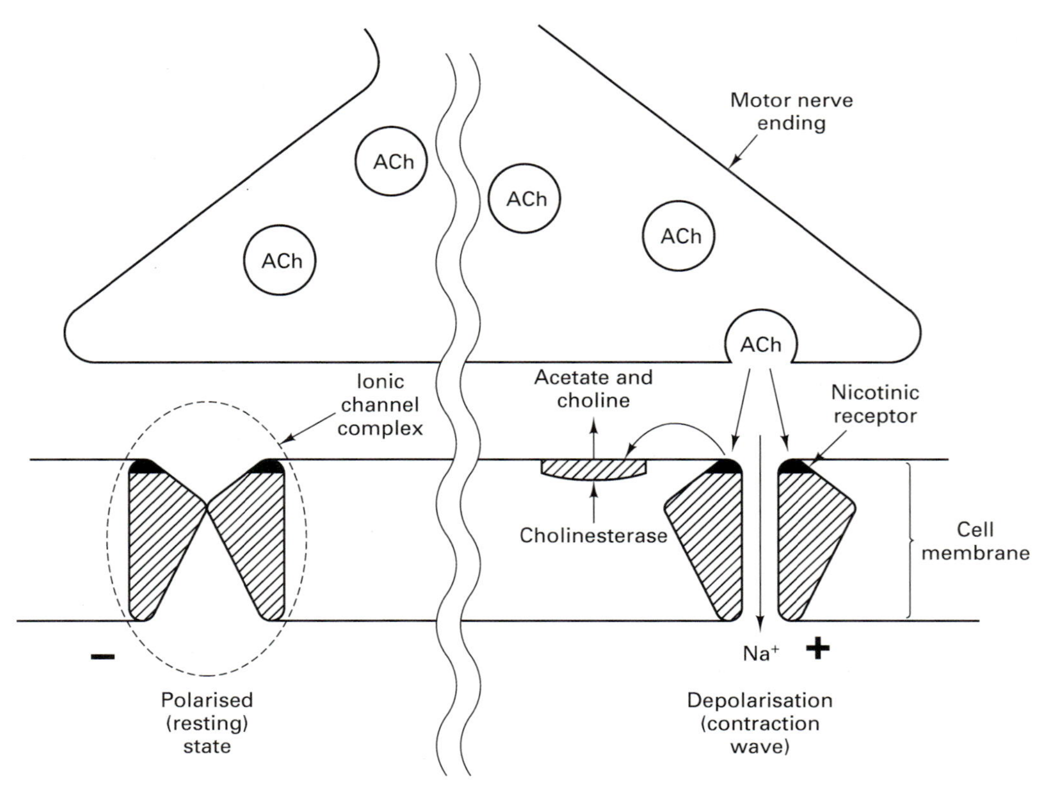

Fig. 2.2 Representation of the neuromuscular junction with the muscle in a resting state (left) and undergoing depolarisation with consequent contraction (right).

polarised (resting) state. When stimulated, electrical excitement takes the form of a wave of depolarisation which passes along the cell. Depolarisation means that the membrane allows a positive charge to pass from the outside of the cell membrane to the cell interior. Thus, the potential difference between the inside and outside of the cell is abolished during electrical excitation. The chemical and electrical similarities to the process of neural transmission (see Ch. 17) will be obvious.

In the muscle fibre, therefore, when acetylcholine reaches cholinergic receptors on its surface, the muscle becomes depolarised. The cholinergic receptors on the surface of voluntary muscle are of the *nicotinic* type. They consist of pentameric proteins which occupy the full thickness of the cell membrane and are connected directly to the Na^+ and K^+ ion channels. When acetylcholine binds to the ligand site on the receptor protein, the latter changes shape and thus opens the Na^+ and K^+ channels. Depolarisation results. Electrical excitation of a muscle fibre is, therefore, a wave of depolarisation. This spreads along the length of the fibre which, as a consequence, contracts.

One short burst of nerve impulses in the motor axon leads to a brief release of acetylcholine over the muscle fibre. One action potential releases about 100 vesicles of acetylcholine from the nerve terminal. The subsequent contraction of the muscle is short lived because acetylcholine is rapidly removed (hydrolysed) by an enzyme, acetylcholinesterase, to form acetate and choline. Acetate is oxidised to form carbon dioxide and water. Some of the choline is taken up again into nerve endings for resynthesis of acetylcholine. Stimulation leads only to a single contraction. Even when the muscle is kept in a depolarised state it relaxes after the initial contraction.

The sequence of events in the initiation of muscular contraction is summarised in Table 2.1.

Table 2.1 Summary of events in the initiation of muscle contraction

1. The motor nerve cell body or its dendrites are stimulated by another neurone in the central nervous system
2. The wave of excitation (depolarisation) travels from the central nervous system in the axon of a motor nerve which terminates in the motor end-plates on the surface of striated muscle fibres
3. At the nerve terminal in the motor end-plate, the zone of depolarisation causes the transmitter (acetylcholine) to be released into the gap between nerve and muscle
4. Acetylcholine diffuses across the gap, binds to cholinergic receptors in the muscle cell membrane and triggers the opening of ion channels
5. Opening of the Na^+ and K^+ ion channels causes a wave of depolarisation to spread over the entire muscle
6. Depolarisation is followed by contraction, but it is short lived because acetylcholine is hydrolysed by cholinesterase

Muscle relaxant drugs

During surgery, reflex contraction of abdominal and other muscles needs to be blocked. Paralysis of muscles during general anaesthesia can be produced by drugs which interfere with the normal stimulation of the acetylcholine receptor on the surface of the muscle. During treatment with these paralysing drugs, the muscles of respiration are as severely affected as other striated muscle. The patient therefore has respiratory paralysis and respiration must always be maintained artificially.

The term 'muscle relaxants' is euphemistically applied to these drugs, but in fact they are muscle *paralysing* agents.

Muscle relaxants comprise two groups:

1. Non-depolarising
2. Depolarising drugs.

Non-depolarising muscle relaxants (competitive blockers)

Non-depolarising muscle relaxants act by binding to the cholinergic receptors on the surface of the muscle in the region of the motor end-plate. They therefore prevent access of acetylcholine to the receptors and thus prevent depolarisation in the muscle (Fig. 2.3). Since a wave of depolarisation must pass over the muscle to induce contraction, the muscle does not contract and remains in the relaxed state. This type of drug effect is known as *competitive antagonism* because the muscle relaxant is competing with acetylcholine for access to the receptor on the muscle. A substance such as acetylcholine, which binds to a receptor and then stimulates it, is termed an *agonist*,

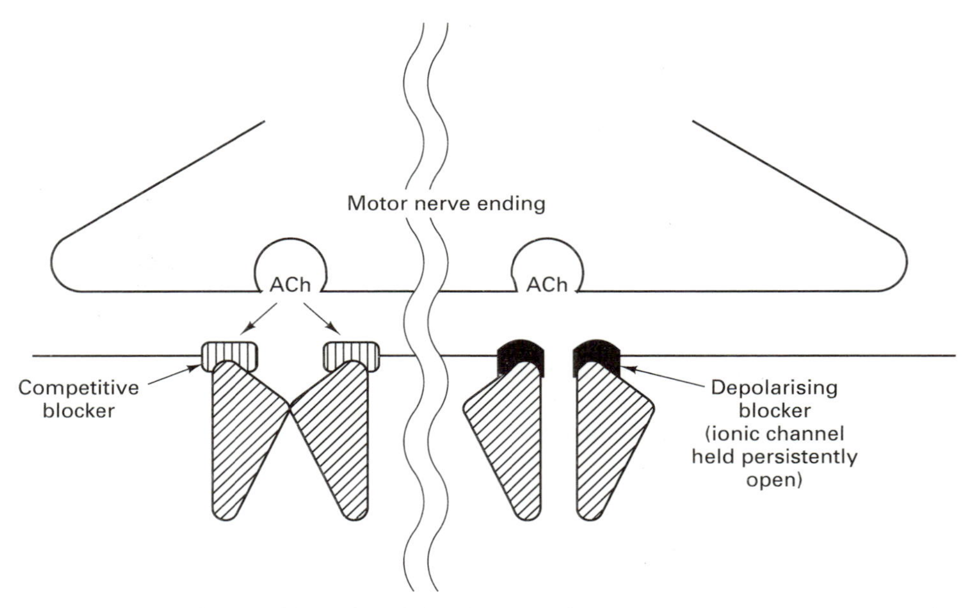

Fig. 2.3 Action of competitive (left) and depolarising (right) neuromuscular blocking agents on the ion channel complexes of muscle cell membrane.

while a substance which binds to a receptor and then has no action except to prevent agonists from reaching the receptor is an *antagonist*.

The action of these neuromuscular blockers can in turn be antagonised by a cholinesterase inhibitor, such as neostigmine, which raises the concentration of acetylcholine around the cholinergic receptor.

An early and typical example of a non-depolarising muscle relaxant is *tubocurarine*. It is an extract of curare, a South American arrow poison. Tubocurarine is given by injection, starts to act within 3–5 min and is effective for about 30 min. Tubocurarine is a weak ganglion blocker and thus produces hypotension. It often also causes erythematous rashes by inducing histamine release. *Alcuronium* is similar to tubocurarine, and other preferred muscle relaxants are shown in Table 2.2.

Depolarising muscle relaxants (non-competitive blockers)

Suxamethonium is the only currently used depolarising muscle relaxant and acts in an unusual way. Having some agonist activity, it binds to the muscle receptors to cause depolarisation. However, unlike acetylcholine which produces very short-lived depolarisation, depolarising muscle relaxants cause depolarisation of the muscle, which persists for several minutes. During this time, the muscle cannot be further depolarised or respond to acetylcholine (Fig. 2.3).

Depolarising agents produce more rapid and complete muscle relaxation than do the non-depolarising group, but unlike the latter their

Table 2.2 Currently used muscle relaxants

Drug	Advantages and limitations
Atracurium	Elimination does not depend on enzyme action. Can therefore be used in liver and kidney failure. Acts for 15–25 min
Vecuronium	Low toxicity. Does not liberate histamine. Acts for 20–30 min
Pancuronium	Does not cause ganglion blockade or significant changes in blood pressure
Gallamine	Rapid onset and recovery, but causes undesirable tachycardia by its vagolytic action. Contraindicated in patients with renal disease

action cannot be terminated by giving an anti-cholinesterase or any other drug.

When suxamethonium is given there is initial twitching of the muscles as depolarisation spreads over the muscle fibres. As mentioned earlier, muscle can only contract once following a single wave of depolarisation and, even when depolarisation is maintained, the muscle then relaxes. A single intravenous injection of suxamethonium produces muscular paralysis for about 5 min. The effect of the drug is terminated by the action of *plasma pseudocholinesterase* which hydrolyses the drug and abolishes its pharmacological activity.

The action of suxamethonium is greatly prolonged – often for many hours – in patients who have an inherited deficiency of plasma pseudocholinesterase. During this period of paralysis, respiration must be maintained artificially until the respiratory muscles recover. An anticholinesterase (which blocks hydrolysis of acetylcholine) will not accelerate recovery and could theoretically slow it by increasing depolarisation at the motor end-plate.

Clinical applications of muscle relaxants

Since paralysis of voluntary muscle is always accompanied by respiratory paralysis, it is inevitably terrifying. Muscle relaxants must therefore usually be given under general anaesthesia and always accompanied by assisted (intermittent positive pressure) respiration.

Important uses of muscle relaxants are summarised in Table 2.3.

Table 2.3 Clinical uses of muscle relaxants

1. Relaxation of laryngeal muscles to aid endotracheal intubation
2. Relaxation of abdominal muscles, to gain access to the viscera, or of limb muscles when a joint has to be manipulated
3. To relax persistent spasm of the larynx (rarely)
4. To counter the violent convulsions of electroconvulsive therapy used in the treatment of severe depression (Ch. 3)
5. Suppression of the patient's efforts to breathe when mechanically assisted ventilation is carried out. Without a muscle relaxant there is a tendency to fight the action of the ventilator
6. Relaxation of muscle spasm in tetanus to allow assisted ventilation to be given

THE AUTONOMIC NERVOUS SYSTEM

The axons of nerves which leave the spinal cord to form the autonomic nervous system have their cell bodies in the lateral grey horns. These efferent axons then terminate in autonomic ganglia where they excite the nerve cells of autonomic nerves to supply most of the structures in the body which are not under voluntary control. These include digestive and sweat glands, the heart and blood vessels, and the smooth muscle of the alimentary and genitourinary systems.

There are two peripheral junctions in the autonomic outflows:

1. A nerve–nerve junction in the autonomic ganglion
2. A neuroeffector junction at the point of nerve supply to the organ.

At both junctions there is a gap of about 20 nm with no electrical continuity. The chemical transmitter at the nerve–nerve junction (the synapse), in both the *sympathetic* and the *parasympathetic* systems, in the autonomic ganglia and at the neuroeffector junction of the parasympathetic system is acetylcholine. But at most neuroeffector junctions of the sympathetic system the transmitter is *noradrenaline* (Fig. 2.4).

The autonomic nervous outflow is divided into two functional divisions: the sympathetic and parasympathetic nervous systems. Activation of the sympathetic system is associated with increased physical and emotional activity and brought into heightened function during fright, fight and flight. The parasympathetic system is brought into use during more sedate ('vegetative') activities such as digestion, sleep and contraction of the smooth muscles of the gut and bladder.

THE SYMPATHETIC NERVOUS SYSTEM

Nerve cells in the lateral grey horns of the spinal cord in segments T1 to L2 give off axons which leave the cord with each efferent nerve. The axons terminate in the sympathetic ganglia where they form a synapse with a nerve cell, the axons of which form the sympathetic nerves travelling to organs under sympathetic control (Fig. 2.4).

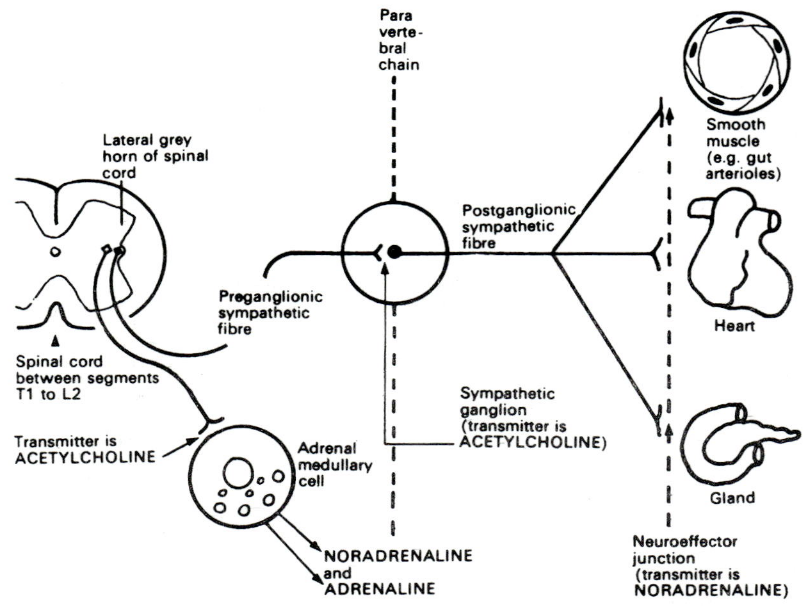

Fig. 2.4 Diagram of sympathetic nervous system to show the main connections and the sites of release of the different chemical mediators.

Another part of the sympathetic outflow is the nerve to the adrenal medulla, which has no synapse along its course. From a developmental point of view, the adrenal medullary cells are analogous to the nerve cell bodies in the sympathetic ganglion and, like them, are stimulated by nerves arising in the lateral horn of the cord.

As mentioned earlier, the chemical transmitter substance in the sympathetic ganglia is *acetylcholine*, but in most sites the transmitter in the neuroeffector junction is *noradrenaline*. The exceptions are the nerves to the adrenal medullary cells and to the sweat glands which are cholinergic. The adrenal medulla secretes both adrenaline and noradrenaline.

Fight, fright or flight

The concept of the sympathetic nervous system as mediating the responses to an emergency is useful. When violent action is anticipated or performed the cardiovascular, respiratory and skeletal muscle systems need to respond appropriately.

Important responses of the body to sympathetic stimulation in response to an emergency therefore include:

1. Raised cardiac output to increase blood supply to the muscles to enable them to act more vigorously
2. Vasodilatation in the skeletal muscles which provide the action
3. Dilatation of the bronchi and faster rate of respiration to maximise oxygen intake
4. Central stimulation (sensations of anger or panic) and dilatation of the pupils.

To compensate for the diversion of blood to the more active parts, blood flow to the skin and viscera is limited by contraction of the smooth muscles of their arterioles. Production of digestive secretions (including salivation) and peristalsis also decrease and sphincters close.

Sympathetic activity therefore prepares the body for violent action and sympathomimetic drugs produce these effects to a greater or lesser degree and with varying degrees of selectivity.

Sympathomimetic agonist drugs and receptors

Sympathomimetic drugs are those which produce some or all of the effects of sympathetic activation.

The main examples are the natural products *noradrenaline* and *adrenaline*. At the neuroeffector junction, the released noradrenaline diffuses across the gap and stimulates specific receptors in the target cells. The effects of a sympathetic transmitter (adrenaline or noradrenaline) binding and then activating these postjunctional receptors are:

1. Increased force and rate of the heartbeat
2. Increased velocity of conduction down the atrioventricular bundle (bundle of His)
3. Increased excitability of the myocardium
4. Vasodilatation in the myocardium and in voluntary (striated) muscle
5. Vasoconstriction in skin and viscera
6. Bronchodilatation
7. Central stimulation.

Injected noradrenaline does not produce all these different effects with the same degree of intensity. Other sympathomimetic drugs have selective actions to produce only a few of these effects.

The selective action of sympathomimetic drugs depends on the fact that there are five groups of sympathetic (adrenergic) receptors. Sympathomimetic drugs can therefore act on one or several of these receptors at the same time. These different receptors can also be blocked selectively by another group of drugs, the adrenergic blocking agents (described later).

One important aspect of these subdivisions of sympathomimetic activity is that many (e.g. vasoconstriction or bronchodilatation) are sometimes useful, while others (e.g. increased myocardial excitability) can be dangerous to susceptible patients.

The five types of adrenergic activity are:

α_1 actions:
1. Contraction of some type of smooth muscle including certain blood vessels
2. Relaxation of intestinal muscle.

α_2 actions:
1. Decreased release of noradrenaline from nerves by stimulating prejunctional receptors
2. Contraction of vascular smooth muscle in some regions (unconfirmed)
3. Inhibition of insulin release from the pancreatic islet cells.

β_1 actions:
1. Increased rate of heartbeat
2. Increased rate of conduction down the A-V bundle
3. Increased myocardial excitability
4. Increased force of contraction of the heart.

β_2 actions:
1. Bronchodilatation
2. Vasodilatation in the myocardium
3. Vasodilatation in voluntary muscles.

β_3 actions:
1. Lipolysis in adipose tissue.

Prejunctional (inhibitory) receptors. As noted above, α_2 receptors are *prejunctional*. They are within the cell membranes of nerve endings which release noradrenaline. By a feedback mechanism, release of noradrenaline into the synaptic cleft stimulates prejunctional receptors. This *inhibits* further release of noradrenaline and shortens its action. Blockade of prejunctional receptors therefore causes *release* of noradrenaline (Fig. 2.5).

An α receptor blocking drug, such as *phentolamine* (which blocks both pre- and postjunctional receptors), produces initial dilatation of arterioles, but this action is quickly weakened or terminated because of blockade of the prejunctional α receptors. This leads to an outpouring of noradrenaline which overcomes the initial dilatation of the blood vessels.

Phentolamine therefore has only a brief action as an antihypertensive drug. *Prazosin*, by contrast, is a selective postjunctional α receptor blocker and, having no significant prejunctional receptor blocking action, has no effect on noradrenaline release. It therefore causes prolonged vasodilatation and is a useful antihypertensive drug (Table 2.4).

Adrenaline (one of the adrenal medullary hormones) injected subcutaneously produces α, β_1 and β_2 actions, all of similar intensity. It therefore causes tachycardia and increased force of contraction of the heart (causing raised systolic blood pressure), vasodilatation in muscles (which tends to lower the diastolic blood pressure), and bronchodilatation.

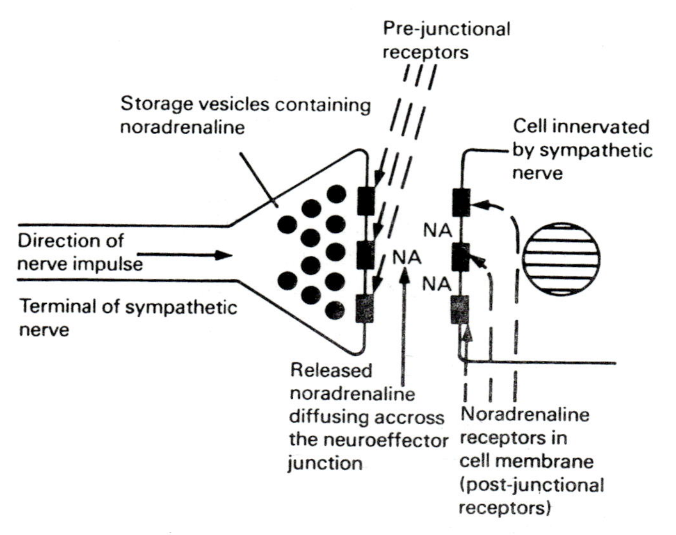

Fig. 2.5 At a sympathetic (adrenergic) nerve ending, noradrenaline released from the storage vesicles diffuses across the synaptic cleft to reach specific receptors on target cells, i.e. those innervated by the sympathetic nervous system. The stimulation of prejunctional noradrenaline receptors inhibits further release of transmitter.

Large doses of adrenaline heighten the excitability of the myocardium and can cause dangerous cardiac arrhythmias. Adrenaline is rarely given intravenously, because a sudden increase in β_1 stimulation of the heart can induce ventricular fibrillation. Fibrillation means that there is no effective ventricular contraction and, therefore, there is total loss of cardiac output. If uncorrected, death follows in a few minutes.

Subcutaneous injection of *noradrenaline* produces all these actions, but the α_1 effects are much stronger than the β_1 or β_2 actions. Thus, noradrenaline mainly causes constriction of the arterioles in the skin and viscera. This raises the peripheral resistance in the vascular system and thus raises the blood pressure – particularly the diastolic component. The rise in blood pressure usually causes reflex slowing of the heart.

Table 2.4 Drugs acting on pre- and post-junctional α receptors

Drug	Action on prejunctional a receptor	Action on postjunctional a receptor	Result of drug action
Phenoxybenzamine Phentolamine Tolazoline	Blockade ∴ more NA released	Blockade ∴ vasodilatation	Weak vasodilator ∴ little or no hypotension
Prazosin	No effect	Blockade ∴ vasodilatation	Strong vasodilator ∴ considerable antihypertensive action
Clonidine Methyldopa	Powerful stimulation ∴ reduced NA release	Weak stimulation ∴ tendency to vasoconstriction	Net result is vasodilatation and hypotension because NA not released

NA, noradrenaline.

Isoprenaline has only β_1 and β_2 effects and has no α activity. Since it stimulates β_1 and β_2 receptors only, isoprenaline produces tachycardia and increased force of contraction of the heart (β_1 effects) and bronchodilatation (β_2 effects). This has the danger that an overdose can heighten the excitability of the myocardium excessively to cause ventricular fibrillation. Isoprenaline and noradrenaline are equally active in stimulating β_3 receptors and are more powerful than adrenaline in this lipolytic action.

Salbutamol is even more selective. It stimulates β_2 receptors only and has very little action on β_1 receptors. Thus it produces bronchodilatation with little tachycardia or increase in excitability and is widely used for asthma (Ch. 6) as there is little danger of ventricular fibrillation (Table 2.5).

Central effects of sympathomimetic agents

Sympathomimetic drugs cause central stimulation – an alerting effect in-keeping with the flight, fright and fight actions of the sympathetic system. Thus, adrenaline causes sensations of anxiety or panic. *Amphetamines* and more especially *cocaine* produce sensations of alertness or elation which is so pleasurable that they are highly addictive. They are, as a consequence, Controlled Drugs (Ch. 4). Appetite suppressants such as *diethylpropion* have a similar but milder effect. All sympathomimetic agents induce wakefulness, and amphetamines have been widely used in the past, for example, by students working (as usual) at the last moment for examinations or by truck drivers who want to complete a long journey without resting. However, noradrenaline has no significant effects on mood.

Table 2.5 Directly and indirectly acting sympathomimetic drugs

1. *Directly acting:*
   Noradrenaline – α activity stronger than b activity
   Adrenaline – α, β_1 and β_2 activity
   Isoprenaline – β_1 and β_2 activity
   Salbutamol – β_2 activity
2. *Indirectly acting:*
   Cocaine
   Amphetamine (mainly stimulation of the CNS and only weak peripheral actions)
3. *Mixed direct and indirect acting:*
   Ephedrine

Directly and indirectly acting sympathomimetic agents

Many of the drugs mentioned so far – noradrenaline, adrenaline, isoprenaline and salbutamol – act directly on α and/or β receptors. They are therefore called 'directly acting sympathomimetic agents'.

Another group of drugs such as the amphetamines has an indirect sympathomimetic action. They do not stimulate α and β receptors but enter the storage vesicles to displace noradrenaline which then leaves the nerve ending. The transmitter crosses the gap and stimulates the α and β receptors. In this way, such drugs lead only indirectly to receptor activation.

Ephedrine is a drug which has both indirect and direct sympathomimetic activity. The classification of sympathomimetic drugs is summarised in Table 2.5.

Directly acting sympathomimetic drugs

Noradrenaline. Noradrenaline causes visceral and cutaneous vasoconstriction. When given intravenously, it almost immediately raises the blood pressure. For this reason it has been used in the treatment of shock, but has the disadvantage that the intense vasoconstriction reduces the blood supply to vital organs. Shocked patients with peripheral circulatory failure are not, therefore, treated in this way because the aim of the treatment is to increase blood flow to vital organs such as the kidneys.

Noradrenaline has been used in some local anaesthetic solutions to prolong their duration of action by producing vasoconstriction around the site of injection. However, it has no advantages for this purpose and has caused several deaths from acute hypertension.

Adrenaline. Adrenaline has been used in the past as a bronchodilator for treating asthmatic attacks. After subcutaneous injection (the correct route of administration in most cases), there is not only effective bronchodilatation but also a rise in the systolic blood pressure and heart rate. As a result, adrenaline is no longer used for asthma now that selective β_2 agonists such as salbutamol are available. Adrenaline is still given for anaphylaxis but should not be given intravenously because of the danger of cardiac arrhythmias except in dire emergency.

Adrenaline is widely used as a vasoconstrictor agent incorporated with local anaesthetics to prolong their action, and over many decades of use, has proved to be remarkably safe.

Isoprenaline. Isoprenaline is another bronchodilator drug. It is absorbed through the oral mucosa and thus directly enters systemic capillaries and so avoids breakdown in the liver. Isoprenaline has been widely used for asthma by inhalation. This route of administration delivers a high concentration of the drug immediately to the airways, while relatively little reaches the rest of the body. Nevertheless, some patients have given themselves excessive amounts and died suddenly – probably because of ventricular fibrillation due to massive β_1 stimulation. Now that more selective agents are available, isoprenaline is no longer used for asthma.

Isoprenaline may be used to treat cardiac arrhythmias when a higher rate of initiation of the cardiac impulse or accelerated A-V conduction is needed, or to treat loss of consciousness due to excessive bradycardia or heart block.

Salbutamol. Salbutamol is one of the drugs of choice in the day-to-day management of bronchial asthma. Salbutamol is a selective β_2 stimulator – it produces bronchodilatation without significantly increasing cardiac excitability.

It is usually given by inhalation of an aerosol or of a powder from a special dispenser (Rotahaler), but can also be given orally (it is absorbed from the upper part of the small intestine), or intravenously. Intravenous injection produces an almost immediate response and is useful for the management of acute asthmatic attacks, when the intense brochospasm prevents effective inhalation of an aerosol.

Indirectly acting sympathomimetic drugs

As noted earlier, sympathomimetic agents have a stimulant effect on the CNS. Cocaine and amphetamine cause wakefulness and elation as their predominant effect.

Cocaine. Cocaine is a central stimulant but, uniquely, is also a potent local anaesthetic agent which is strongly sympathomimetic by its indirect α and β effects. It displaces stores of noradrenaline from the sympathetic nerve endings and blocks their reuptake. Cocaine is therefore an effective vasoconstrictor and has similar effects on the heart to adrenaline. Overdose may therefore cause sudden death, particularly from ventricular fibrillation. Because of this risk cocaine is not given by injection except by some addicts.

Cocaine therefore has a remarkable assortment of properties in that it is:

1. A potent, (indirectly acting) sympathomimetic agent, and hence a vasoconstrictor
2. A potent local and surface anaesthetic
3. A strong central stimulant
4. A drug of dependence because of its euphoriant effects.

Amphetamine. Amphetamine has weak peripheral sympathomimetic activity. It usually produces only slight bronchodilatation, tachycardia and hypertension. Its main action is on the brain as a central stimulant. It accelerates mental activity, suppresses sensations of sleepiness and fatigue, and produces excitement, euphoria and anorexia.

Amphetamine has been used in the past to suppress appetite in the hope of controlling obesity. Unfortunately, the drug is powerfully addictive and its effect on appetite only transient. Because of its high addictive potential, amphetamine is used very little in clinical practice and is a Controlled Drug.

Sympathomimetic drugs with both direct and indirect actions

Ephedrine. Ephedrine has two actions: it displaces stores of noradrenaline from sympathetic nerve endings, and also stimulates α and β receptors, as does adrenaline.

Ephedrine can be given orally for the treatment of asthma, but is no longer the drug of choice. It is occasionally given by injection to maintain the blood pressure during a spinal anaesthetic.

Ephedrine may be used in nose drops for hay fever and in dentistry, to reduce congestion and oedema of the nasal mucosa, and thus improve drainage from the maxillary antrum. This may be useful if, for example, the antrum is exposed to infection via an oroantral fistula.

Adrenoreceptor (adrenergic) blockers

The idea of a division of the results of sympathetic stimulation into α and β effects is confirmed by the fact that these effects can be selectively blocked by different drugs.

Drugs such as *phentolamine* and *thymoxamine* bind to and block α receptors, leaving β activity mainly unaffected. They are therefore termed 'α blockers'.

β-blocking drugs block β receptors, but some have additional actions. Important examples are *propranolol* and *oxprenolol.*

α receptor blockers

Phentolamine binds reversibly to α receptors. This short-acting drug has been used in the diagnosis and management of phaeochromocytoma. This tumour of the adrenal medulla secretes adrenaline and noradrenaline. It causes hypertension which is reversed by phentolamine.

Phentolamine and other α blockers are used in an attempt to improve blood flow to the tissues in obstructive peripheral vascular disease. In shock, α blockers may, by themselves, lower blood pressure further so that in practice blood, plasma or dextran is also given intravenously to replace the circulating fluid volume and restore the blood pressure.

Thymoxamine is a long-acting α blocker used in the treatment of hypertension due to phaeochromocytoma.

Prazosin is a selective, postjunctional α receptor blocker. It is used for the treatment of hypertension (Ch. 5).

Uses of α adrenoreceptor blocking drugs

These include the treatment of:

1. *Hypertension* due to:
    a. Overdose of noradrenaline or potentiation of pressor amines (particularly by tyramine in cheese) in patients receiving monoamine oxidase inhibitors (see Ch. 3)
    b. Essential hypertension
2. *Peripheral vascular disease.*

Essential hypertension. The older α blockers were not usually suitable, as their hypotensive effects did not persist and side-effects were troublesome. Side-effects included tachycardia, postural hypotension and gastrointestinal actions, such as diarrhoea, as a result of unopposed parasympathetic activity. However, drugs such as labetalol which possess both α and β adrenoceptor properties are useful hypotensive agents. The pure α_1 adrenoceptor blocker prazosin has no action on prejunctional α receptors (Table 2.5). It is an effective vasodilator and is also valuable in the treatment of essential hypertension.

Peripheral vascular disease. α blocking agents such as thymoxamine may be used for relief of spasm of peripheral vessels in Raynaud's disease. Their use to improve the circulation to promote the healing of chronic ulceration of the skin as a complication of varicose veins is rarely successful.

β receptor blockers

Propranolol blocks both β_1 and β_2 receptors. Because of its action on β_1 receptors it diminishes sympathetic drive to the heart. Thus, the tachycardia and the greater cardiac work of exercise are blocked. These effects benefit patients with angina pectoris. Such patients have restricted blood flow to the myocardium, so that exercise, which raises the oxygen needs of the myocardium, causes pain in the chest. Propranolol dampens the response of the heart to exercise and thus prevents the pain of angina.

Propranolol is also used to block background sympathetic tone which otherwise enhances the excitability of the heart. The ability of the drug to lessen myocardial excitability makes it useful for the treatment of cardiac arrhythmias such as atrial and ventricular tachycardias and extrasystoles.

Propranolol also blocks both β_2 receptors and background sympathetic tone which dilates the bronchi. Asthmatic patients rely on relaxation of the bronchial muscle to maintain a free airway so that a β_2 blocker causes a dangerous bronchospasm in them.

Atenolol and *metoprolol* are selective β_1 blockers and have similar actions and uses to propranolol in cardiovascular disease. Because they have relatively little β_2 blocking action they may be somewhat less dangerous for asthmatic patients, but nevertheless are sufficiently so to produce dangerous bronchospasm in some patients.

The β blockers are widely used for the treatment of hypertension. This is partly by decreasing the stroke volume of the heart, but there is also a central action on the nervous control of blood pressure, a reduction in renin output by the kidney and diminished release of noradrenaline from sympathetic nerves.

Table 2.6 Some uses of β blockers

Angina pectoris
Hypertension
Arrhythmias
Acute and secondary management of myocardial infarction
Anxiety states with strong sympathetic manifestations
Thyrotoxicosis
Hypertrophic cardiomyopathy and some other heart diseases
Migraine prophylaxis
Essential tremor
Open angle glaucoma
Alcohol and narcotic withdrawal
Intra-operatively to control arrhythmias due to halothane

Uses of β blocking agents

The main applications can be summarised as:

1. *Angina pectoris*. β blockers diminish sympathetic drive to the heart, particularly during exercise, and lessen cardiac effort.
2. *Essential hypertension*. β blockers diminish sympathetic tone and decrease cardiac output, but possibly also have a central action on nervous control of blood pressure.
3. *Cardiac arrhythmias*. β blockers reduce cardiac excitability. This may be useful during general anaesthesia with halothane which sensitises the myocardium to catecholamines such as adrenaline. β blockers may also be effective in controlling arrhythmias after myocardial infarction and improve survival by reducing the risk of reinfarction.
4. *Anxiety*. When characterised by obvious sympathetic overactivity (dry mouth, palpitations, tremor), anxiety can disable speakers and musicians who are giving public performances, and generally responds better to β blockers than to benzodiazepines.

In addition to these important applications, β blockers have a remarkable range of activities, a few of which are discussed in later chapters, which are summarised in Table 2.6. However, it should be noted that individual β blockers vary significantly in their effectiveness in these different applications.

Sympathetic blockade in the treatment of hypertension

Peripheral resistance, and hence blood pressure, can be lowered by reducing sympathetic tone, i.e. by diminishing its vasoconstrictor action on the arterioles. This effect may be predominantly:

1. Central – clonidine and methyldopa act centrally but also have important peripheral effects (Table 2.4); β blockers may also act partly on the CNS
2. At the arteriole, e.g. prazosin
3. At the adrenergic nerve ending, e.g. guanethidine – β blockers possibly lessen transmitter release.

These effects are discussed in more detail in Chapter 5.

Appetite suppressants (anorectics)

Anorectics are drugs used to suppress appetite (i.e. induce anorexia) in order to help the obese lose weight. They are discussed here as most of them are sympathomimetic and related chemically to the amphetamines.

Obesity is one of the current major problems in medicine, particularly because of its association with or contribution to diabetes, hypertension, atherosclerosis and ischaemic heart disease. Although obese persons may not necessarily have a greater calorie intake than thin ones, the only way by which they can safely and reliably lose weight is by eating (and drinking) less and by taking more exercise. This is more easily said than done, since an uncommon degree of self-discipline is needed to remain persistently faithful to a restricted and boring diet.

Sympathomimetic drugs, particularly the amphetamines, suppress appetite. Amphetamines and other somewhat similar drugs, such as diethylpropion, are addictive and are Controlled Drugs. They may cause mild euphoria, insomnia, 'edginess', or tachycardia in some patients.

Fluorinated amphetamines such as fenfluramine have the opposite side-effects. They have a sedative action on the CNS and their main disadvantages are drowsiness and sometimes depression. However, patients are less likely to become dependent and suffer insomnia. In addition, unlike the amphetamines, fenfluramine does not antagonise antihypertensive therapy. This is important as obesity and hypertension are often associated.

The appetite-suppressant effect of both these types of drug is real, but most patients quite quickly acquire tolerance and the effect is relatively transient. Needless to say, anorectics are completely ineffective when patients do not also restrict their diet. Anorectics have little more than a temporary effect, but they can be used for a short time to help with dietary re-education. Fenfluramine, however, has been used for periods of at least 6 months with significant and sustained loss of weight.

THE PARASYMPATHETIC NERVOUS SYSTEM

The general arrangement of neurones in the parasympathetic nervous system is similar to that in the sympathetic system (Fig. 2.6).

The parasympathetic nerve fibres leave the CNS with some of the cranial nerves (e.g. the nerves to the ciliary muscle and iris travel with the third cranial nerve; the vagus mainly carries parasympathetic fibres to the thoracic and abdominal viscera), and with the sacral nerves from segments S2 and S3. The parasympathetic ganglia are generally closely associated with the organs which they innervate, and thus the postganglionic nerve fibres are very short. The neurotransmitter chemical in both the parasympathetic ganglion and at the neuroeffector junction is acetylcholine. The types of chemical mediator acting in the voluntary and autonomic nervous systems are summarised in Figure 2.7.

Muscarinic and nicotinic effects. At the neuroeffector junction of the parasympathetic system, acetylcholine is said to exert *muscarinic* actions because these sites are also stimulated by

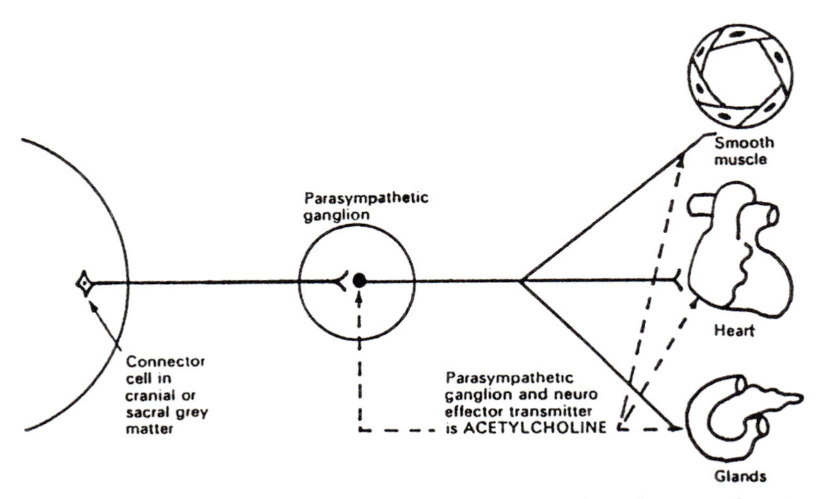

Fig. 2.6 The parasympathetic nervous sytem. This shows the main connections and that acetylcholine acts as the transmitter at both the ganglion and neuroeffector junctions.

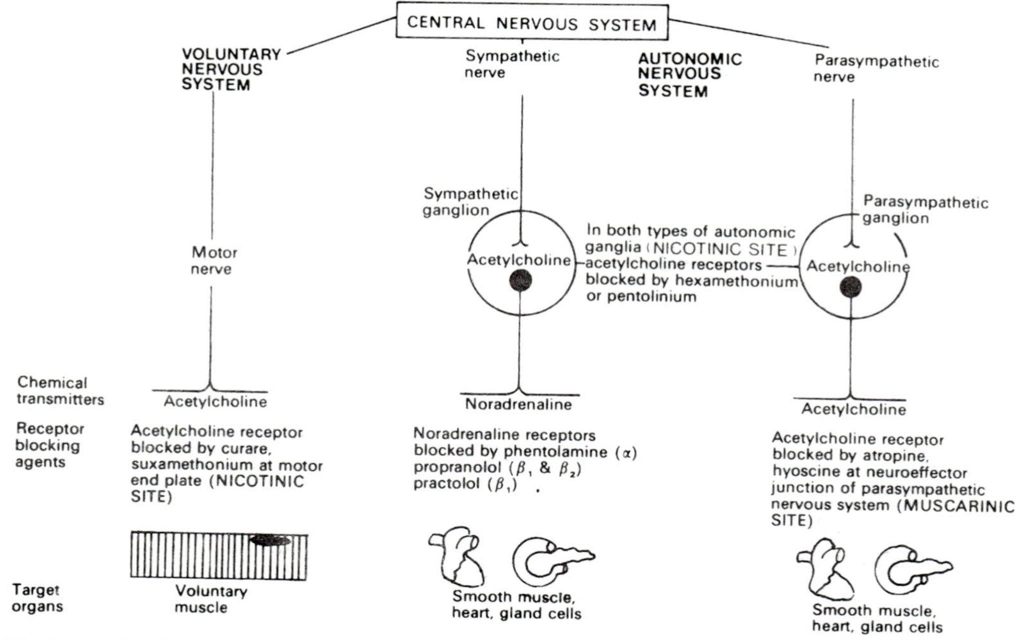

Fig. 2.7 This diagram summarises the types of chemical mediator released in both the voluntary and the autonomic nervous systems. In addition, the different blocking agents and their sites of action are shown.

the toxin, muscarine (from the poisonous toadstool *Amanita muscaria*). The effects of acetylcholine at the sympathetic and parasympathetic ganglia and at the motor end-plate of voluntary muscle are called *nicotinic* because in low concentrations nicotine also stimulates these sites. In high concentration nicotine blocks transmission across these junctions. The importance of these distinctions is that, although acetylcholine is the chemical transmitter in these different situations, its muscarinic effects are blocked by atropine while its nicotinic effects are not.

The nicotinic receptor is a protein which is closely attached to ion channels in the cell membrane, as described earlier. The muscarinic receptor is also a membrane protein, but acts only indirectly to open ion (Na^+ and K^+) channels via a regulatory protein (G protein) and production of a second messenger, guanosine nucleotide. The main differences between these two types of cholinergic receptors are summarised in Table 2.7.

At all sites under normal conditions the action of acetylcholine is brief because it is destroyed by the enzyme *acetylcholinesterase*. This is in contrast to the termination of the action of noradrenaline, which is actively taken up again into the sympathetic nerve endings and is thus removed from the receptor targets.

Parasympathomimetic drugs

Acetylcholine is a parasympathomimetic drug, but it is not used clinically because it is almost immediately destroyed by cholinesterase in the blood and tissues. Instead, *anticholinesterases* are

Table 2.7 Features of nicotinic and muscarinic receptors in the parasympathetic system

Nicotinic receptors	Muscarinic receptors
Present at neuromuscular junction (also at autonomic ganglia and CNS)	Present at neuroeffector junction in the parasympathetic system
Open Na^+ and K^+ channels in milliseconds to cause depolarisation	G-protein-coupled reaction giving a slower response. May be excitatory or inhibitory
Blocked by muscle relaxants	
Not blocked by atropine	Blocked by atropine

usually used to inhibit the enzymes which normally destroy acetylcholine. Thus, the action of acetylcholine which has been physiologically released is greatly prolonged.

Pilocarpine is used to constrict the pupil to relieve glaucoma (raised introcular pressure). It is not hydrolysed by cholinesterase and acts for 3–4 h. Pilocarpine has been suggested to be effective for improving salivation in those with dry mouth, but side-effects such as sweating and colic may be troublesome.

Carbachol has actions similar to those of acetylcholine, but is not destroyed by cholinesterase. When given by injection it strengthens smooth muscle tone in the gut and bladder. It is used to initiate peristalsis after an operation and to treat an atonic bladder. Carbachol is also used to expel gas from the large intestine before an X-ray examination of the abdomen.

Anticholinesterases (Table 2.8)

Physostigmine

Physostigmine is a reversible inhibitor of cholinesterase and an important use for it, or one of its analogues such as pyridostigmine, is for treatment of myasthenia gravis. The latter is characterised by increasing muscle weakness and excessive tendency to fatigue. This is caused by loss of acetylcholine receptors in the motor end-plate due to autoantibodies to them. Anticholinesterases raise the concentration of acetylcholine in the region of the receptors and thus strengthen muscular power.

Table 2.8 Summary of actions and uses of cholinergic drugs and anticholinesterases

1. Acetylcholine is the chemical transmitter at all ganglia and endings of the autonomic nervous system with the single exception of adrenergic endings of the sympathetic system
2. Acetylcholine has a wide variety of effects, but is too unselective in its actions and too rapidly destroyed by cholinesterase to be useful clinically
3. Cholinergic agents such as pilocarpine and its analogues have been used for such purposes as increasing salivary secretion, but widespread unselective actions (direct cholinergic effects) make their use impractical
4. Other choline esters such as carbachol are resistant to cholinesterase and have more selective actions. For example, they may be used to stimulate bowel or bladder action after surgery
5. Anticholinesterases are used in medicine principally as antidotes to competitive neuromuscular blocking agents and to treat myasthenia gravis

Physostigmine eye drops are used to constrict the pupil. When this happens, fluid can more readily drain from the anterior chamber and reduce intraocular pressure. Physostigmine is therefore used to lower the excessive intraocular pressure characteristic of glaucoma.

Anticholinesterases, such as pyridostigmine can also be used in an attempt to increase salivary secretion in diseases of these glands, such as Sjögren's syndrome. However, other cholinergic effects of these drugs (particularly physostigmine), such as nausea, diarrhoea and bradycardia are often troublesome.

Another use of anticholinesterases is to reverse the action of a non-depolarising muscle relaxant such as tubocurarine.

Organophosphorus pesticides

Chemicals such as di-isopropylfluorophosphonate (DFP), are *irreversible* inhibitors of cholinesterase. They form the basis of the chemical weapons known as nerve gases, and of some pesticides. They are quickly absorbed through the skin and mucous membranes. Even a small amount applied to the conjunctival sac can produce systemic effects such as increased salivary and bronchial secretions, bronchospasm, colic and diarrhoea. However, the main effect is twitching followed by muscular paralysis due to the enhanced nicotinic action of acetylcholine, and death from respiratory paralysis.

Parasympathetic blocking drugs (antimuscarinic agents)

Atropine

Atropine* together with hyoscyamine and hyoscine, is derived from solanaceous plants – particularly Deadly Nightshade, the berries of which are poisonous because of these substances.

*Atropine was used by sixteenth-century ladies to dilate the pupils and produce 'sparkling eyes'; hence its older name, Belladonna (lit. fair lady). Atropine was also valued as a poison and its name derives from Atropos (one of the Fates of Greek mythology) whose job was to cut the thread of life.

The atropine group of drugs antagonises the actions of acetylcholine at *muscarinic* sites only. At these sites, they act by competing with acetylcholine for cholinergic receptors. This is therefore another example of competitive drug antagonism. Thus, the atropine group of drugs blocks the action of acetylcholine on the heart, on glands and on smooth muscle, but does *not* affect transmission in the autonomic ganglia or at the motor end-plate of voluntary muscle (Figs 2.7 and 2.10).

The actions and uses of atropine, or atropine-like drugs are summarised in Table 2.9.

Dilatation of the pupil by antimuscarinic drugs is by abolishing parasympathetic-mediated pupillary constrictor tone. At the same time, the ciliary muscle (also under parasympathetic control) is paralysed and the patient cannot accommodate the lens for near vision. These effects can be prolonged so that similar but shorter-acting drugs, such as homatropine, tropicamide or cyclopentolate may be preferred. Alternatively the action of atropine can be reversed in the eye by the local instillation of physostigmine eye drops.

Table 2.9 Actions and uses of antimuscarinic drugs

1. As premedication to diminish salivary and bronchial secretions during anaesthesia
2. To diminish vagal slowing of the heart during induction of anaesthesia*
3. To reverse excessive slowing of the heart (sinus bradycardia), particularly after myocardial infarction (see Ch. 5)
4. To induce bronchodilatation in asthma. Atropine itself is little used for this purpose but isopropyl atropine (*ipratropium*) and *oxitropium* are, for some patients, effective and useful bronchodilators with less drying effect on bronchial secretions than atropine
5. To reduce bronchial secretions and bronchospasm in patients being treated with an anticholinesterase such as physostigmine for myasthenia gravis
6. To dilate the pupil (by local instillation into the conjunctival sac) to facilitate ophthalmoscopic examination of the retina
7. To moderate excessive central cholinergic activity and hence reduce muscle spasm in parkinsonism (Ch. 3)
8. To relieve peptic ulcer. For this purpose the selective (gastric) antimuscarinic drug *pirenzepine* is very effective in blocking parasympathetically mediated acid secretion Ch. 12)

* The effectiveness or even the need for atropine for this purpose nowadays is questionable.

Atropine and related drugs are contraindicated in glaucoma, since they block drainage from the anterior chamber of the eye and further increase intraocular pressure.

Hyoscine

Hyoscine has identical peripheral actions to atropine but, while atropine is a central stimulant, hyoscine is a depressant. It causes drowsiness and inhibits the vomiting centre. Hyoscine is thus a valuable drug as a premedication before general anaesthesia. Not only does it reduce salivary and bronchial secretions (and therefore lessens the risk of pulmonary complications), it also lessens the apprehension of patients being brought to the anaesthetic room. This in turn reduces the amount of anaesthetic necessary to produce general anaesthesia and also lessens the risk of vomiting. The antiemetic properties of hyoscine also make it effective for preventing travel sickness.

Antihistamines, such as promethazine, cyclizine an diphenhydramine, happen also to have hyoscine-like properties. Hence they are also useful for managing motion sickness, but most of them also cause drowsiness and a dry mouth.

Actions of acetylcholine and its antagonists

As shown in Figure 2.8, drugs with an anticholinergic action do not block all its activities and different types of drugs act at different sites in a selective fashion as follows:

1. Ganglion blocking agents. These block transmission at sympathetic ganglia and quickly lower blood pressure. Parasympathetic activity is also blocked to cause such effects as depressed salivary secretion, constipation and retention of urine. An example is *trimetaphan* used to provide controlled hypotension during surgery (Ch. 5).

2. Anticholinergic agents. This term is loosely used for antimuscarinic drugs. They act at *postganglionic*, cholinergic (mainly parasympathetic) nerve endings and include atropine and drugs with atropine-like actions. Such drugs block the muscarinic actions of acetylcholine for the purposes shown in Table 2.9. Some of these agents,

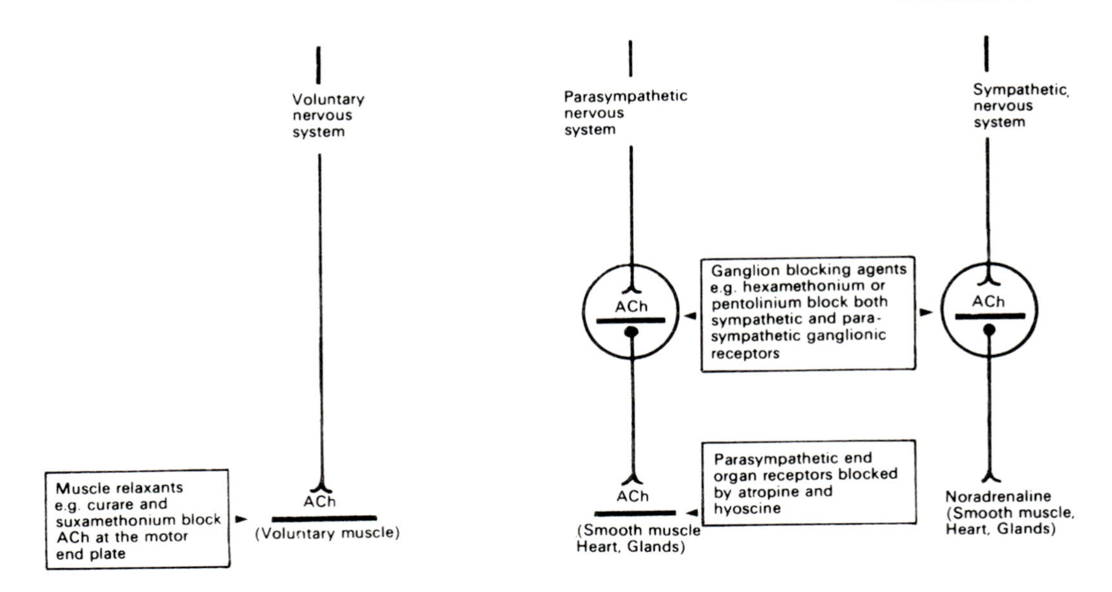

Fig. 2.8 Receptor blockade of acetylcholine (ACh) in different parts of the nervous system by different drugs.

such as hyoscine, also depress the CNS and thus cause sedation and suppress the vomiting reflex.

*3. **Competitive neuromuscular blocking agents.*** Acetylcholine is the chemical transmitter at the neuromuscular junction. This so-called nicotinic action is *not* antagonised by atropine. Curare and related drugs block this action of acetylcholine by combining with (competing successfully for) the specific receptors on the motor end-plate. The effect can only be reversed by promoting the build-up of a sufficient concentration of acetylcholine. This is done by using an anticholinesterase to prevent the destruction of normally produced acetylcholine.

Table 2.10 Summary of actions of acetylcholine as an autonomic transmitter and of acetylcholine blocking drugs

Acetylcholine is the chemical transmitter at:

1. *All autonomic ganglia*, whether sympathetic or parasympathetic
2. *All parasympathetic nerve endings* – also sympathetic nerve endings controlling sweat glands and vasodilator fibres
3. *Neuromuscular end-plates*

Different types of drugs with anticholinergic actions which act on different receptors include:

1. *Ganglion blocking drugs* for lowering blood pressure
2. *Antimuscarinic drugs* used particularly to
   a. Depress digestive, including salivary, secretions
   b. Relax smooth muscle of the gut and bronchioles
   c. Depress vagal activity and increase heart rate
   d. Block muscarinic receptors in the brain to mitigate the severity of parkinsonism (Ch. 3)
3. *Competitive neuromuscular blocking agents* – these combat the nicotinic actions of acetylcholine at the motor end-plate to cause muscle paralysis

Effects of autonomic drugs on salivary function

Salivary secretion is stimulated by parasympathetic activity and is inhibited by sympathetic stimulation, as exemplified by the dry mouth of acute anxiety. In addition, salivary secretion can be diminished as a result of dehydration (itself occasionally caused by drugs, particularly the potent diuretics) or disease of the glands themselves.

Causes of drug-induced xerostomia are listed in Chapter 13 but are also summarised in Table 2.11.

Table 2.11 Causes of drug-induced xerostomia

Drugs with antimuscarinic effects, including:
Atropine and its analogues
Tricyclic antidepressants
Phenothiazines
Antihistamines
Sympathomimetic drugs including:
Ephedrine and other sympathomimetic drugs in so-called 'cold cures'
Decongestants and bronchodilators
Amphetamines

Hypersalivation is not a clinical problem, unless there is dysphagia or impaired neuromuscular function to cause dribbling, as any excess is normally swallowed. Drugs which increase salivary secretion (sialagogues) may be needed if the glands are diseased and the amount of functional tissue reduced. Unfortunately the only effective sialagogues are the cholinesterase inhibitors (physostigmine and its analogues) which also increase the activity of all organs with muscarinic nerve endings, such as the gastrointestinal tract, with diarrhoea as the main side-effect, as discussed earlier. When such drugs are given (particularly for the treatment of myasthenia gravis), atropine or an analogue must, therefore, also be given.

3. The nervous system
II. Depressants of cerebral function and some other centrally acting drugs

Depressants of the CNS are among the most widely used drugs both medically and non-medically. Most of the drugs of dependence (apart from cocaine, amphetamine and related drugs) are CNS depressants and, conversely, most types of CNS depressant are addictive to some degree.

Alcohol is the archetype of all sedatives, hypnotics and general anaesthetic agents and is also the most widely used drug of dependence. The main action of alcohol, namely progressive, non-selective depression of the CNS, is essentially the same as that of barbiturates and anaesthetic agents.

Alcohol as a general CNS depressant

There is almost unlimited opportunity to observe the effects of alcohol, which illustrates clearly the actions of a typical CNS depressant. The apparent differences between the effects of anaesthetic agents and sedatives such as barbiturates on the one hand and alcohol on the other, depend mainly on dose and rate of uptake. All, in large enough doses, cause unconsciousness and eventually respiratory depression and death. In smaller doses, sleep is promoted if circumstances are favourable and alcohol is often spoken of euphemistically as a 'night cap'.

In moderate doses both barbiturates and alcohol relieve anxiety.* This relief of anxiety by alcohol, as with barbiturates, is at the cost of blunting other mental faculties. Under appropriate social circumstances (in pubs or at parties) small amounts of alcohol and other sedating drugs first depress the higher centres and, by blunting anxiety and inhibitions, usually produce a pleasant brightening of mood and conversation – an almost essential requirement to alleviate the hideous boredom of most social occasions. Initially, at least, a congenial atmosphere develops and, as more drink goes down, tongues are loosened and talk becomes noisier. For this reason, alcohol is widely regarded as a 'stimulant'. This is a dangerous misconception since the unselective depressant action of alcohol on the CNS causes both rapid deterioration of skill and judgement, and also such loss of insight that drinkers believe their performance to be improved. As more drink goes down, therefore, speech becomes slurred due to deterioration of muscular control, moods become unpredictable (but generally worsen) and movements become uncoordinated.

The consequences of these effects of alcohol in terms of motor accidents alone have been disastrous. In many, aggression is released and expressed as violent arguments, fighting or lethal car driving. Eventually, if enough drink is taken and if vomiting does not supervene, the hypnotic action of alcohol becomes overwhelming and is marked traditionally by the guest (or host) sliding under the table.

Death due to acute alcohol overdose can happen when an enterprising individual decides to swallow in quick succession (often for a bet or bravado) two or more bottles of neat whisky or gin – a bottle usually contains 750 ml of approximately 40% ethanol. Death can result from de-

* 'Dutch courage' is a nickname for this property of alcohol, though the term does not refer to any lack of courage on the part of the Dutch. It was probably because of the introduction of Hollands (Dutch gin).

pression of the respiratory centre or, more often, from aspiration of vomit.

Unlike alcohol, general anaesthetic agents are given rapidly, in relatively high doses, and by a route (inhalation or intravenous) ensuring rapid absorption. Nevertheless, small doses of general anaesthetics are just as intoxicating as alcohol. Nitrous oxide (laughing gas) in particular can cause wild euphoria, as can ether. Both agents were used as intoxicants soon after the discovery of their anaesthetic properties and 'ether revels' were a remarkable feature of an otherwise puritanical social scene in nineteenth-century USA. Chloroform was introduced as an anaesthetic agent in 1847, by Sir James Simpson after experimenting with a wide variety of substances which he and his colleagues tried out on themselves. When chloroform was tried, 'Immediately an unwonted hilarity seized the party: they became bright-eyed, very happy and loquacious – expatiating on the delicious aroma of the new fluid. The conversation was of unusual intelligence and quite charmed the listeners . . .'. There was a sudden crash as the experimenters suddenly lost consciousness. The similarities between the effects on Simpson and his friends of chloroform and those of alcohol will be only too obvious.

Alcohol has also been used as an anaesthetic agent but has severe limitations. It is insufficiently volatile to be useful as an inhalational agent and the anaesthetic dose is close to that which causes respiratory depression. However, it is mildly analgesic and this effect of alcohol often causes a drunk to be unaware of injuries, and analgesia is enhanced by its anxiolytic effects. Thus, the drunk may not feel pain so sharply and is also less concerned about such pain as he or she feels: this represents the first stage of general anaesthesia (Ch. 18).

In view of its desirable properties, it is hardly surprising that alcohol is so heavily used and can lead to dependence. Attempts at prohibition have generally failed. Punitive taxation also does not discourage consumption, which steadily rises. Most governments have, therefore, taken advantage of the situation to use alcohol as a source of enormous revenue. The public cannot do without alcohol and the State cannot do without the revenue. So for these and other reasons alcohol is an almost inseparable feature of our culture.

Alcohol is a potent drug of dependence by virtue of its power to blunt anxiety and to induce a pleasantly stuporous state. The ready availability and social acceptability of alcohol also contribute to its wide use as a drug of dependence.

Withdrawal can have severe effects on the confirmed alcoholic and continued heavy consumption can damage health in various ways. Alcohol is nevertheless a permitted drug of dependence as yet, and dependence is on a huge scale.

Alcohol therefore has actions typical of many unselective CNS depressants, namely:

1. Progressive depression of higher centres, coordination and consciousness, culminating in coma
2. Respiratory depression
3. Anxiolytic
4. Mildly analgesic
5. Addictive.

Alcohol has virtually no uses in medicine, apart from being an effective skin antiseptic. Its 'strengthening' and 'tonic' properties are illusory, or no more than subjective. Belief in such effects is, however, widely held and sedulously encouraged by the brewers and distillers. 'Tonic wine' is itself a contributory cause of chronic alcoholism.

Types of CNS depressant

Depressants of the CNS have varying degrees of selectivity of action on different aspects of brain function and are of the following types:

Anxiolytics. Anxiolytic drugs are used to lessen feelings of tension and to alleviate anxiety, ideally without causing drowsiness. In practice, the benzodiazepines, which are the most widely used anxiolytics, usually cause some degree of sedation. The terms 'sedative' and 'tranquilliser' should be avoided.

Hypnotics. Hypnotics are used to induce sleep, but in smaller doses are often used as anxiolytics. Barbiturates were the main hypnotics used, but have been replaced by the benzodiazepines which are safer in overdose and are possibly less addictive.

Opioid (narcotic) analgesics. Opioids are the most potent analgesics by their action on the CNS. They are also anxiolytic and hypnotic, and in larger doses induce stupor (narcosis). The opioids are also one of the main groups of abused drugs because of their pleasurable anxiolytic effects (Ch. 4).

General anaesthetics. General anaesthetics rapidly induce unconsciousness deep enough to resist arousal by pain, but ideally without significant depression of the respiratory and cardiac centres. Ideally also, recovery quickly follows withdrawal (Ch. 18).

Other centrally acting drugs

Most of these drugs have some central depressant effect but this is only a side-effect of their main action. They include the following:

Drugs used for Parkinson's disease. Antiparkinsonian drugs are given to correct the imbalance between central dopaminic and cholinergic activity which causes the disorders of movement characteristic of Parkinson's disease and related disorders.

Antidepressants. Antidepressants are used to counter the lowering of mood and misery characteristic of depression, mainly by raising levels of amines in brain synapses.

Antipsychotics. Drugs such as the phenothiazines are used to suppress psychotic excited states such as schizophrenia and mania. 'Neuroleptic' (lit. 'mind grasping') is an alternative but unsatisfactory term sometimes used for this group of drugs.

ANXIOLYTIC DRUGS

Anxiety is fear. The essential difference between physiological anxiety and anxiety neurosis is the disparity between the severity of the response in relation to the cause. Suddenly meeting an angry cobra in one's bed would be likely to provoke some anxiety – undeniably, a physiological response. By contrast, panic when confronted by a pigeon or having to leave the house to go shopping are inappropriate responses and could justifiably be termed an anxiety neurosis. Such a neurosis may also manifest itself as feelings of anxiety or tension in the absence of any recognisable external precipitating factor.

Anxiety provoked by the prospect of dental treatment is almost universal, but ranges from controllable apprehension to a phobia which makes treatment impossible. It is obviously impossible to draw a line between normal and neurotic responses in such circumstances. Anxiety neurosis is very common and often difficult to treat. Psychotherapy (particularly listening patiently and sympathetically to the patient) may be helpful, but there is little objective evidence of its effectiveness. Psychoanalysis is of even more questionable value.

The manifestations of anxiety are not only sensations of fear, but also the peripheral manifestations of excessive sympathetic activity. There may therefore be a dry mouth, rapid forceful beating of the heart (palpitations), rapid breathing, tremor and sweating.

The drugs (anxiolytics) most widely used for the short-term treatment of anxiety are the benzodiazepines such as *diazepam*. Anxiety may be associated with depression, but anxiolytics are *not* antidepressive drugs. They may occasionally make depression worse or at least more obvious by their releasing action and should not be given for the long-term treatment of anxiety.

Psychotic agitation and hyperactivity are features of schizophrenia. These and other symptoms of this disease need to be treated with the antipsychotics such as the phenothiazines described later. The terms 'minor tranquillisers' for such drugs as the benzodiazepines and 'major tranquillisers' for such drugs as the phenothiazines, have been an unnecessary source of confusion by lumping together groups of drugs having totally different properties and toxic effects, and used for completely different types of disease. These terms should be avoided.

Benzodiazepines

Mode of action. Benzodiazepines act on the limbic system in the brain, where they potentiate the inhibitory neurotransmitter γ-aminobutyric acid (GABA); there are GABA-benzodiazepine receptor complexes in the brain. GABA is released from neurones in the CNS into the synaptic cleft. It binds to the GABA receptor and reduces the excitability of the adjacent excitatory neurone by increasing its permeability to chloride ions.

Closely associated with the GABA receptor is the benzodiazepine receptor, where benzodiazepines potentiate the inhibitory action of GABA by increasing permeability to chloride ions and further decreasing the excitability of the neurone (Fig. 3.1). The action of benzodiazepines can be reversed by the benzodiazepine antagonist, *flumazenil*. The latter acts by binding strongly to the benzodiazepine receptor and displacing benzodiazepine molecules. Potentiation of the inhibitory action of GABA is thus reversed.

Clinical uses. The benzodiazepines are effective anxiolytics which are considerably less sedating than their predecessors the barbiturates, though large doses can cause drowsiness. Individual susceptibility also varies widely and a satisfactory dosage regime has to be established for each patient.

Examples of benzodiazepines are *diazepam*, *midazolam* and *temazepam*. They differ mainly in their duration of action.

Benzodiazepines are effective for treating the central and peripheral manifestations of the anxiety state. Muscle tension and palpitations, as well as feelings of fear, may be suppressed. However, tolerance and dependence can develop within 4 weeks.

In dentistry, diazepam or midazolam are widely used for intravenous sedation (Ch. 18). Diazepam or flunitrazepam are frequently also used as premedication for general anaesthesia.

β Blockers

β-blocking drugs, such as propranolol and oxprenolol, may be more useful than benzodiazepines for patients whose symptoms of anxiety are mainly peripheral. For example, palpitations (awareness of rapid or forceful beating of the heart) may be suppressed by blockers of β adrenergic (sympathetic) activity. Tremor is also diminished.

Antidepressants

Tricyclic or monoamine oxidase inhibitor antidepressants are sometimes used by specialists for patients with chronic anxiety and for those who suffer from panic attacks or from phobic anxiety.

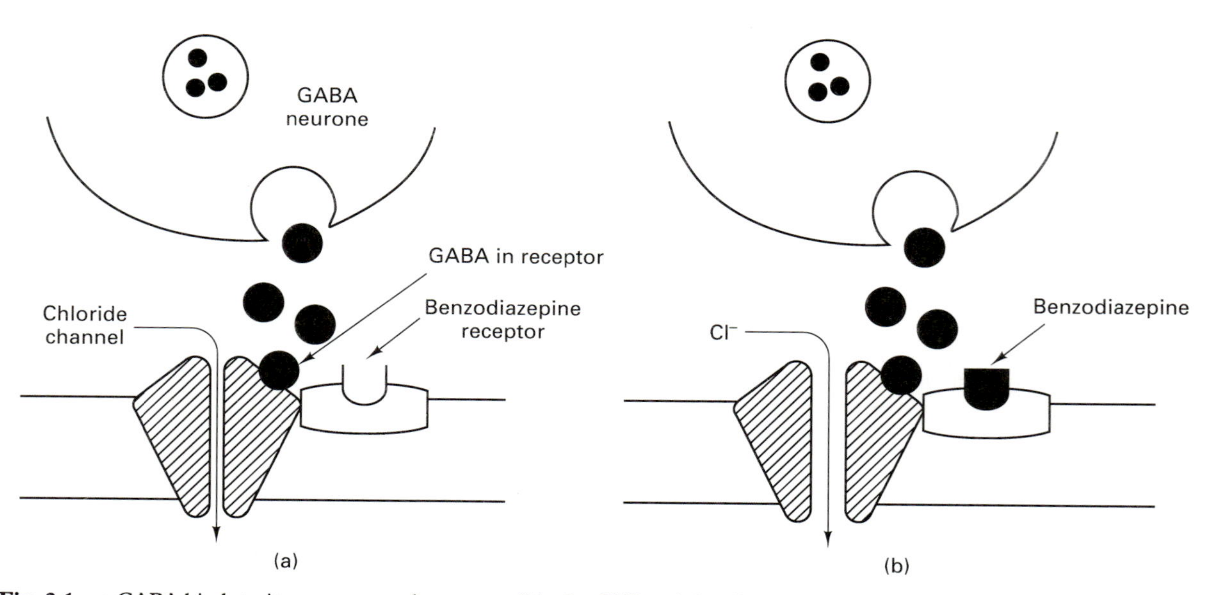

Fig. 3.1 **a** GABA binds to its receptor on the target cell in the CNS and, by allowing the inflow of chloride ions, reduces its excitability. **b** A benzodiazepine binds to a receptor closely related to the GABA receptor. When this happens the inflow of chloride ions is greatly enhanced and the inhibitory effect of GABA is intensified.

Other aspects of the management of anxiety

Complications of anxiety, particularly difficulty in falling asleep and disturbed sleep, may require specific treatment. In such cases benzodiazepines are used as hypnotics, as discussed below.

Acute panic attacks may punctuate the course of anxiety. These may be precipitated by a trivial stimulus or may be the result of confrontation with a 'phobic situation', such as visiting the dentist.

HYPNOTICS

Hypnotics are drugs that induce a state of sleep which is similar in depth to physiological sleep, in that the subject can be roused by external stimuli. However, this sleep is not the same as normal sleep – rapid eye movement (REM) sleep is suppressed and there is diminished dreaming. The physiological importance of REM sleep is not known.

There is no doubt that hypnotics are overprescribed. Little harm can come from not sleeping; when the need for sleep is great, falling asleep should be irresistible. In general, it is preferable if possible, to resist the temptation to prescribe hypnotic drugs – fatigue is a much safer hypnotic. On the other hand, tiredness caused by lack of sleep makes emotional problems and performance of exacting tasks more unmanageable. The use of a hypnotic drug may be justified during admission to hospital before an operation or before a stressful dental procedure, but once the threat has been resolved, the drug should be stopped. Depression and chronic anxiety states are also common and often interfere with sleep.

Hypnotics are not generally analgesic, and some of them, such as the largely obsolete barbiturates, potentiate sensitivity to pain. If pain prevents sleep an analgesic should be given.

There are several different types of hypnotic in general use. These include:

1. Benzodiazepines
2. Chloral hydrate
3. Chlormethiazole
4. Antihistamines
5. Barbiturates.

Of these the benzodiazepines are by far the most widely used.

Benzodiazepines

The mode of action of benzodiazepines has been described above. Earlier hypnotics were non-specific depressants of the CNS and in overdose could cause medullary paralysis. By contrast, the main action of benzodiazepines is to suppress anxiety, but they usually also cause some drowsiness and, in appropriate circumstances (a warm bed, darkness and quiet), induce sleep. Their effect on respiratory function in normal persons is negligible.

A great variety of benzodiazepines is now available but they differ mainly in their duration of action and to a slight degree in other properties.

Nitrazepam is one of the hypnotics of choice. It has a half-life of about 24 h and thus its sedating action may persist well into the next day. *Diazepam* has a half-life of 20–50 h but also has active metabolites which persist longer. It can thus cause more prolonged hangover than nitrazepam. *Flurazepam* itself has a short half-life but, like diazepam, has a metabolite which is a powerful hypnotic with an even longer half-life. *Temazepam*, by contrast, has a short half-life and no active metabolites, and is therefore a useful hypnotic.

The advantages of benzodiazepines as hypnotics are summarized in Table 3.1.

Respiratory depression by oral benzodiazepines is normally insignificant and overdose does not cause progressive depression of respiration. Hence, the risk of successful suicide is so slight as

Table 3.1 Advantages of benzodiazepines

1. Respiratory depression with normal doses is insignificant in healthy patients
2. Overdose does not cause severe or progressive depression of respiration
3. The potential for dependence is less than that of barbiturates
4. In the elderly, benzodiazepines are less likely to cause nocturnal confusion
5. After-effects ('hangover') may be less than with other hypnotics
6. Potentiation by other sedating agents is the only important drug interaction

to have raised doubts as to whether it is even possible.*

Respiratory depression due to benzodiazepines is only important in patients with chronic respiratory disease and impaired oxygen exchange. Most deaths ascribed to benzodiazepines have therefore either been in patients with chronic lung disease or as a result of taking alcohol or other drugs at the same time.

The addictive potential of benzodiazepines is relatively low, though benzodiazepine dependence may be seriously disabling for many weeks.

The after-effects of benzodiazepines also tend to be slight. Many patients experience no subjective after-effects.** In fact, most patients have slightly depressed mental acuity for a few hours after waking. Careful testing shows that reaction times are usually prolonged for several hours after waking, especially when long-acting benzodiazepines have been taken.

The effects of benzodiazepines may come on very quickly and they should be taken immediately before going to bed – not in the bath and certainly not in the car while driving home in the evening.

Chloral hydrate and trichloroethanol

Chloral hydrate has been in use since the nineteenth century. It was the first synthetic hypnotic, is relatively safe, and in normal doses does not cause significant respiratory depression. It has an unpleasant taste and is a gastric irritant. However, these disadvantages lessen the chances of overdose, which causes depression of respiration, the heart and the vasomotor centre.

Chloral is quickly absorbed from the gastrointestinal tract and converted into trichloroethanol which is the active metabolite. *Triclofos* is an ester of trichloroethanol and has similar actions to and the advantages of chloral hydrate. Triclofos has the additional advantages of not causing gastric irritation and is a tablet not a liquid.

Chlormethiazole

Chlormethiazole (Heminevrin) is an effective hypnotic with a short duration of action. It can cause cardiovascular and respiratory depression in large doses.

Zopiclone

Zopiclone is not structurally related to the benzodiazepines but has a similar type of action on the GABA receptors. Its disadvantages are persistent sedation, nausea and a bitter taste.

Antihistamines

Promethazine like many drugs of this group, is also a sedative and hypnotic. It may be used in children, particularly if sleep is disturbed by itching. The main objections to promethazine are the prolonged hangover of persistent drowsiness, potentiation by alcohol, respiratory depression and fits.

Barbiturates

The intermediate acting barbiturates are powerful hypnotics but their use is now largely obsolete. Examples are amylobarbitone, pentobarbitone and quinalbarbitone, but they have a high addictive potential and are therefore Controlled Drugs. Barbiturates can also cause excitement and confusion in the elderly and depress respiration. As with most hypnotic drugs, after-effects often persist for several hours after waking. These include loss of mental acuity, drowsiness and headache.

The respiratory depression caused by barbiturates made them effective and commonly used agents of suicide. In patients with emphysema or chest infections they may also precipitate respir-

---

* A man in the USA is known to have taken 2000 mg of diazepam (2 mg is a normal dose). He was hospitalised but remained responsive and not disorientated, and was discharged apparently none the worse for wear after 48 h. Two weeks later, he was still excreting the metabolite desmethyldiazepam.

** A remarkable confirmation of this property was that temazepam was widely used by aircrew to enable them to sleep, whenever off duty, during the Falklands campaign. They were able to fly 6 h after taking the hypnotic without any evidence of impaired performance. However, this should not be used as encouragement to fly highly complex aircraft in combat after taking a hypnotic!

atory failure, even in normal doses. The cerebral depressant action of barbiturates is further enhanced by taking antihistamines or alcohol. Barbiturates also have the disadvantage of causing enzyme induction in the liver and interacting with other drugs such as anticoagulants.

Barbiturates are therefore only used by specialists as hypnotics for intractable insomnia. The dangers of barbiturates as hypnotics are summarised in Table 3.2.

Table 3.2 Dangers of barbiturate hypnotics

1. High addictive potential
2. Potent respiratory depressants
3. Frequent use for self-poisoning
4. Can cause confusion or fits in the elderly
5. Sometimes prolonged after-effects
6. Dangerous potentiation by alcohol and other sedating drugs
7. Interactions with other drugs, particularly by enzyme induction in the liver

Management of barbiturate poisoning

The main aim is to restore spontaneous respiration. There is no specific antagonist, but there is no need to try to hasten recovery of consciousness.

The stomach should be washed out to remove undissolved tablets and (if possible) allow their identification. This, however, can be dangerous unless a cuffed endotracheal tube is used to prevent gastric contents from getting into the airway.

Intermittent positive-pressure ventilation is the treatment of choice once spontaneous respiration has failed.

Forced alkaline diuresis can be used to help remove the drug from the body. The plasma level of the barbiturate should be assayed if possible and, if very high, dialysis may be necessary to get rid of the drug.

Analeptics (CNS and respiratory stimulants) such as doxapram may be dangerous and should not be used, as the measures outlined above are safer and more effective.

Opioids

Opioids include morphine and its derivatives and synthetic analogues. They are strongly sedating but only used as hypnotics in patients with otherwise uncontrollable pain. Therefore they are predominantly used as potent centrally acting analgesics (Ch. 4).

ANTICONVULSANTS

Epilepsy is not a single disease but can be a sign of several disorders characterised by paroxysmal dysfunction produced by abnormal electrical discharges in the brain. But in many cases no cause can be found.

Although no single biochemical trigger can usually be identified (apart from such factors as hypocalcaemia and hypoglycaemia), the threshold for initiation of an epileptic fit can be manipulated by drugs. These act by modifying brain transmitters. The neurotransmitters glutamate and aspartate are excitatory and involved in fast synaptic transmission by regulating the permeability of ion channels. Opposing such stimulatory influences are inhibitory transmitters such as γ-aminobutyric acid (GABA) and glycine. Many of the antiepileptic drugs such as phenytoin, phenobarbitone, benzodiazepines, vigabatrin and valproate act in various ways to enhance the action of GABA (Fig. 3.2). The benzodiazepines enhance the response of the chloride channel to GABA by prolonging their opening, while valproate and vigabatrin enhance GABA's action by blocking its metabolic breakdown.

There are several forms of epilepsy. The best known is major epilepsy, of which the most common type is tonic–clonic (grand mal). In the latter, consciousness is lost, quickly followed by uncoordinated motor activity, typically with rigidity, then jerking and slow recovery of consciousness. Minor epilepsy includes petit mal, in which the patient, usually a child, suffers very brief lapses of consciousness ('absences') and rapidly recovers without complete loss of postural muscular control.

Drugs commonly given to control tonic–clonic epilepsy are carbamazepine, phenytoin, sodium valproate and phenobarbitone.

Carbamazepine

Carbamazepine is the drug of choice for tonic–

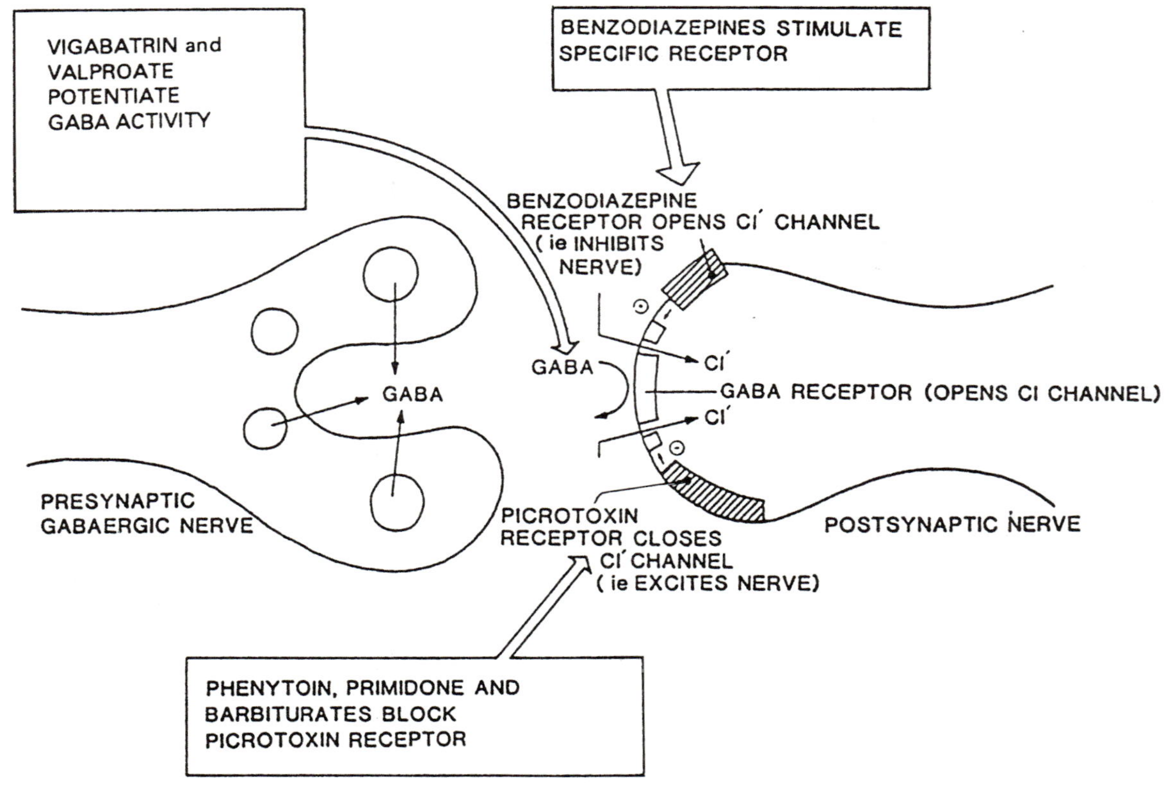

Fig. 3.2 Anticonvulsant drugs and the γ-aminobutyric acid (GABA) receptor complex. (Reproduced with permission from *Aids to Pharmacology*.)

clonic fits. It is well absorbed when given orally and is 75% protein bound. Its half-life is 25–60 h, but this falls to about 10 h in long-term use because of enzyme induction. Its toxic effects include sedation, ataxia, slurred speech, hyponatraemia and water intoxication, but these are rarely troublesome. It is also an enzyme inducer and can cause mild, reversible leucopenia.

In addition to its use for epilepsy, carbamazepine is the most effective drug for the control of trigeminal neuralgia (see Ch. 4).

Phenytoin

Phenytoin is effective and has long been used for tonic–clonic epilepsy, focal fits and psychomotor epilepsy. However, its many toxic effects (summarised in Table 3.3) have led to its gradual replacement by carbamazepine or sodium valproate. Many of these toxic effects result from long-term use, but this is unavoidable in epilepsy.

Sodium valproate

Valproate is effective in all types of epilepsy and

Table 3.3 Toxic effects of phenytoin

1. In large doses, nystagmus, ataxia and possible cerebellar damage
2. Gingival hyperplasia, thickening of facial features and hypertrichosis
3. Folic acid deficiency frequently and, rarely, macrocytic anaemia
4. Enhanced catabolism of vitamin D causing hypocalcaemia and histological signs of osteomalacia*
5. Lymphadenopathy with lymphoma-like changes histologically
6. Slightly enhanced risk of lymphoma
7. Allergic reactions – rashes, lupus-erythomatosus-like disease

* Osteomalacia is usually subclinical but can rarely cause florid rickets or osteomalacia. Vitamin D should be given if there is clinical evidence of bone disease.

can give excellent control of major and many forms of minor epilepsy. Minor gastrointestinal disturbances and temporary hair loss seem to be the main side-effects, but the drug is usually well tolerated. The effectiveness of drugs in the control of epilepsy is notoriously difficult to assess; nevertheless, sodium valproate appears to be a useful drug with the advantage that it usually seems to make patients more alert rather than drowsy. In small children, high doses of valproate occasionally cause liver failure.

Phenobarbitone

Phenobarbitone is an effective anticonvulsant but its use has greatly declined because of serious disadvantages summarized in Table 3.4.

Primidone is effective in major epilepsy, but often causes sedation and cerebellar-type ataxia.

Table 3.4 Disadvantages of phenobarbitone as an antiepileptic

1. Usually excessively sedating when therapeutic blood levels are attained
2. Rebound hyperexcitability of the motor cortex and severe fits result from sudden withdrawal of the drug
3. Enzyme induction accelerates the metabolism of numerous other drugs
4. Paradoxical excitement in some children

Petit mal

Ethosuximide or valproate may be used, but ethosuximide is the drug of choice and side-effects are not usually serious.

Benzodiazepines (particularly clonazepam) are effective in petit mal and some other forms of epilepsy, but are mainly used as intravenous injections for status epilepticus.

Status epilepticus

Status epilepticus is a condition in which fits recur without regaining consciousness or until the patient dies. Intravenous diazepam or clonazepam is usually effective, but may have to be repeated at intervals to prevent further fits. Alternatives are intravenous chlormethiazole or intramuscular paraldehyde.

PARKINSON'S DISEASE AND PARKINSONISM

Parkinson's disease mainly affects the elderly and is characterised by rigidity, akinesia (poverty of movement), tremor, a mask-like facies and excessive salivation. This neurological syndrome is a disorder of the extrapyramidal system which normally governs the quality and smoothness of voluntary movement. The lesions may be the result of arteriosclerosis or past encephalitis, but in many cases no cause can be found.

Normal function of the extrapyramidal system depends on a balanced action of excitatory and inhibitory components. The excitatory transmitter is acetylcholine, while the inhibitory transmitter is dopamine. In parkinsonism the inhibitory component is deficient and the concentration of dopamine in the basal ganglia may be low. The chemical basis of parkinsonism is confirmed by the effects of drugs which induce the disease by the following actions:

1. Deplete dopamine stores (e.g. reserpine)
2. Block dopamine receptors (e.g. phenothiazines)
3. Interfere with dopamine synthesis (e.g. methyldopa)
4. Selective toxic effects on the nigrostriatal pathway (MPTP).

MPTP (methylphenyltetrahydropyridine) is a synthetic, illegally made pethidine-like drug which was discovered as a result of finding an addict in a state of extreme parkinsonian rigidity.

The aim of treatment of Parkinson's disease is to restore the balance between excitation and inhibition, either by supplementing dopaminergic activity with a drug such as levodopa or weakening cholinergic activity with an anticholinergic drug – an antimuscarinic, atropine-like agent (Fig. 3.3).

Atropine-like drugs used for the treatment of parkinsonism include benzhexol and orphenadrine. These drugs have similar actions to atropine and hyoscine: they may have weaker peripheral

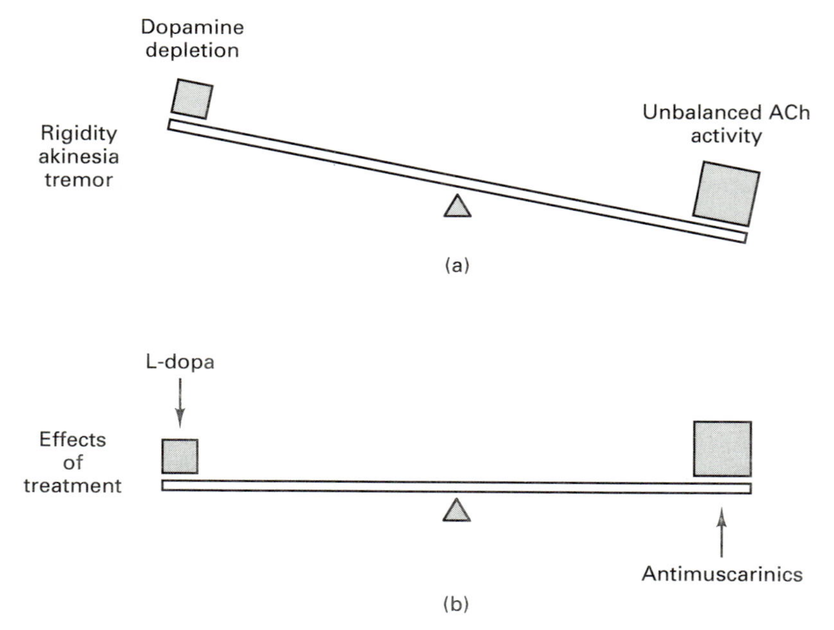

Fig. 3.3 **a** Parkinson's disease. Dopamine depletion is unable to counter the excitatory transmitter acetylcholine (ACh). **b** Levodopa (L-dopa) may modify the dopamine depletion in Parkinson's disease, or antimuscarinic agents such as benzhexol can counter the unbalanced central cholinergic effects on muscle control.

actions but similar central antiparkinsonian activity. Nevertheless, dry mouth and constipation are common, and urinary retention and glaucoma can also be precipitated. These drugs are effective in lessening the rigidity but not the tremor of parkinsonism; they may be used to supplement the actions of levodopa.

Levodopa

Levodopa, a dopamine-like drug, induces a good response in about two-thirds of patients with Parkinson's disease. It ameliorates all the components of the syndrome. Levodopa (L-dopa) is absorbed from the intestine, enters the brain from the circulation and is then converted to dopamine. The most common toxic effects are nausea, vomiting and postural hypotension. Excessive doses, however, can cause involuntary movements which may be more troublesome than the original disease.

Decarboxylase in the nervous system converts levodopa to dopamine. Smaller doses of levodopa are therefore effective and less toxic if a decarboxylase inhibitor is given simultaneously. Such inhibitors include *benserazide* and *carbidopa.*

Overall, levodopa in combination with benserazide or carbidopa are the most effective drugs for Parkinson's disease, but may not be of permanent benefit. Eventually, the duration of benefit may become shorter after each dose.

Amantadine is an antiviral drug which was found by chance to have antiparkinsonian activity. It potentiates dopamine release from neuronal stores.

Bromocriptine stimulates surviving dopamine receptors. It has the same adverse effects as levodopa and can also cause nausea, postural hypotension and involuntary movements. It is given when levodopa cannot be tolerated or is no longer effective.

Selegiline is a monoamine-oxidase-B inhibitor which inhibits the breakdown of dopamine centrally. It is used to improve control of severe Parkinson's disease, with levodopa plus a decarboxylase inhibitor. If given early, selegiline slows the progress of the disease. Selegiline differs from the monoamine-oxidase-A inhibitor antidepressants by its lack of hypertensive response to tyramine (see below).

Parkinsonism and dopamine receptor blockers

The pathogenesis of Parkinson's disease suggests that drugs which block dopamine receptors can have parkinsonian effects. The phenothiazine antipsychotics are the main cause of this side-effect and can cause dyskinesia (involuntary face and body movements) including parkinsonism. An irreversible consequence of long-term antipsychotic treatment is *tardive dyskinesia* characterised by grotesque and uncontrollable grimacing and jaw movements.

Metoclopramide, an antiemetic, achieves its effects partly by blocking dopamine receptors in the vomiting centre (the 'chemoreceptor trigger zone'). It can cause dyskinesia and, in particular, trismus.

In the control of drug-induced parkinsonism, anticholinergic drugs are used. Levodopa and other dopaminic agents are contraindicated.

NEUROSES AND PSYCHOSES

Neuroses and psychoses, particularly anxiety and depression, are some of the most common diseases seen in clinical practice. As a consequence, enormous quantities of psychoactive drugs, particularly anxiolytics and antidepressants, are prescribed. Although they are probably greatly overused, it must be accepted that such drugs can make life tolerable for many people. Psychoactive drugs do not of course remove patients' basic problems (indeed this is often impossible), but treatment with appropriate drugs may at least enable patients to face their difficulties and, with sympathy and support from their doctor or family, help them to seek some solution.

DEPRESSION AND ANTIDEPRESSIVE AGENTS

In normal persons, variations of mood are usually related to external events and are not socially disabling. By contrast, the depressed patient suffers dramatic lowering of the spirits, misery, hopelessness and despair quite disproportionate to the life situation. Work may become impossible and death by suicide may be felt to be preferable. A 'nervous breakdown' is usually severe, disabling depression. An attack of depression may last for weeks, months or even years and then characteristically lifts. Patients usually have repeated attacks of depression, but a few swing rapidly from depression to elation or mania. The phenomenon of such swings of mood is called cyclothymia and the depressive diseases are called the manic–depressive psychoses. Depression is, however, by far the most common state.

Chemical basis for the drug treatment of depression

There is substantial evidence that mood depends on chemical events in the brain and, in particular, on the levels of cerebral amine transmitters. Low cerebral amine levels appears to be the mechanism of production of depression. The amines involved in abnormal mood changes have not been firmly identified. Many antidepressants enhance the activity of noradrenaline and 5-HT (5-hydroxytriptamine, serotonin). Some of the more recent antidepressants have a specific potentiating effect on 5-HT, but little or no action on noradrenaline (see Table 3.6). Thus 5-HT may indirectly activate the limbic system, which is concerned with the expression of emotion.

Supportive evidence is provided by, for example, the effects of the hypotensive drug reserpine. Reserpine depletes cerebral amines (including noradrenaline) and at the same time causes depression. Recovery of normal levels of cerebral amines after stopping the drug is accompanied by recovery of normal mood.

The only site of action of chemical transmitters in the nervous system is the receptor area on the cell membrane of the neurone. This indicates that amines, released into the synaptic cleft, are able to stimulate receptors and thus influence mood. The stored amine in the presynaptic neurone is pharmacologically inactive. The most important route by which released amine is removed from the synaptic cleft is by reuptake into the presynaptic nerve storage vesicles. The tricyclic antidepressant drugs block this reuptake mechanism and, by raising the concentration of amine in the synaptic cleft, enhance and prolong stimulation of the receptors. Other antidepressant drugs probably also act by raising the levels of cerebral amine transmitters.

Clearly, there must also be central mechanisms which trigger these chemical events as it is only too evident that external events, such as bereavement, can precipitate depression.

Drugs are used extensively in the treatment of depression. Psychotherapy can be given, though its value is questionable, but some techniques such as cognitive therapy may be effective.

There are several types of antidepressant drug:

1. Monoamine oxidase inhibitors (familiarly known as the MAOIs) such as phenelzine
2. Tricyclic antidepressants such as imipramine, amitriptyline and related drugs
3. 'Second-generation' antidepressant drugs, with miscellaneous structures, such as mianserin, viloxazine, trazodone and fluoxetine.

Monoamine oxidase inhibitors (MAOIs)

These drugs inhibit a wide range of oxidative enzymes, including brain monoamine oxidase. If any noradrenaline leaks out of the vesicles into the cytoplasm it is normally destroyed by the enzyme monoamine oxidase. This enzyme maintains low levels of noradrenaline in the neuronal cytoplasm outside the vesicles. The result of inhibiting this enzyme with MAOI drugs is that there is a rise in the quantity of noradrenaline and 5-HT stored within nerve endings. Thus, when a nerve impulse arrives, more noradrenaline and 5-HT are available for release and the postsynaptic receptors are more strongly stimulated. This is possibly the basis of their antidepressive activity.

Toxic effects

1. Interactions with foods. The main hazard is the severe interactions of MAOIs with indirectly acting sympathomimetic agents which, surprisingly, are present in many foods. Tyramine, in cheese and other foods, is one such agent. If such a food is eaten by a normal person, the tyramine is oxidised by amine oxidase enzymes in the gut wall and in the liver. In patients being treated with MAOIs, ingested tyramine raises tyramine levels throughout the body. Tyramine acts as an indirectly acting sympathomimetic agent – it enters storage vesicles in the adrenergic nerve ending and liberates noradrenaline by displacement. The free noradrenaline diffuses across neuroeffector junctions and causes vasoconstriction. Since blood pressure depends partly on the state of arteriolar tone, the blood pressure rises. Furthermore, persons treated with MAOIs have considerably enlarged noradrenaline stores. Thus the hypertensive action of tyramine is very great and the rise in blood pressure may be severe enough to cause a cerebral haemorrhage and even death.

Cheese is rich in tyramine. The most serious, and occasionally fatal, reactions of this type are caused by cheeses such as Camembert, Stilton, Brie or matured Cheddar in which microbial activity has converted tyrosine to tyramine. Other foods which may contain vasoactive amines include broad beans (the second most dangerous food on this list) which contain dopamine, while yeast extracts contain histamine. Ripe bananas, Chianti, beer and some other alcoholic drinks containing yeast by-products have also caused hypertensive attacks in patients taking MAOIs. In general, reactions with these substances are less severe than with cheese.

A hypertensive crisis such as that caused by interaction between an MAOI and tyramine can be treated by giving an α blocker, such as intravenous phentolamine.

2. Interactions with sympathomimetic drugs. As indicated above, MAOIs can interact with sympathomimetic agents of the *indirectly acting* type. This has led to unjustifiable confusion and the belief that they interact with all sympathomimetic agents. However, this is not the case, and MAOIs do *not* interact with the vasoconstrictors adrenaline or noradrenaline since they are directly acting sympathomimetic agents.

If this seems inconsistent with what has been said earlier concerning the destruction of noradrenaline in the CNS by MAOIs, the situation may be summarised as follows:

1. Noradrenaline is destroyed within the cytoplasm of the cells of the nervous system by MAO.
2. Injected noradrenaline is mainly removed from the circulation by reuptake into the nervous system.
3. Monoamine oxidase inhibitors do *not* inhibit removal of noradrenaline from the circulation by this uptake mechanism. In effect, therefore, MAOI drugs, although inhibiting the destruction of noradrenaline *within* the central nervous system, play no significant role in the removal of noradrenaline from the circulation and hence on its circulatory effects.
4. Residual noradrenaline (or adrenaline), not taken up into the nervous system, is destroyed by another enzyme, namely COMT (catechol-*O*-methyl transferase). This takes place within the cytoplasm of other cells, including smooth muscle and glands.
5. During treatment with MAOI drugs noradrenaline accumulates in greater than normal quantities in the cells (see (1) above). Under these circumstances, *indirectly acting* sympathomimetic agents can displace excessive amounts of noradrenaline from the sympathetic terminals and in this way cause acute hypertension.

3. Interactions with opioids. Drugs which are normally metabolised by oxidation have a more intensive or long-lasting effect in patients taking MAOIs. Morphine and pethidine are examples of drugs handled in this way and, if administered to a patient receiving MAOIs, the interaction can cause prolonged unconsciousness with deep respiratory depression. Interactions with pethidine can be particularly dangerous and can result in severe respiratory depression or, alternatively, excitation, delirium, hyperpyrexia and convulsions which can be fatal.

4. Interactions with other drugs. When given in combination with tricyclic antidepressants, MAOIs can give rise to excitement, confusion and hyperpyrexia. Nevertheless, MAOIs and tricyclic antidepressants are occasionally given together for the treatment of severe depression, under specialist supervision.

MAOIs can also interact with the hypotensive drug methyldopa to produce excitement and confusion.

Some MAOIs, particularly phenelzine, lower the blood pressure and, therefore, enhance the effect of many hypotensive agents. By contrast, the hypotensive effect of guanethidine is reduced.

Uses of MAOI in depression

MAOIs take 1–3 weeks to become effective, and it is usual to continue treatment for at least 4 weeks before assessing the response. The effects persist for at least 2 weeks and during this period after stopping MAOI there can be a serious drug or food reaction.

If adequate precautions are taken with the kinds of food eaten (especially avoidance of cheese) and against administration of interacting drugs, the MAOIs appear generally to be safe and effective. However, the precise indications for the use of MAOIs in depression remain somewhat controversial and the number of foods and drugs with which they can interact remains as a limitation on their use.

Tricyclic antidepressants

The most widely used tricyclic antidepressant drugs are *imipramine*, *dothiepin* and *amitriptyline*. These are similar drugs except that imipramine is mildly stimulating and can cause insomnia, while amitriptyline is sedating and may cause drowsiness. Their antidepressant activity does not start immediately, there being a latent period of 1–3 weeks before the mood improves. Side-effects are common, particularly dry mouth, constipation and postural hypotension.

Imipramine and amitriptyline are usually given in gradually increasing doses until the optimal response is attained. This dose is then maintained for several months; the drug is then gradually withdrawn. In about half the patients so treated the attack of depression is terminated.

Amitriptyline was probably the most widely used of the tricyclic antidepressants and is often used as a standard against which newer agents are tested. *Prothiaden* is another widely used tricyclic which has additional anxiolytic activity,

Table 3.5 Toxic effects of tricyclic antidepressants

1. *Antimuscarinic.* Tricyclic antidepressants are strongly antimuscarinic and dry mouth caused by amitriptyline can be so severe as occasionally to lead to ascending parotitis. Other effects are constipation, tachycardia and paralysis of accommodation
2. *Cardiotoxic.* Dysrhythmias particularly in the elderly can be fatal
3. *CNS.* Amitriptyline is sedating but imipramine is mildly stimulant. There can be sleep disturbances or, occasionally fits
4. Interactions with sympathomimetic agents (largely theoretical)

but *lofepramine* has considerably weaker antimuscarinic effects.

The toxic effects of tricyclic antidepressants are summarised in Table 3.5.

Tricyclic antidepressants and local anaesthetics

Tricyclic antidepressants have been shown to enhance the effects of adrenaline, but only in some bizarre experiments in which volunteers (pretreated with tricyclics) were given adrenaline in enormous doses by continuous *intravenous* (!) infusion for no less than 25 min. The main effect was then to produce a rise in systolic but a fall in diastolic blood pressure. In practical terms the amount of adrenaline in local anaesthetic solutions for dental purposes is too small to produce this effect and there is *no clinical evidence of interactions between tricyclic antidepressants and adrenaline in local anaesthetic solutions.* However, this myth of dangerous interactions between dental local anaesthetics and tricyclic antidepressants is still widely believed, partly because it is perpetuated by 'experts' who presumably have never read the relevant report.

Uptake-blocking of noradrenaline by tricyclics is also mainly central, as discussed below.

Adrenergic uptake blockers and adrenergic receptor blockers

As mentioned earlier, noradrenaline, once released, is removed from the synaptic cleft by *uptake* into the presynaptic nerve storage vesicles. Uptake of amines such as noradrenaline is blocked by tricyclic antidepressants, particularly in the CNS. Relief of depression by such drugs is attributed to this mechanism. However, tricyclic antidepressants have relatively little effect on sympathetic activity in the rest of the body. Nevertheless, drugs such as tricyclic antidepressants may be described as 'adrenergic uptake blockers' and this may cause confusion with 'adrenergic *receptor* blockers' which are drugs which have a quite different action.

Adrenergic receptor blockers are the α and β blockers such as phentolamine and propanolol, respectively. The β blockers, widely used for angina or to lower blood pressure, also have central activity, but their difference from the 'adrenergic uptake blockers' is shown by the fact that they can actually *cause* depression.

'Second-generation' antidepressants

Amitriptyline remains the standard by which other antidepressants are judged. Nevertheless, its unpleasant antimuscarinic effects and the risk of more dangerous toxic effects have led to the development of other, possibly safer, antidepressants.

Newer antidepressants include mianserin, viloxazine, trazodone and fluoxetine. They are not tricyclic in structure but have similar properties in that they enhance the actions of amine transmitters in the brain. Some of them act on 5-HT receptors or block its reuptake (Table 3.6). They have little antimuscarinic activity and are safer in overdose. They are also less toxic to the heart, but mianserin can cause postural hypotension, dizziness and, rarely, agranulocytosis. Fluoxetine, a 5-HT reuptake blocker is currently

Table 3.6 Some 5-hydroxytryptamine receptors and antidepressive drugs acting on them

Target receptor or action	Drugs and main effects	Clinical uses
5-HT_{1A} receptors	Lithium – agonist	Control of manic depression
5-HT_{1C} receptors	Mianserin – antagonist	Antidepressant
5-HT uptake	Fluoxetine and fluvoxamine – block reuptake	Antidepressants

regarded as one of the most effective antidepressants.

Electroconvulsive therapy

Electroconvulsive therapy (ECT) is a non-drug treatment used for severe depression with a strong risk of suicide.* The patient is anaesthetised and given a short-acting muscle relaxant such as suxamethonium. An electric current (250–500 mA at up to 150 V) is then applied across the temples for not more than 1 s; but for the muscle relaxant, this would cause violent convulsions. This procedure is repeated once or twice weekly for about 5 weeks.

ECT was for a long time given empirically and without objective substantiation of its benefits.** However, controlled trials of ECT suggest that it raises cerebral amine levels and is one of the most effective treatments for severe depression where there is a risk of suicide.

Amphetamines

Amphetamines elevate mood but have no place in the treatment of depression. They produce elation in individuals who are not depressed, and are addictive. The amphetamine Ecstasy (Ch. 4), enhances 5-HT release. Depressed patients usually do not respond at all to amphetamines or may transiently improve and then relapse into a state worse than before.

Hypomania

Hypomania is abnormal elation. The patient is overactive mentally and physically and feels euphoric and confident. The patient therefore feels extremely well and has no complaints, but his anxious and often exhausted relatives bring, or try to bring, him to the physician.

This illness can lead to many social complications such as starting (but not finishing) too many projects, taking out hire-purchase agreements and simultaneously attempting overambitious entertainment programmes. Hypomania is usually self-limiting and a more normal mood may emerge quite suddenly or the mood may equally suddenly plunge into depression. Quite often the mood swings rapidly and repeatedly from one extreme to the other (cyclothymia). Although hypomania is the opposite side of the coin to depression, it is very much less common.

An episode of hypomania can usually be terminated by giving an antipsychotic such as chlorpromazine or haloperidol. The dose has to be adjusted to the patients' response – too much may swing the mood to depression.

Lithium salts are 5-HT_{1A} receptor agonists and have the remarkable property of stabilising mood. They are particularly successful in cyclothymia and may be effective in preventing repeated attacks of hypomania or depression. The dose has to be controlled by monitoring the blood levels of lithium. High blood levels may lead to intestinal disturbances, involuntary movements and cardiac arrhythmias. The risk of arrhythmias is greatly enhanced by general anaesthetics.

Carbamazepine may be used in place of lithium when the latter is contraindicated or not tolerated.

SCHIZOPHRENIA AND ANTIPSYCHOTIC DRUGS

Schizophrenia is a truly appalling mental illness suffered by nearly 1% of the population. In everyday speech it is 'madness' and is quite unlike disorders such as depression which are a recognisable, if exaggerated, disturbance of mood.

Schizophrenia predominantly affects personality, but it is incorrect to call it split personality; it is rather a disintegration of personality. The idea that schizophrenic persons can become two quite separate individuals like Dr Jekyll and Mr Hyde, each behaving rationally but unaware of the other, is the creation of a novelist. In life, schizophrenics become progressively more out of touch with or completely inaccessible to others, while their responses to everyday situations become totally inappropriate. Patients may have

* Depression and suicide: the Catch-22 of antidepressant treatment is that without such treatment the patient may commit suicide, but some patients are so determined upon self-destruction that they use the antidepressant drug as the agent for suicide.

** Some psychiatrists even believed that it was more effective when given without an anaesthetic. This probably tells us more about those psychiatrists than the alleged benefits of the treatment.

auditory hallucinations and delusions of persecution. They may feel that others are controlling their thoughts and actions. This delusion that thoughts or actions are being controlled by outside human or physical influences is a form of paranoia. They may also feel that their thoughts are being blocked. There may be bizarre bursts of excitement, or prolonged periods of statue-like immobility. Multiple, irrational murders are typical but rare schizophrenic acts.

Without treatment, few patients were able to live outside long-stay mental hospitals and it was mainly because of schizophrenia that strait-jackets and padded cells had to be used. However, the introduction of chlorpromazine enabled many of these patients to live at home and even resume some kind of work. Even more impressive, the early stages of the disease were completely arrested and deterioration prevented. Patients are now given antipsychotics for 1 or 2 years and these usually prevent both acute episodes and relapse of the illness.

The efficacy of antipsychotic drugs parallels their ability to block dopamine (D_2) receptors. Dopamine is a neurotransmitter with many actions. In the limbic system of the brain, it is concerned with the expression and memory of emotional experiences. There is some evidence that dopamine and serotonin levels are abnormally raised in schizophrenia. This may explain how drugs which block dopamine and other amine receptors are beneficial in psychotic states such as schizophrenia. However, blockade of dopamine receptors causes adverse effects and, in particular, parkinsonism and other disorders of movement, as discussed earlier.

The antipsychotics include several groups of drugs, of which the most important are the phenothiazines.

Phenothiazine antipsychotics

The phenothiazines include *chlorpromazine*, *trifluoperazine* and *fluphenazine*. Their central effects include diminished emotional responsiveness to external stimuli, sedation (in large doses), inhibition of hypothalamic activity causing hypothermia and hypotension, and depression of the vomiting centre. The antipsychotics potentiate the action of other cerebral depressants such as alcohol or the barbiturates, but also usefully potentiate the action of analgesics. The latter effect is therapeutically valuable for severe pain.

Phenothiazines* are also weak muscle relaxants peripherally and block the actions of the catecholamines.

Phenothiazines are used for acute schizophrenia, in the long-term management of chronic schizophrenia, and in many forms of excited psychotic states including senile confusion, drug withdrawal syndromes, delirium and hypomania.

Fluphenazine enanthate is given by deep intramuscular injection at intervals of up to 28 days in the long-term treatment of schizophrenia because patients cannot be relied upon to continue to take tablets.

Phenothiazines such as chlorpromazine or trifluoperazine are also used to suppress vomiting of central origin.

Other groups of antipsychotics are butyrophenones and thioxanthines, such as thiothixine.

Adverse effects

These are summarised in Table 3.7.

Tardive dyskineisa. This serious toxic effect develops in about 30% of patients, particularly after long-term administration of phenothiazines.

Table 3.7 Toxic effects of phenothiazines and other antipsychotics

1. Antimuscarinic effects such as dry mouth
2. Postural hypotension
3. Tremor of a parkinsonian type
4. Chlorpromazine occasionally causes a reversible type of intrahepatic jaundice
5. Involuntary facial movements
6. Pigmentation of the oral mucosa
7. Tardive dyskinesia

* One of the writers was once taken to see the vast stockyards of Fort Worth, Texas, in the company of a psychiatrist from nearby Dallas. A large advertisement hoarding extolling the virtues of a particular phenothiazine stood over the cattle pens and was a source of considerable puzzlement to both of us, who were unaware that phenothiazines were originally introduced to treat worm infestations.

There are involuntary movements which typically involve the face. Repeated grimacing and chewing movements may be so violent that biting causes scarring and deformity of the tongue. Other parts of the body may be involved, including the limbs and muscles of respiration. Other antipsychotics, such as haloperidol (a butyrophenone), and the antiemetics metoclopramide and domperidone can also cause tardive dyskinesia. This terrible complication may be irreversible and may even worsen when the drug is withdrawn.

Some more recently developed antipsychotics appear to have more specific effects with relatively little tendency to cause extrapyramidal toxicity such as parkinsonism. These drugs include pimozide and, more recently, sulpiride.

Butyrophenones and other antipsychotics

The main example is *haloperidol* which has actions similar to those of the piperazine group of phenothiazines and thus causes less sedation than older phenothiazines. It causes mild hypotension, but depresses the blood pressure less than do the phenothiazines. Haloperidol is sometimes used as a premedicating agent before surgery, but causes some respiratory depression.

Clozapine, belonging to yet another chemical group, is reserved for disease resistant to other antipsychotics. It is sedating but has weaker antimuscarinic effects than the phenothiazines and may have less risk of causing tardive dyskinesia. However, it can cause agranulocytosis and, occasionally, fatal myocarditis.

4. The nervous system III. Analgesics and drug dependence

NON-STEROIDAL ANTI-INFLAMMATORY DRUGS AND OTHER NON-OPIOID ANALGESICS

Drugs such as aspirin are often referred to as 'minor' analgesics. This implies that they are useful only for the management of mild pain, but understates their effectiveness. They are effective for very painful conditions such as rheumatoid arthritis, other forms of skeletal disease and cancer, and are particularly useful for dental pain which is typically inflammatory. They are less potent analgesics than the opioids such as morphine but many of the 'minor' analgesics are in fact at least as effective as some of the opioids that are given by mouth.

Non-steroidal anti-inflammatory drugs (NSAIDs) are so-called because they alleviate pain by blocking the formation of inflammatory mediators, as do corticosteroids (Ch. 10). However, NSAIDs lack many of the troublesome side-effects of corticosteroids.

Aspirin is the archetype, and still one of the most useful of the many NSAIDs of which the following, apart from paracetamol, are examples:

1. Aspirin and other salicylates
2. Paracetamol
3. Pyrazolones
4. Mefenamates
5. Indomethacin and related drugs
6. Propionic acid derivatives and related drugs.

Aspirin

Aspirin is acetylsalicylic acid. It is mainly absorbed from the small intestine, but some is absorbed from the stomach. The main site of its action is in the peripheral tissues, where it has an anti-inflammatory effect. This is the main analgesic action of aspirin; any central (thalamic) inhibitory action is controversial.

One of the important chemical mediators of pain and inflammation in injured or diseased tissues is the prostaglandins, a group of lipid substances. Aspirin and other NSAIDs block the synthesis of prostaglandin E_2 (PGE_2), and hence diminish peripheral manifestations of tissue injury. Thus pain, some of the swelling and impaired function of inflamed tissues are lessened.

Aspirin and other NSAIDs exert their main actions by inhibiting a single step in prostaglandin synthesis by blocking the enzyme cyclo-oxygenase (Fig. 4.1); thus cyclic endoperoxides fail to form from arachidonic acid. One consequence is that in areas of tissue damage production of various prostaglandins (PGD_2, PGE_2 and $PGF_{2\alpha}$) is inhibited. These prostaglandins are mediators of vasodilatation, swelling and pain in inflamed tissues.

Aspirin is antipyretic by its action on the hypothalamus. This is probably also due to inhibition of synthesis of prostaglandin, which is a mediator of the febrile response to infections.

Gastric irritation. This is a common and important side-effect of aspirin and other NSAIDs. The particles of aspirin in particular are especially damaging, but this effect can be lessened by taking buffered aspirin, or by taking it with food.

More important, NSAIDs interfere with the mechanisms by which the gastric mucosa is protected from its own acid/pepsin secretions (Ch. 12). Protection by proliferation of the epithelial lining cells and mucus secretion is mediated by gastric

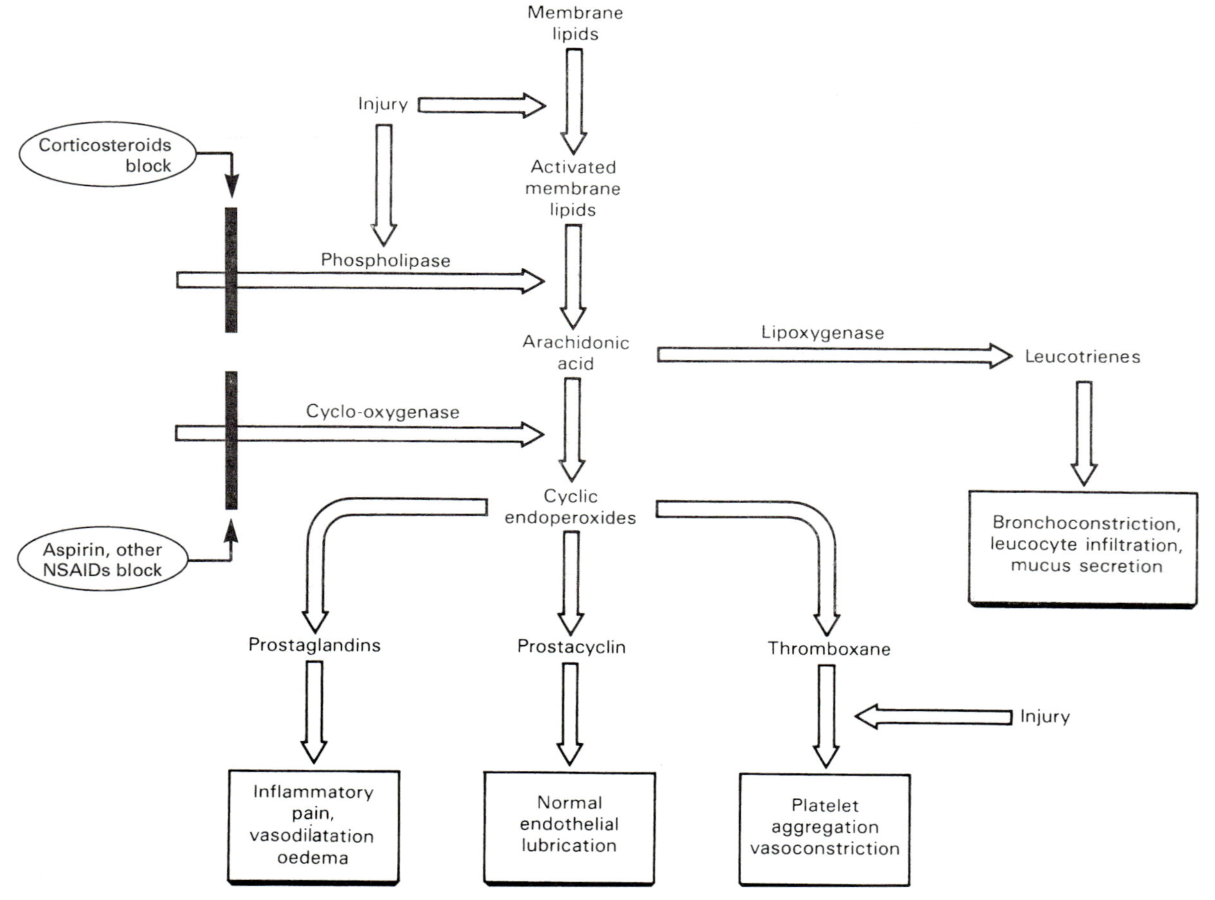

Fig. 4.1 Sites of action of aspirin and of other agents blocking the synthesis of mediators of inflammation.

prostaglandins. This protection may be lost when NSAIDs block prostaglandin production. Gastric erosions caused by these actions frequently bleed – sometimes torrentially. Even in the absence of any clinical evidence of gastric irritation, about 70% of people taking aspirin regularly lose up to 10 ml of blood a day and this is detectable in the faeces. Bleeding is aggravated by taking alcohol and diminished by simultaneous administration of alkalis, or using buffered aspirin. Other anti-inflammatory agents are also gastric irritants.

Interference with haemostasis. In addition to its gastric irritant effect, aspirin impairs haemostasis mainly by blocking thromboxane production and by interfering with platelet aggregation. Even in normal doses aspirin prolongs the bleeding time. As a consequence aspirin-induced gastric bleeding is one of the most common single causes of emergency admission for acute haematemesis. In most cases, bleeding is subclinical, but aspirin should not be given to a patient with a known haemorrhagic tendency (such as haemophilia or as a result of anticoagulant therapy) or with a history suggestive of peptic ulceration (indigestion or epigastric pain).

However, advantage can be taken of this action of aspirin to impair platelet adhesion and aggregation to lessen the risk of thrombus formation in arteries. Aspirin is therefore given to lessen the risks from myocardial infarction (Chs 5 and 7).

Allergy. Aspirin can occasionally cause allergic reactions, including bronchospasm and urticaria, and should not be given to patients with a history of bronchial asthma. Rashes (petechial or erythematous, but sometimes mimicking measles or scarlet fever) are another type of allergic reaction.

Salicylism. Large doses of aspirin cause tinnitus and temporary deafness. Moderate overdose causes nausea, vomiting, abdominal pain and stimulation of the respiratory centre. Increased rate and depth of respiration ultimately lead to respiratory alkalosis, due to rapid excretion of carbon dioxide via the lungs.

Reye's syndrome.* Reye's syndrome is a rare combination of liver and brain damage which usually presents as deepening drowsiness and can be fatal. It particularly affects young children. Its pathogenesis is unknown but it can follow viral infections such as chickenpox and there is an association with the administration of aspirin. Aspirin is therefore contraindicated for children under 12 years, particularly if febrile.

Depression of renal function. Renal function declines after prolonged exposure to high doses of aspirin and analgesic nephropathy may persist after withdrawal of the drug.

Drug interactions. As can be predicted, aspirin has additive effects with other gastric irritants and anticoagulants. It also potentiates hypoglycaemic drugs and, by causing salt and water retention, aspirin and other NSAIDs antagonise diuretics and hypotensive drugs.

Aggravation of gout. Moderate doses of aspirin depress urate excretion and antagonise uricosuric drugs.

Metabolic acidosis. Overdose of aspirin causes respiratory alkalosis which leads to an intracellular acidosis that can be fatal. Being so easily available, aspirin is a common means of self-poisoning and accounts for about 200 suicides a year in Britain.

All the above factors (Table 4.1) suggest that aspirin is a dangerous drug. In fact, it is estimated that at least 2000 tons (6000 million tablets) are taken each year in Britain and many patients (such as those with arthritis) have taken considerable quantities of aspirin every day for years on end. The frequency of toxic reactions is remarkably low considering the scale of use.

*Reye was an Australian pathologist of German parentage. For those who care about such matters, the correct pronunciation is probably therefore 'Rye' rather than 'Ray'.

Table 4.1 Toxic effects of aspirin

1. Gastric irritation and bleeding
2. Aggravation of bleeding disorders
3. Allergy
4. Salicylism
5. Reye's syndrome
6. Depression of renal function with prolonged, high doses
7. Interactions with other drugs
8. Aggravation of gout
9. Fatal metabolic acidosis in overdose

With reasonable care aspirin is a safe and effective drug. After nearly a century aspirin has not been superseded as a general-purpose analgesic and has been shown to have other beneficial effects.

The properties of aspirin illustrate well the very long period sometimes required to discover the many facets of a single drug's activities. It was introduced in 1899, its mode of action as an analgesic was not elucidated until the 1970s, its ability to lessen the mortality from myocardial infarction was not confirmed until the 1990s, and now (1994) it also appears significantly to lessen the risk of colorectal cancer.

Paracetamol

Paracetamol is antipyretic and analgesic but has no anti-inflammatory effect. Its mode of action appears to be essentially similar to that of other NSAIDs, namely, inhibition of prostaglandin synthesis, but this action appears to be central. There is no significant peripheral inhibition of prostaglandin production so that the gastric irritant effect is absent.

The main toxic effect of paracetamol is hepatic damage and liver failure in overdose. This can be particularly dangerous because overdose of paracetamol may not lead to symptoms of liver damage for several days. The liver damage is then difficult to treat and more likely to be fatal than the effects of aspirin poisoning.

Paracetamol taken in therapeutic doses for occasional use seems otherwise to be safe and it is a useful alternative to aspirin for patients with gastric ulceration or who react to aspirin in other ways.

In view of the risk of Reye's syndrome with

aspirin, paracetamol is the analgesic recommended for children under 12 years.

Treatment of paracetamol overdose. Overdose of paracetamol overloads the normal hepatic metabolic pathway and detoxification of products of the minor pathway by glutathione is overwhelmed. The liver is damaged by formation of a reactive metabolite that covalently binds sulphydryl groups in cell membrane enzymes once hepatic glutathione has been depleted.

The principles of treatment are to lessen paracetamol absorption by gastric washout if seen within 4 h of the overdose, and to prevent liver damage by providing sulphydryl groups to allow synthesis of glutathione.

Ideally, acetylcysteine should be given by intravenous infusion. Oral methionine can also be effective but absorption is unreliable, particularly if the patient is vomiting. The decision to give either of these drugs is based on plasma paracetamol levels and a prolonged INR (international normalised ratio; prothrombin time), but liver damage is likely to be advanced or irreversible if more than 24 h have elapsed after the overdose.

Other anti-inflammatory analgesics

These drugs have a potent anti-inflammatory action. They are useful only for pain due to inflammation, particularly rheumatic disorders. In spite of these newer potent anti-inflammatory actions, aspirin remains a useful and effective drug for arthritis, although it may be necessary to give large doses. Even large doses, however, may not necessarily cause more severe side-effects than the newer NSAIDs. There are now very many of these drugs, as shown in Table 4.2.

Phenylbutazone and oxyphenbutazone

Phenylbutazone and its analogues are pyrazolone derivatives and potent anti-inflammatory analgesics. The main metabolite of phenylbutazone is oxyphenbutazone which is also an anti-inflammatory analgesic and is used in eye ointments. Both are gastric irritants and can precipitate severe gastric haemorrhage. They also cause sodium and water retention which can aggravate hypertension and congestive cardiac failure.

Phenylbutazone and oxyphenbutazone were widely used in the treatment of osteoarthritis, rheumatoid arthritis, phlebitis, gout and ankylosing spondylitis, but are toxic to the bone marrow. They are prone to cause leucopenia and agranulocytosis or aplastic anaemia, and have been estimated to have caused more than 1000 deaths in Britain. Since phenylbutazone and oxyphenbutazone have no major advantages over other NSAIDs to compensate for their dangers, they are restricted to specialist use.

Indomethacin

Indomethacin is a strong anti-inflammatory analgesic which is mainly used in the treatment of inflammatory joint disease. A common side-effect of this drug is headache. Like many other anti-inflammatory drugs, indomethacin can cause gastric irritation, ulceration and haemorrhage. Indomethacin can rarely cause agranulocytosis.

Ibuprofen, ketoprofen, fenoprofen, naproxen, flurbiprofen, and fenbufen

These anti-inflammatory agents are widely used in the management of rheumatic diseases. They are as effective as aspirin but usually cause less gastric irritation and are useful when aspirin cannot be tolerated. Nevertheless, there is very wide individual variation in susceptibility to gastric irritation from different drugs in this group. Their success in rheumatic diseases appears to be solely due to their anti-inflammatory action, as they have no central analgesic activity.

Since most dental pain is inflammatory, aspirin and the propionic acid derivatives, such as ibuprofen, are usually the drugs of choice and are likely to be the most effective.

Ibuprofen is the NSAID least likely to cause toxic effects and is frequently the first choice, despite the fact that it is a weaker anti-inflammatory analgesic than the others in this group.

Minor opioid analgesics

These include propoxyphene, which is related

Table 4.2 Non-steroidal anti-inflammatory drugs (NSAIDs)

Approved name	Trade name	Tolerability	Clinical usefulness
Aspirin Soluble aspirin	 Disprin Solprin Palaprim	Excellent for acute pain. Large doses cause gastric irritation in prolonged use	Very useful. Effective antipyretic, analgesic and anti-inflammatory. Contraindicated in childhood
Aloxiprin Benorylate Sustained release aspirin	Benoral	Better tolerated than plain aspirin in prolonged use	
Diflunisal	Dolobid	Less irritant to stomach	Similar to aspirin
Pyrazalones			
Phenylbutazone Oxyphenbutazone	Butazolidin Butacote Tanderil Tandacote	Rashes and gastrointestinal disturbances common Agranulocytosis*	Effective but, because of toxicity, use is reserved mainly for ankylosing spondylitis. Highly effective anti-inflammatory agents
Azapropazone	Rheumox		Effective analgesic and anti-inflammatory agent
Fenamates			
Mefenamic acid	Ponstan	Diarrhoea common	Analgesic, but weak anti-inflammatory properties
Indomethacin group			
Indomethacin	Indocid Mobilan Imbrilon	Headache common	Highly effective anti-inflammatory agents
Sulindac	Clinoral	Gastrointestinal disturbances fairly common	
Propionic acid derivatives and similar drugs			
Ibuprofen Ketoprofen	Brufen Orudis	Little gastric irritation	Mild analgesic, and anti-inflammatory
Naproxen Flurbiprofen Fenoprofen Diclofenac Fenbufen Piroxicam Tolmetin	Naprosyn Synflex Froben Fenopron Progesic Voltarol Lederfen Feldene Tolectin	Moderate-mild gastric irritant	Moderate-powerful analgesic and anti-inflammatory agents

*Phenylbutazone was the most common cause of drug-related marrow depression in the UK.

to methadone, and codeine. These drugs are discussed with the opioids to which they are related.

Analgesic combinations

Dose-dependent toxic effects in the treatment of pain can sometimes be overcome by using several drugs together in small doses. Thus, in treating mild to moderate pain, aspirin, paracetamol and codeine, or paracetamol and dihydrocodeine may have stronger analgesic effects. It is, however, difficult to assess the potency of analgesic agents objectively and it is possible that the effectiveness of analgesic mixtures is due to the high total amount of analgesic used.

MANAGEMENT OF SPECIAL TYPES OF PAIN

Pain due to inflammation

Acute pulpitis and periapical periodontitis are the main causes of severe dental pain. Ideally, immediate elimination of the cause of the pain by appropriate dental treatment is the best course of action. Otherwise, aspirin in adequate doses or one of the propionic acid derivatives ('profens') is most likely to be effective for this type of dental pain.

The mode of action of anti-inflammatory analgesics is such that they are most effective in preventing the onset of inflammatory pain, rather than countering the effects of prostaglandins already formed. Whenever possible, therefore, these drugs should be given when pain is anticipated. Thus, after a difficult third molar extraction, aspirin or other NSAID should be given before the local anaesthetic starts to wear off.

Occasionally intense toothache-like pain can be caused by herpes zoster when it affects the posterior horn cells of the second and third divisions of the trigeminal nerve. Analgesics are helpful but use of an antiviral agent is also necessary. *Acyclovir* (Ch. 15) by mouth, or in severe cases by intravenous injection, should be given at the earliest possible moment and should significantly shorten the illness.

Trigeminal neuralgia

Trigeminal neuralgia is an acute paroxysmal pain often of unbearable severity and typically precipitated by touching or chilling a trigger zone on the face or in the mouth. There is no peripheral disease and the most effective drugs are *anticonvulsants*. *Carbamazepine* is the drug of choice but phenytoin is also moderately effective. Another anticonvulsant, the benzodiazepine clonazepam, is sometimes also effective and can be used if carbamazepine cannot be tolerated, but it is more sedating.

The effectiveness of anticonvulsants in trigeminal neuralgia may be related to the fact that the latter may be a sensory counterpart to epilepsy. Sudden electrical discharges in the brain can trigger violent muscular activity (epilepsy) or pain (trigeminal neuralgia). Anticonvulsants probably act mainly by reducing the spread of excitation and responsiveness of neurones in the brain and may therefore affect sensory as well as motor cortical cells.

Anticonvulsants are not of course analgesics and have no effect on an attack once it has started or on other types of pain. These drugs are only effective for trigeminal neuralgia if given long-term and will usually then control the frequency and severity of attacks. Cases where there has been no beneficial response is sometimes due to the fact that carbamazepine has been mistakenly used as an analgesic when an attack has started.

Migraine and migrainous neuralgia

Classical migraine is characterised by a sequence of events which typically starts with an aura (warning) often consisting of an hallucination of a zig-zag pattern of flickering light (a 'fortification spectrum'). This is followed by photophobia, nausea and intense headache of one side of the head (hemicrania) which may persist for several hours. The headache appears to be due to dilatation and stretching of vessels at or near the base of the brain, thus, many cases respond to drugs such as ergotamine or sumatriptan which have a vasoconstrictor action.

Mild migraine can be managed by use of simple analgesics, and the majority of attacks are controlled by aspirin or paracetamol. If nausea is severe, absorption of analgesics is improved by giving metoclopramide. Resistant migraine is treated with *ergotamine*. This has to be given early to be effective. Oral absorption is variable and severe migraine can often only be controlled by ergotamine given by subcutaneous injection. An alternative is to inhale ergotamine powder from an aerosol inhaler (Medihaler); this is much more reliable than oral administration.

Sumatriptan is effective in the great majority of cases of classical migraine and in an unknown proportion of cases of atypical migraine. It stimulates 5-HT_{1D} serotonin receptors (Table 4.3) and causes constriction of cerebral arteries. It can sometimes also cause serious toxic effects by constricting coronary arteries and precipitating ischaemic heart disease.

Table 4.3 Some important 5-hydroxytryptamine receptors and drugs acting on them

Target receptor or action	Drugs and main effects	Clinical uses
5-HT_{1A} receptors	Lithium – agonist	Control of manic depression
5-HT_{1C} receptors	Mianserin – antagonist	Antidepressant
5-HT_{1D} receptors	Sumatriptan – agonist (vasoconstricts)	Migraine
5-HT_2 receptors	LSD - partial agonist	Abuse only (hallucinogenic)
5-$HT_{1\&2}$ receptors	Methysergide and pizotifen – antagonists	Migraine prophylaxis
5-HT_3 receptors	Ondansetron, granesetron and tropisteron – antagonists	Control of vomiting, especially that due to chemotherapy
5-HT uptake	Fluoxetine and fluvoxamine – block reuptake	Antidepressant
5-HT release	Fenfluramine–enhances release and blocks reuptake	Appetite suppression
	MDMA (Ecstasy)–enhances release	Abuse (central stimulant and hallucinogen)

LSD, lysergic acid diethylamide.

Prophylaxis of migraine

Pizotifen is an antihistamine chemically related to the tricyclic antidepressants and has antiserotinergic activity. It is effective for prevention of attacks but can cause weight gain and drowsiness.

NSAIDs can also be effective prophylactics for migraine, but side-effects may be unacceptable.

β-Blockers are effective. Their use is limited mainly by their contraindications, particularly asthma or heart failure and their interaction with ergotamine.

Methysergide is also effective but has dangerous side-effects, namely retroperitoneal, endocardial and pleural fibrosis so that it is restricted to specialist use in hospital.

Migrainous neuralgia (cluster headache)

This variant of migraine can be mistaken for dental pain, since it is localised to the maxilla deep to and around the eye on one side. Young adults are mainly affected and, apart from the site, migrainous neuralgia differs from classical migraine in that the attacks may recur regularly at the same time, day after day, for weeks. One typical feature is that the attacks are often at night. Then there may be a complete remission for one to several months and the disease usually improves or ceases altogether in later middle age. Another characteristic feature of migrainous neuralgia is visible vascular changes such as reddening of the conjunctiva of the affected side, sometimes with oedematous swelling of the face which may be sufficient to close the eye. There is no aura or nausea, but the condition is managed as for classical migraine with sumatriptan or ergotamine. It is an uncommon cause of facial pain and in a rare variant of this disorder the pain is felt in the mandible and is known as 'lower-half headache'.

Spasm of voluntary muscle

Muscle spasm (tension headache) is a common cause of headache, particularly of the occipital region. Muscle spasm is probably also the main cause of the pain of so-called 'temporomandibular pain-dysfunction syndrome'. Anxiety and tension seem to play a large part and anxiolytic drugs, particularly diazepam which also has a mild muscle relaxant action, may help some patients.

Ischaemic muscle pain – myocardial infarction

Myocardial infarction is one of the most severe kinds of pain that can be experienced. It occasionally presents diagnostic difficulties in dental surgery when the pain is referred to the lower jaw. The pain of myocardial infarction can only be managed by giving potent analgesics such as intravenous morphine or nitrous oxide and oxygen (see Chs 5 and 19).

Pain as a symptom of depression

A minority of depressed patients have physical rather than psychic symptoms. One of these is *atypical facial pain* often affecting the upper jaw. It is frequently described as severe or unbearable, aching in character, is unremittent and of very long duration. The pain may sometimes be dramatically relieved by giving an antidepressant. Inevitably, however, it is difficult to exclude an organic cause with absolute certainty and a psychiatrist's opinion should be sought.

THE OPIOIDS

The terms *narcotic analgesic, major analgesic* and *opioid* are used interchangeably, but opioid is preferable. The group includes morphine, codeine and their derivatives, and synthetic morphine-like drugs. They are potent analgesics, particularly when given by injection. They are also cough and respiratory depressants, and inhibitors of intestinal motility. Tolerance develops with all these drugs. After repeated administration the dose has to be raised to maintain the same level of effect, and dependence can result.

The opioids are most effective against severe pain, particularly of visceral or skeletal origin, such as myocardial infarction, deep bone pain or post-operative pain, and the pain of advanced cancer. The accompanying emotional reaction to pain is also lessened or abolished. The tendency to cause dependence, however, restricts the use of these drugs to the relief of pain which is either non-recurrent or is caused by terminal cancer.

Dependence on the opioids readily develops and most of them therefore are Controlled Drugs (Ch. 14).

Enkephalins and endorphins

Natural peptides (enkephalins and endorphins) are present in the brain and have properties mimicking those of morphine. The enkephalins react with specific opioid receptors in the brain and cord and these receptors are also the targets for opioids (Fig. 4.2). The enkephalins are probably released during pain or other stressful events and by stimulating their receptors raise the pain threshold and help the individual to adapt. Stimulation of these receptors by drugs raises the pain threshold and also induces feelings of relaxation or, alternatively, of dysphoria according to which receptors are stimulated (Table 4.4). Opioid antagonists also bind to these same receptors and prevent access of analgesics, thus stopping their actions.

Opioids

The main types are:

1. Morphine and its derivatives, such as heroin
2. Codeine and its derivatives, such as dihydrocodeine
3. Pethidine
4. Propylamines, such as methadone and propoxyphene
5. Benzomorphans, such as pentazocine and phenazocine.

Morphine

Morphine is a natural opioid readily obtained, together with other opioids such as codeine, from the juice of the unripe seed pods of the oriental poppy (*Papaver somniferum*).

Administration of morphine is usually by injection. It is also absorbed through the intestinal, nasal and respiratory epithelia, but less completely. Shortly after an injection there may be a brief phase of excitement. In the normal (non-addicted) person this is followed by sedation and sleepiness. If the subject was previously in pain, then the relief brings euphoria. Morphine has a strong anxiolytic action and, in addicts particularly, produces euphoria and feelings of self-confidence and relaxation.

After morphine has been given a variety of unpleasant stimuli such as pain become less effective in eliciting withdrawal reflexes and feelings of apprehension – both the sensation of pain is diminished and the emotional response to pain is also suppressed.

Toxic effects. As shown in Table 4.5, morphine is mainly a depressant of brain function but also has some central stimulant effects which are, occasionally, the dominant response.

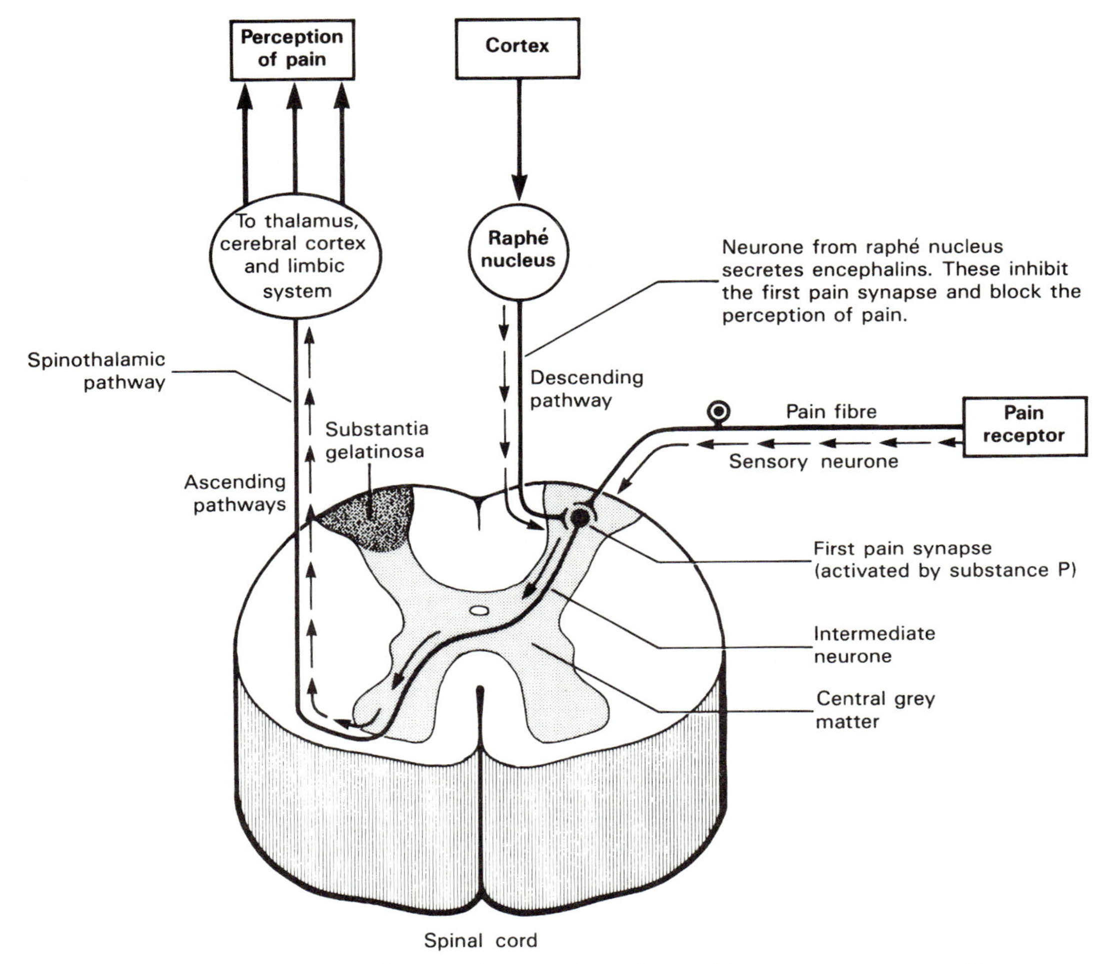

Fig. 4.2 First pain synapse in the substantia gelatinosa of the spinal cord. The synapse is stimulated by pain fibres (via substance P). The synapse is blocked by encephalins secreted by descending neurones.

Morphine depresses the rate and depth of respiration by decreasing the sensitivity of the respiratory centre to carbon dioxide. Because of this respiratory effect, opioids are particularly dangerous in patients suffering from lung diseases such as chronic bronchitis, asthma and pneumonia.

An added hazard to patients with asthma is that morphine releases histamine by a direct action on mast cells. This causes bronchoconstriction and mucosal oedema, which aggravate the respiratory difficulties of patients with asthma.

Table 4.4 Important opioid receptor types

Receptor type	Effect of receptor stimulation	Examples of agonists
μ	Mediates brain analgesia; respiratory depression; euphoria and dependence	Morphine (buprenorphine is a partial agonist)
κ	Mediates spinal analgesia; sedation	Morphine; pentazocine
δ	Dysphoria; hallucinations	Pentazocine

Table 4.5 Actions of morphine

Central
1. Stereospecific stimulation of opioid brain receptors
2. Analgesia
3. Depression of anxiety and other emotional responses to pain
4. Depression of consciousness and coma in overdose
5. Depression of respiration
6. Depression of cough
7. Vomiting due to stimulation of chemoreceptor trigger zone
8. Constriction of pupils
9. Physical and psychological dependence
10. Tolerance (increasing amounts of opioids required to achieve the same results, as a result of a central effect)

Peripheral
1. Constipation (due to smooth muscle spasm – partly a result of stimulation of cholinergic activity in gut wall ganglia)
2. Contraction of smooth muscle of the sphincter of Oddi and ureters
3. Bronchospasm in asthmatics, flushing and arteriolar vasodilatation due to histamine release. Vasodilatation contributes to the hypotensive effects of morphine
4. Fall in cardiac output and blood pressure due to lowered sympathetic discharge and arteriolar dilatation

The central sedative (and possibly analgesic) actions of morphine are potentiated by antipsychotics such as chlorpromazine and any other sedating drug. These effects are generally undesirable but may occasionally be exploited. It may be helpful, for example, to damp down the excessive respiratory activity and consequent load on the heart in left ventricular failure.

Morphine stimulates the brainstem chemoreceptor trigger zone, which activates the vomiting centre, but individual susceptibility to this side-effect varies widely. For the pain of myocardial infarction, intravenous morphine is the drug of choice, but administration of the antiemetic *cyclizine* at the same time is advisable. In a few susceptible individuals the motor system is stimulated and this may lead to convulsions. The pupils are also constricted by stimulation of the midbrain. Eye signs are important in the assessment of head injuries and a fixed dilated pupil is indicative of raised intraocular pressure. Morphine can disguise this change and, since it is also a respiratory depressant, is strictly contraindicated after head injuries.

Peripherally, morphine increases the tone of smooth muscle in the ureters, gall bladder and intestine. This may (theoretically) aggravate colic, but prolonged use certainly causes constipation by inhibiting peristalsis in the colon. Morphine in very low concentrations is therefore used in mixtures to stop diarrhoea.

Morphine dependence and abuse

Morphine is one of the longest established drugs of abuse and dependence (addiction). It can induce both physical and psychological dependence if given for 3–4 weeks or more and, as discussed later, an addict can develop serious physical and mental withdrawal reactions when the drug is stopped.

Diamorphine (heroin)

Heroin is diacetylmorphine; *diamorphine* is the approved name. It is regarded by some as being more powerfully analgesic than morphine, but objective evidence for a clinically significant difference is hard to establish. However, diamorphine appears to be more highly addictive; certainly the withdrawal syndrome is the most severe of any of the opioids. In Britain the use diamorphine is mainly restricted to is relieving exceptionally severe pain, particularly in the terminal stages of cancer. For this purpose the greater solubility of diamorphine over morphine allows injection in a smaller volume. This is an important advantage for an emaciated patient.

Codeine

Codeine (methylmorphine) is a natural opioid. Although it shows all the main pharmacologic actions of morphine, it is a very much weaker analgesic. When given subcutaneously the estimated potency of codeine is only a twelfth of that of morphine (weight for weight). Nevertheless, it is not feasible to try to get the same analgesic response as to morphine, as large doses of codeine cause unpleasant side-effects. In practice, codeine is usually given in doses of up to 20 mg orally with other analgesics such as aspirin. Codeine is used for the treatment of moderate pain, for the symptomatic treatment of diarrhoea and particularly for suppression of cough. In these doses, it causes little or no sedation or euphoria. It is not significantly addictive, but drug abuse is not unknown.

Dihydrocodeine is said to have approximately twice the analgesic effect of codeine. It possesses all the main characteristics of morphine, but its effectiveness is midway between that of morphine and codeine. In practice, it may be effective in the treatment of moderately severe pain that is not relieved by codeine. Drug dependence is rare and when it does develop withdrawal symptoms are not severe. The main side-effects with normal doses are dizziness and constipation.

Pethidine

Pethidine is a synthetic opioid which has many of the actions of morphine, but also has some atropine-like properties in that it relaxes the smooth muscle of the ureters. However, some constipation is common because of spasm of intestinal muscle.

Pethidine is a potent analgesic (100 mg of pethidine produces the same effect as 10 mg of morphine) and, unlike codeine, pethidine can if necessary be given in doses of several hundred milligrams to get the required response. Respiration and cough are depressed. The drug is more likely than morphine to cause dizziness and vomiting, but the pupils are not constricted. Euphoria, sedation and addictive potential are similar to those of morphine. As mentioned in Chapter 3, monoamine oxidase inhibitors can give rise to a particularly severe interaction with pethidine. In some cases, as with morphine, central depression is enhanced and the patient goes into coma, but in other cases there is hyperpyrexia and convulsions which can be fatal.

Methadone

Methadone is a synthetic analgesic which has very similar potency and pharmacological properties to morphine. It is effective by mouth. Like morphine, it causes smooth muscle spasm. There is, however, an important difference: though dependence can develop, methadone has less addictive potential than morphine and pethidine. As a consequence, methadone is used to wean addicts off morphine or heroin.

Dextropropoxyphene

Dextropropoxyphene is a methadone derivative, but not a potent analgesic. Its side-effects are similar to those of codeine. Thus in high doses drowsiness, constipation, abdominal pain and nausea are common.

Dextropropoxyphene is considerably less effective when taken by mouth than after subcutaneous injection. Although it is a popular analgesic, some trials have found that propoxyphene has little or no detectable analgesic effect when taken by mouth. In proprietary preparations propoxyphene is often combined with another analgesic such as paracetamol as in co-proxamol and its enormous popularity is almost certainly not due to its potency as an analgesic, but rather because of the effect of the opioid component (propoxyphene) on mood.

Toxic effects. The abuse potential of dextropropoxyphene is less than that of pethidine, because high doses and parenteral administration can cause unpleasant psychotic reactions. Nevertheless, co-proxamol has become widely used as a drug of dependence and withdrawal signs have been described even in an infant born to a woman regularly treated with this drug during pregnancy.

Self-poisoning is another hazard. Partly as a result of its ready availability, acute overdosage of propoxyphene is now common. This leads to rapid fluctuation between coma and convulsions together with cardiac and respiratory depression. Co-proxamol is a popular analgesic and in the form of Distalgesic has been widely used for self-poisoning. It is hepatotoxic as a consequence of the paracetamol content, in addition to its effects on the nervous system caused by the propoxyphene content. Sudden cardiac or respiratory arrest is a danger even when the patient's condition seems satisfactory. Acute cardiorespiratory depression and pulmonary oedema are important causes of death, but if these hazards are survived acute liver failure often develops. At one time,

Distalgesic was the most common cause of death in cases of drug overdosage referred to a forensic laboratory. The amount of fatal overdose is estimated to be within the range of 20–30 tablets, but in nearly 50% of cases alcohol had been taken in addition.

Phenazocine

Phenazocine is a potent analgesic and is about three times as active as morphine. It is otherwise similar to pentazocine. Drug dependence develops slowly, but the withdrawal syndrome is prolonged.

Pentazocine is a potent analgesic when given by injection. Weight for weight pentazocine is about a third as effective as morphine. The actions of pentazocine and morphine are qualitatively similar, but in doses which produce equal degrees of analgesia and respiratory depression pentazocine causes less sedation – indeed, it can cause unpleasant hallucinations and anxiety (the dysphoric syndrome). This considerably lessens but does not abolish the risk of drug dependence.

Despite earlier hopes, pentazocine is not a particularly safe analgesic. It has most of the toxic effects of morphine and, in particular, also causes respiratory depression and has been widely abused.

Because pentazocine is a partial antagonist it is contraindicated in opioid addicts in whom it may produce withdrawal syndromes.

Nalbuphine

Nalbuphine is an opioid which is given by injection and appears to be as effective as morphine for pain control but with fewer side-effects and less potential for abuse. Nalbuphine causes respiratory depression, but the latter does not progress beyond a certain level with increasing dosage ('ceiling effect'). Nalbuphine also appears to be less prone to cause nausea than morphine. It is therefore useful for perioperative analgesia.

Other potent analgesics

A great variety of analgesics, some of which are not opioid in nature, is now available. Their main features are shown in Table 4.6.

Buprenorphine, for example, is an exceedingly potent analgesic, which is usually administered sublingually, but can also be given by injection and acts for 6–8 h.

The main adverse effects are nausea, drowsiness and dizziness. Respiratory depression is rare but, when it happens, is resistant to reversal by naloxone.

Analgesic potency

Analgesic potency is in some ways a misleading term. All that it means is that, weight for weight and given by the same route, drugs differ in their ability to reduce the sensation of pain. This difference is of little clinical importance. For example, if morphine is believed to possess five times the potency of pethidine, then 100 mg of pethidine can be given to achieve the same degree of analgesia as that produced by 10 mg of morphine. Of much greater practical importance is the acceptable ceiling effect of analgesics. This refers to the greatest degree of analgesia that can be obtained with the highest dose which can be comfortably tolerated. For example, morphine is about 12 times more active than codeine, but 240 mg of codeine cannot be used instead of 20 mg of morphine because approximately 80–120 mg of codeine causes unacceptable sedation, nausea, abdominal pain and vomiting in most patients.

The opioids share many important qualities and, particularly when given by injection, are unrivalled for the relief of severe pain. However, many of the opioids, such as codeine, dextropropoxyphene and pentazocine when given by mouth may not be significantly more effective than anti-inflammatory analgesics, and in some situations are less so.

Pain is a subjective phenomenon and difficult to measure precisely. Because of this it is impossible to be dogmatic about the potency of analgesic drugs. Some work, for instance, has claimed to demonstrate that even morphine does not influence the pain threshold but merely lessens the emotional response to pain. In practice, the main guide is the patient's description of how much the drug has eased their discomfort.

Table 4.6 Properties of other major analgesics

Approved name	Proprietary name	Analgesic potency	Dependence liability	Special features
Dextromoramide	Palfium	Equivalent to morphine	Similar to morphine	Duration of action 4 h. Useful drug for severe pain
Codeine (methyl ester of morphine)	in Codis Pharmidone Pardale Panadeine Sonalgin Solpadeine Veganin	One-tenth analgesia of morphine (converted to morphine in brain; some morphine also present in plasma)	Rare	For mild pain and symptomatic treatment of cough and diarrhoea
Dihydrocodeine	DF 118	Equivalent to codeine	Rare	Mild to moderate pain only. Also cough suppression
Diphenoxylate	Combined with atropine in Lomotil		Possible but risk negligible with short-term use	Can cause euphoria. Use limited to treatment of diarrhoea
Dipipanone	Diconal (10 mg with cyclizine 30 mg)	25 mg equivalent to 10 mg morphine	Similar to morphine	Frequently abused powerful analgesic which can be given orally
Ethoheptazine	Combined with aspirin and meprobamate in Equagesic	Equivalent of codeine	None	For mild to moderate pain
Levorphanol	Dromoran	3–4 times that of morphine	Similar to morphine	Only clinically available member of the morphinan series. No advantages over morphine
Nalbuphine	Nubain	Similar to morphine	Less potential for abuse	Less nausea
Pethidine	Pamergan	Half that of morphine	Similar to morphine	Has some atropine-like activity
Phenazocine	Prinadol Narphen	3–4 times that of morphine	Similar to morphine	For moderate to severe pain. Well absorbed orally
Pentazocine	Fortral	About half as effective as morphine	Low. Produces dysphoria	Opiate antagonist with strong agonist properties. Well absorbed from intestine or s.c. or i.m. injection. Can precipitate withdrawal syndrome in opiate addicts
Buprenorphine	Temgesic	15 times as effective as morphine	Appears to be low	Powerful and equal opiate antagonist and agonist properties. Overdose responds poorly to naloxone
Other potent analgesics				
Nefopam	Acupan	Somewhat less potent than morphine	Not yet demonstrated	No response to naloxone
Meptazinol	Meptid	Similar potency to pethidine	Not yet demonstrated	Less sedating and less respiratory depression than morphine. Given by injection

i.m., Intramuscular; s.c., subcutaneous.

Opioid antagonists

Respiratory depression is the cause of death after overdose of morphine or its derivatives. Respiratory depression from this cause can often be treated effectively with *naloxone*. Naloxone is an opioid antagonist with no agonist activity. It precipitates withdrawal symptoms when given to an addict but dependence on naloxone can develop. It is also effective against pentazocine overdose. Naloxone is the antagonist of choice in most cases of opioid overdose, but is relatively ineffective for buprenorphine poisoning.

Naloxone has no beneficial effect on overdose of other depressants such as barbiturates or general anaesthetics and in large doses will itself cause dangerous respiratory depression. Accurate diagnosis of the cause of respiratory depression is therefore essential before naloxone is given.

Some of the newer opioids such as pentazocine and buprenorphine are opioid antagonists but also partial opioid agonists and thus have both agonist and antagonist properties. Thus these drugs antagonise the action of morphine and can, for example, precipitate withdrawal symptoms in opioid addicts; nevertheless, they are potent analgesics.

Uses of opioids in dentistry

The main application of opioids in dentistry is for severe postoperative pain unresponsive to anti-inflammatory analgesics. The problem of addiction is negligible here, as it is likely to be a single short course of treatment.

Morphine remains the drug of choice in the initial care of a patient who has had a myocardial infarction because of its valuable sedating as well as its analgesic effect. However, morphine is unlikely to be kept in the dental surgery.

As mentioned earlier, opioids are absolutely contraindicated for head-injured patients because they may conceal important pupillary signs and because of their respiratory depressant effect.

DRUG DEPENDENCE AND ABUSE

'Drug abuse' can be defined as self-administration for non-medical purposes. The term is not precise and alcohol in particular is not usually regarded as a drug of dependence, even though it is powerfully addictive. Dependence is compulsive drug use without regard for the consequences. There are usually severe physical or psychological effects if the drug is stopped (withdrawal syndrome).

Drugs of abuse fall into three main groups, namely:

1. Opioids, alcohol and other CNS depressants
2. CNS stimulants such as cocaine
3. Hallucinogens.

Despite the different effects of these groups of drugs they all induce changes in mood or perception that are pleasurable to the addict. The overall extent and effects of drug abuse are impossible to quantify accurately. Deaths and drug hauls by police or customs officers give only a glimpse of the problem.

Alcohol

Alcohol abuse has long been the most common form of drug dependence. Dependence on alcohol causes the most serious drug-related effects in many countries, particularly because of its contribution to violence and road traffic accidents. Up to 5% of British adults may be dependent on alcohol and 15% of American adults have abused or continue to abuse alcohol.

The term 'alcoholism' is frequently used for chronic dependence. It has no precise definition but describes consumption of alcohol to such a degree as to cause deterioration in social behaviour or physical illness, with difficulty in or adverse effects from withdrawal.

The causes of alcohol dependence are obscure, but a genetic factor is involved. Other risk factors are ready availability of alcohol and domestic or work-related stresses.

Alcohol is frequently an important, if not the main, causal factor in over 25% of road traffic accidents and also in many other accidents or assaults. Many patients with maxillofacial or head injuries have been drinking. The difficulties in recognising whether a patient has been taking alcohol have been shown in hospital surveys where over 30% of casualty patients have been found to have blood alcohol levels over 80 mg/100 ml. Medical staff underestimated the true extent of the problem by nearly 20%, despite being alerted to it.

Signs suggestive of recent excessive drinking include slurred speech, a smell of alcohol on the breath, signs of self-neglect and an evasive, truculent, overboisterous or facetious attitude. Alternatively, there may be anxiety sometimes with tremor of the hands. Neither social class nor educational level seems to confer immunity. There is a high prevalence of alcoholism amongst vagrants as well as among doctors.

Laboratory abnormalities include raised blood levels of alcohol, γ-glutamyl transpeptidase and of other hepatic enzymes. Macrocytosis alone is one of the earliest signs of alcoholism and folate deficiency without obvious cause is also suggestive. Later, macrocytic anaemia may develop (Table 4.7).

Teratogenic effects are seen when pregnant women take large quantities of alcohol. They can produce infants with a characteristic facies, varying degrees of mental defect and other abnormalities.

The mortality rate of alcoholics is several times that of non-drinkers.

Dental aspects of alcohol abuse

The most common oral effect is neglect leading to advanced dental disease. Folate deficiency may cause glossitis or, simetimes, angular stomatitis or recurrent aphthae. Cirrhosis may cause bleeding tendencies. Sialosis (bilateral painless swelling of the parotids or other major salivary glands) may occasionally result. However, one of the most important dental complications of excessive alcohol intake is maxillofacial trauma and head injuries. In head-injured patients, unconsciousness is frequently due at least in part to alcohol itself.

Alcoholic cirrhosis slows the metabolism of many drugs and general anaesthesia should be avoided. If the patient has premedicated himself with alcohol, the risk of vomiting and inhalation of vomit is greatly enhanced. Alcoholics are especially prone to aspiration lung abscess. Drug interactions with alcohol which may be important in dental management include:

1. *CNS depressants*. General anaesthetic agents, sedatives or hypnotics have an additive effect with alcohol. Nevertheless, heavy drinkers become tolerant not only of alcohol but also of other sedatives and are notoriously resistant to general anaesthesia. Once liver disease develops the position is reversed and drug metabolism is then impaired and drugs have a disproportionately enhanced effect.

2. *Analgesics*. Aspirin should be avoided since it is more likely in the alcoholic patient to cause gastric erosions and to precipitate bleeding. The hepatotoxic effects of paracetamol are not enhanced and it is probably a safe analgesic in this group.

3. *Antimicrobials*. Metronidazole interacts with alcohol to cause widespread vasodilatation, nausea, vomiting, sweating and palpitations similar to the Antabuse reaction. The effects are unpleasant but rarely dangerous. Intraconazole for fungal infections should be avoided in those with liver damage.

Table 4.7 Toxic effects of alcohol abuse

1. *Gastrointestinal:* gastritis, hepatitis, cirrhosis and pancreatitis, peptic ulcer
2. *Cardiac:* arrhythmias and cardiomyopathy
3. *Nervous system:* cerebral damage and dementia
4. *Bone marrow:* depression of erythropoiesis
5. *Teratogenic effects*

Causes of death among alcoholics:

1. Accidents
2. Suicide
3. Overdose (respiratory depression)
4. Asphyxiation (inhalation of vomit)
5. Bleeding (from oesophageal varices or haemorrhagic gastritis)
6. Liver failure
7. Heart failure
8. Fits after withdrawal

Opioids ('narcotics')

Morphine, diamorphine (heroin) and pethidine are the main examples, but many synthetic opioids are also abused. Abuse of intravenous opioids in many cities has been a potent factor in the spread of AIDS. The enormous use of intravenous heroin is a major drug problem in Britain.

Complications of opioid abuse

Illegal drugs are often adulterated with talc, sucrose, baking soda, quinine or starch. Complications frequently also result from dirty intravenous injection technique as much as from the drug or its adulterants. The drug is often suspended in dirty water – even water from a lavatory pan. Syringes and needles are often reused or shared by several addicts. Venous thromboses are common, but more serious are infective complications such as septicaemia, pneumonia and acute right-sided endocarditis which can cause substantial cardiac damage or be rapidly fatal. Viral hepatitis (B, C or D) is a particularly frequent result of using contaminated injection equipment and from associated hetero- or homosexual promiscuity. Infection with HIV is a growing problem and in certain areas, such as the east of Scotland where well over 50% of heroin addicts were HIV-antibody-positive by early 1987. Intravenous drug abuse is now a major cause of spread of the infection in the USA. The mortality among opioid addicts is 2–6% per annum, usually from overdose. Less often, there may be an anaphylactoid reaction to the opioid or impurities in the preparation. Suicide and assaults are other common causes of death, as is AIDS. The morbidity is also high from other infective complications or malnutrition.

Withdrawal of opioids leads to a syndrome (cold turkey) within about 8 h. Early features include craving for the drug, lacrimation, rhinorrhoea, sweating and persistent yawning. After about 12 h there is a phase of restless tossing sleep (yen) with dilated pupils, tremor, gooseflesh, anorexia, nausea, vomiting, muscle spasms, orgasms, diarrhoea and abdominal pains. Pulse rate and blood pressure also rise. Although withdrawal symptoms subside within about a week, the subject remains intolerant of stress and pain for several weeks.

Medical withdrawal should be gradual and mainly depends on replacement with oral methadone which is less powerfully addictive.

Pentazocine is also an abused drug of dependence, particularly amongst medical and paramedical personnel in the USA. Pentazocine tablets together with an antihistamine (Ts and Blues) have been used intravenously as an alternative to the more expensive heroin. Co-proxamol (because of the dextropropoxyphene) and dipipanone may also be abused.

Abuse of an illicitly manufactured pethidine-like drug (MPDP) has caused specific damage to the substantia nigra of the basal ganglia and extreme parkinsonian rigidity. This, by chance, led to more detailed understanding of Parkinson's disease and a search for other environmental causes (Ch. 3).

Few drugs prescribable by the dental surgeon under National Health Service regulations are likely to appeal to the drug addict who may nevertheless try to obtain pethidine, codeine, pentazocine or co-proxamol. By contrast, medical practitioners may find themselves manipulated with remarkable ingenuity by addicts trying to procure drugs. Simulation of pain is common, prescription pads may be stolen or drug cabinets raided.

Many addicts tolerate pain poorly and local anaesthesia may be inadequate, particularly in those under treatment during the period when they are hypersensitive to pain and stress.

In the established addict, opioids can be legally given for genuine indications such as postoperative pain unresponsive to NSAIDs. Pentazocine, being an opioid antagonist, should not be used as it can precipitate a withdrawal syndrome.

Barbiturates

Barbiturates are readily abused and are therefore Controlled Drugs. Dependence is usually a consequence of their use for insomnia or anxiety. They may be taken orally or, by young addicts in particular, by injection for immediate effect. Many complications, as with opioids, can then result from filthy injection technique. Barbiturates may also be responsible for lethal overdoses when used to adulterate more expensive drugs such as heroin.

Although tolerance to barbiturates grows remarkably quickly, the lethal dose remains the same, and accidental ovredose is a relatively common cause of death, especially if alcohol is also taken.

Immediately after withdrawal, the addict initially improves, but within 12 h a dangerous withdrawal syndrome can develop. Nausea, anxiety, tremor, insomnia, weakness and postural hypotension, are followed by abdominal pain. After 36–48 h there may be fits, coma and death.

Barbiturates induce liver drug-metabolising enzymes and cause resistance to anaesthetics, but also enhance the sedative effects of some drugs.

Benzodiazepines

Abuse of benzodiazepines is a significant hazard but relatively uncommon in relation to the scale of use. Many patients, mainly housewives, claim to have become dependent as a result of having been prescribed benzodiazepines for chronic anxiety. Enormous claims for compensation have been made against the manufacturers or doctors, particularly in the case of triazolam (Halcion).

The onset is typically slow but effects may persist for 8–10 days. Typical effects include insomnia, anxiety, loss of appetite, tremor, perspiration and perceptual disturbances. Sudden withdrawal, particularly of short-acting benzodiazepines, can cause confusion, fits, toxic psychosis or a condition resembling delirium tremens.

Benzodiazepines should only be prescribed for short periods (not more than 2 weeks). In those that have become dependent, withdrawal should be gradual. The benzodiazepine should be changed to diazepam and the dose reduced by fortnightly decrements of 2.5 mg or less. Complete withdrawal may take several weeks or even months.

Unlike other drugs of abuse, benzodiazepines are not, at the time of writing, Controlled Drugs and are virtually harmless in overdose.

Cannabis

Cannabis (marijuana, hashish) is widely abused. It can be taken by many routes but is often smoked. Its effects somewhat resemble those of alcohol, but large doses cause dreams, hallucinations, depersonalisation, and impaired memory and motor function. A striking change is loss of ambition and indifference to external events (apathy syndrome). Abuse of cannabis in adolescence may be followed by dependence on opioids or cocaine.

Withdrawal of cannabis can cause tremor, irritability, insomnia, anorexia and fever. It is controversial whether there are serious medical effects of cannabis abuse. However, chromosomal damage, irreversible neurological impairment, deterioration of personality, bronchitis and interference with sex hormone function are possible consequences.

Conversely, cannabis derivatives (cannabinoids) may be valuable for controlling emesis caused by cytotoxic drugs.

General anaesthetics

Ether and chloroform were abused soon after they were introduced in the nineteenth century, but other agents have become more widely used.

Nitrous oxide, in particular, induces impaired consciousness with a sense of dissociation and often of exhilaration (hence, *laughing gas*). It has all the properties of a drug of dependence, but the effort of carrying the heavy and conspicuous cylinders limits its use. Nevertheless, such is human determination that dental and medical students in the USA have been known to steal large hospital cylinders of nitrous oxide for personal use.

Dependence on nitrous oxide is an occupational hazard of anaesthetists and dental surgeons and occasionally patients have died as a result of drowsiness of an anaesthetist abusing nitrous oxide. Chronic abuse of nitrous oxide can interfere with vitamin B_{12} metabolism and lead to neuropathy but, for unclear reasons, not of anaemia.

Abuse of halothane is a hazard, particularly in the USA. In one remarkable case, a nurse developed skeletal fluorosis, hypertension and renal damage as a consequence of secretly sniffing another fluorinated hydrocarbon anaesthetic, methoxyflurane.

Cocaine

Cocaine is the main example of the central stimulants that include the amphetamines, phenmetrazine and methylphenidate. These drugs have some sympathomimetic activity but, in particular, strongly elevate mood.

Cocaine has become one of the most widely

used drugs of dependence, as a result of its production on an enormous scale in South America. Its production, smuggling and the associated crimes are now a multibillion pound industry for which new markets are constantly being sought.

Cocaine is inhaled, smoked, or injected. Freebase cocaine is made by boiling cocaine hydrochloride with sodium bicarbonate. It is known as *crack*, because the crystals crackle when heated. It acts so rapidly that, when inhaled or smoked, the jolt is similar to that given by intravenous cocaine. Cocaine induces feelings of well-being and heightened mental activity lasting for about an hour. Its social appeal is that the addict is garrulous, witty and the life and soul of the party.

Toxic effects. Cocaine is an indirectly acting sympathomimetic agent with strong central stimulant action. Large doses induce paranoia, hallucinations and tactile delusions. The latter are typically of insects crawling over the skin (formication). Withdrawal leads to an acute phase of depression and craving or sleep, then recurrence of craving but no significant physical effects.

Toxic effects result from sympathomimetic actions and central stimulation. They include angina, coronary spasm, ventricular dysrhythmias, myocardial infarction, cerebrovascular accidents, convulsions and death.

Inhaled cocaine can result in ischaemic necrosis of the nasal septum or, occasionally, perforation of the palate from intense vasoconstrictor action.

Amphetamines

Amphetamines, such as dextroamphetamine, have closely similar central effects to cocaine, but their sympathomimetic effects on the cardiovascular system are comparatively mild. They elevate mood, cause wakefulness and, in large doses, hallucinations.

Amphetamines are taken orally or by intravenous injection and elevate mood for several hours. They have been used in the past by students to remain awake long enough to study their subjects adequately and in the unrealised hope of improving examination results. Truck drivers have also used them to stave off fatigue. Though amphetamines raise mood they are ineffective for the treatment of depression which is worsened when the effects wear off. Amphetamines have been used to suppress appetite to control obesity but, again, the effect is temporary and dependence readily develops. Their only medical indication is for the treatment of narcolepsy (uncontrollable sleep).

Chronic amphetamine toxicity causes restlessness, hyperactivity, loss of appetite and weight, tremor and repetitive movements. Large doses can precipitate a schizophrenia-like psychosis with delusions, hallucinations and paranoid features. This psychotic reaction can persist for many days after the last dose of the drug. Otherwise there is no physical withdrawal syndrome. Overdose can cause convulsions, coma and death, but enormous doses can sometimes be tolerated without apparent harm.

Pure crystalline *methamphetamine* ('ice'), when inhaled, acts almost as rapidly as intravenous cocaine, but has a duration of action of several hours.

Ecstasy (*methylenedeoxymethamphetamine, MDMA*) has similar properties to other amphetamines but is more potently hallucinogenic, possibly because of chemical affinities with mescaline. It can cause permanent brain damage or death.

Amphetamines are relatively easily synthesised. The illicit manufacturing industry is estimated to be worth several *billion* dollars a year in the USA and secret factories have been found in Britain.

Hallucinogens (psychotomimetics, psychotogens)

Psychedelic drugs induce feelings of heightened clarity of sensation, enhanced awareness of sensory input and abnormal perception. They include the indolealkylamines, such as lysergic acid diethylamide (LSD) and psilocybin, phenylethylamines, such as mescaline, phenylisopropylamines, and phencyclidine (PCP) and its derivatives. As mentioned earlier, the amphetamine, MMPD (Ecstasy), is also hallucinogenic; it is widely abused in so-called 'acid house parties'.

LSD (lysergic acid diethylamide) was first synthesised from ergot alkaloids. It acts on 5-HT_2 receptors as a partial agonist. LSD became a favoured drug in the 'swinging 60s' and was even advocated by a few deluded psychiatrists for such alleged benefits as 'opening the doors of perception'. However, such drugs are harmful. Minor effects are often sympathomimetic and include pupil dilatation, tremor, nausea and heightened blood pressure, pulse rate and temperature. LSD can cause major psychotic reactions (hallucinations, flashback effects, prolonged disorders of mood). It also has physiological effects (hyperreflexia, mydriasis, muscular incoordination, seizures).

Overflow from one sense to another (synaesthesia) when, for example, colours are heard, is common. Lability of mood, panic and delusions of magical powers are frequent. Delusions such as believing in an ability to fly are common causes of accidents, assaults and deaths. There is no withdrawal syndrome when psychedelic drugs are stopped, but permanent mental disturbance can follow. Chronic abuse of LSD in particular can cause a persistent schizophrenia-like psychosis.

Dependence is psychological but not physical.

Other abused substances

Substance abuse refers to the abuse of chemicals, particularly organic solvents such as glue or petrol. Solvent sniffing is common, particularly among male teenagers who are predominantly glue-sniffers. The vapour is typically inhaled from glue squeezed into a plastic bag. Other solvents such as petrol can be inhaled from a cloth soaked in it or from aerosol sprays, through a cloth.

Solvent sniffing produces effects somewhat between those of alcohol and an hallucinogen. Common toxic effects include hypoxia, cardiac arrhythmias and sometimes sudden death, liver damage and neurological damage, but vary according to the substance being abused. Chronic abuse of petrol, for example, can cause lead poisoning, anaemia, and cranial nerve palsies. In pregnant women it can have teratogenic effects.

COMPLICATIONS OF DRUG ABUSE

Complications of drug abuse affect the individual and the community. Hazards to the individual can result as much from dirty injection technique or contamination of the drug as from the pharmacological effects of the drug. The main complications are shown in Table 4.8.

Table 4.8 Major complications of drug abuse

1. Infections:
   a. Viral hepatitis (particularly B) and chronic liver disease
   b. Infective endocarditis and cardiac damage
   c. Septicaemia
   d. AIDS
   e. Tetanus (rarely)
   f. Sexually transmitted disease due to promiscuity
2. Overdose with consequences specific to the drug concerned
3. Malnutrition and its consequences
4. Maxillofacial and other injuries from drug-related violence
5. Deaths due to behaviour resulting from delusions
6. Venous thromboses

Hazards to the community include:

1. Crime, often violent, to obtain money for drugs
2. Violence resulting from drug effects
3. Violence among pushers in evading arrest or between gangs
4. Road traffic accidents (especially alcohol)
5. Spread of AIDS and other sexually transmitted diseases

5. The cardiovascular system

Hypertension

Hypertension is abnormally and persistently raised blood pressure. In a minority of patients this may be secondary to kidney or endocrine disease. In over three-quarters of patients the primary cause of raised blood pressure is not known and the disease is called 'essential hypertension'.

It is important to lower a raised blood pressure to avoid complications such as ischaemic heart disease, left ventricular failure, secondary renal damage, cerebral vascular disease and retinal changes. Hypertension and ischaemic heart disease are the most common causes of death in the Western world.

Although there is no evidence that overactivity of the sympathetic nervous system is the major cause of essential hypertension, many drugs which lower a raised blood pressure, block the sympathetic outflow to arteriolar smooth muscle (Fig. 5.1).

The action of drugs in reducing blood pressure is complex and is often the result of action at several sites. Antihypertensive agents fall into the following broad categories:

1. Diuretics
2. Calcium channel blockers
3. β adrenergic blockers
4. α adrenergic blockers

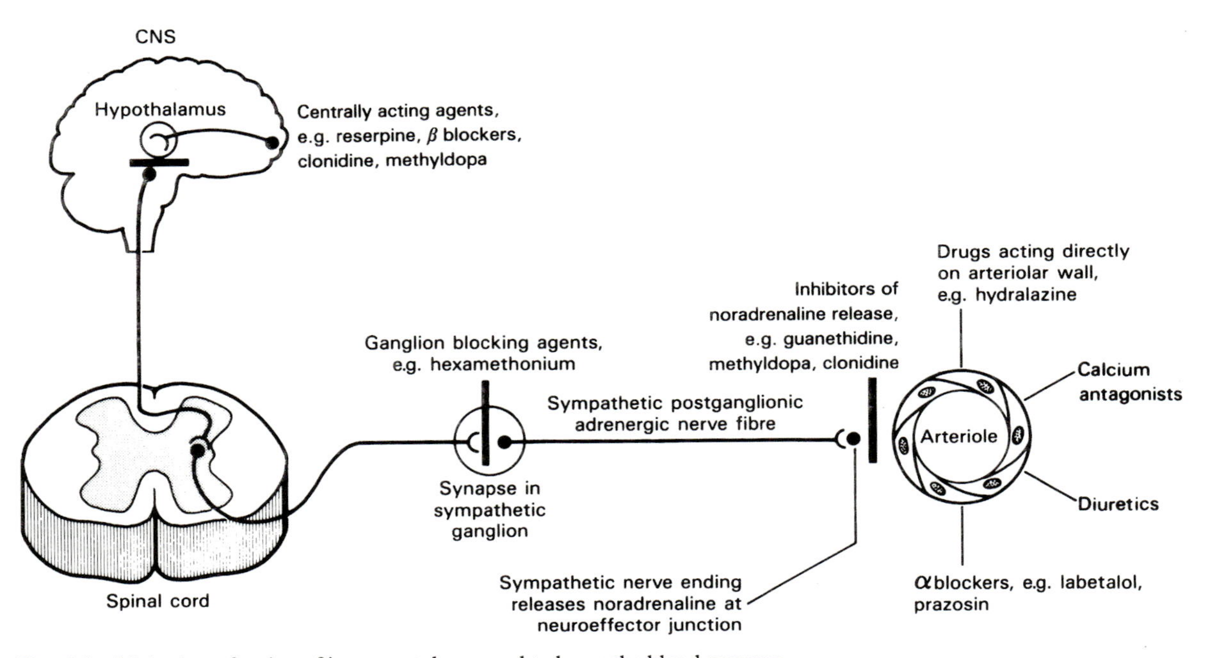

Fig. 5.1 Main sites of action of important drugs used to lower the blood pressure.

5. Vasodilators
6. Angiotensin-converting enzyme inhibitors
7. Others.

Diuretics

The thiazides such as *bendrofluazide* and *cyclopenthiazide* are the first choice for the treatment of mild hypertension, especially in the elderly. Thiazides lower blood pressure by several actions, namely:

1. Vasodilatation
2. Inducing sodium loss
3. Reducing circulating blood volume.

The first two of these actions are the most important.

Calcium channel blockers (calcium antagonists)

This group of drugs includes *verapamil*, *nifedipine* and *diltiazem*. They act by inhibiting the flow of calcium through membranes in cells. Nifedipine acts mainly on peripheral arterioles causing vasodilatation and hence reducing peripheral resistance and lowering the blood pressure. Verapamil is also a useful antihypertensive drug, but also reduces the excitability of the atria and so is used in supraventricular tachycardia. Verapamil, nifedipine and diltiazem dilate coronary arteries and are effective in angina pectoris.

β blockers

β blockers, such as *propranolol*, *oxprenolol*, *metoprolol* and *atenolol*, are valuable for treating hypertension of all grades of severity. They act by several mechanisms, including:

1. Reduced cardiac output
2. Reduced renin release from the kidneys
3. Reduced sympathetic outflow from the CNS
4. Reduced release of noradrenaline from peripheral sympathetic nerves.

β blockers are unusual amongst hypotensive drugs in that they do not cause postural hypotension. At present, β blockers are extensively used in the treatment of hypertension but often cause lassitude and sometimes depression. They can also precipitate incipient heart failure. The β blocker *labetalol* also has some α blocker activity.

β blockers also give better protection than other antihypertensive drugs against recurrences of myocardial infarction.

α adrenergic blockers

Prazosin acts on α_1 receptors in the arteriolar walls and has a vasodilator action. It is a potent antihypertensive with relatively low toxicity. It is widely used for hypertension of all degrees of severity. *Indoramin* is similar.

Other α adrenergic blockers such as *phenoxybenzamine* and *phentolamine* are not normally used for essential hypertension and have many side-effects.

Vasodilator drugs

Vasodilator drugs include the following:

1. *Hydralazine* is useful in the treatment of severe hypertension due to kidney disease because, unlike many other hypotensive drugs, renal blood flow is not reduced. A disadvantage of hydralazine is that it can cause serious autoimmune reactions resembling systemic lupus erythematosus in patients who metabolise the drug slowly. These complications can be prevented by limiting the maximum dose to 200 mg daily.

2. *Diazoxide* is particularly used in severe hypertension when a rapid fall in blood pressure is wanted.

3. *Diuretics* such as the thiazides and also frusemide have, as mentioned earlier, a vasodilator action separate from their diuretic effect and this contributes to their ability to lower blood pressure.

4. *Minoxidil* is a powerful vasodilator used in the specialist treatment of severe hypertension refractory to other drugs. Minoxidil can, however, induce diabetes mellitus and cause hypertrichosis. Application of minoxidil to the scalp is therefore used as a cure for baldness.

Angiotensin-converting enzyme (ACE) inhibitors

Captopril and *enalapril* are examples. Angiotension II is an endogenous vasoconstrictor; it also stimu-

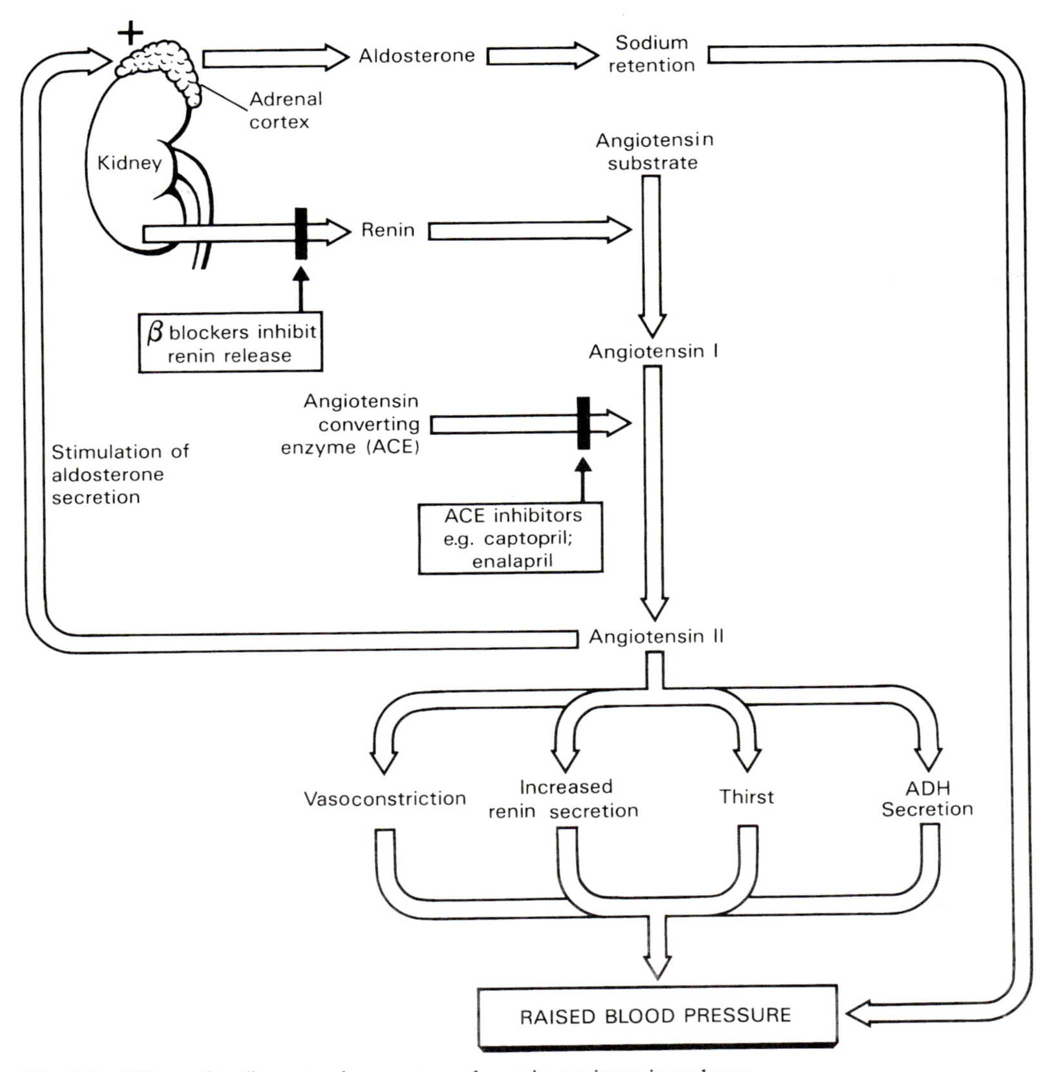

Fig. 5.2 Effects of antihypertensive agents on the renin–angiotensin pathway.

lates aldosterone release from the renal cortex and thus causes sodium retention (Fig. 5.2). These drugs prevent the formation of angiotension II and, therefore, lower blood pressure. Captopril and enalapril are used for moderate and severe refractory hypertension.

Others

Methyldopa. This is centrally acting and a powerful stimulator of α_2 (prejunctional) receptors, thus inhibiting noradrenaline release. It is effective but causes sedation and depression. (Clonidine has a similar action.)

Clonidine and reserpine. These are centrally acting. They are effective but their use is virtually obsolete because of side-effects, particularly depression.

Adrenergic neurone blocking agents. For example, guanethidine and debrisoquine. The main action of these agents is to block the release of noradrenaline from sympathetic junctional nerve endings. They are effective but cause postural hypotension and failure of ejaculation.

General management of essential hypertension

If no primary cause (such as chronic renal disease) can be found, the usual principles of management are as follows:

1. *Body weight.* If the patient is overweight, attempts must be made to bring this back to a reasonable level.
2. *Smoking.* Cigarette smoking should be stopped as it is an important risk factor for atherosclerosis.

Measures (1) and (2) alone may sometimes be sufficient to control mild hypertension.

3. *Relaxation exercises and meditation.*
4. *Reducing alcohol intake.* More than 4–8 units of alcohol (2–4 pints of beer) each day may contribute to raising the blood pressure.
5. *Regular exercise* (such as jogging for 20 min at least three times weekly) may lower blood pressure to some degree.
6. *Lowering dietary salt intake.*
7. *Changing to a vegetarian diet.* In particular a reduction in animal fats may lower blood pressure and reduce any hyperlipidaemia to some extent.
8. *Antihypertensive agents.* If the above measures fail, a thiazide diuretic is given initially. A β blocker or ACE inhibitor can be added if necessary. For severe hypertension more complicated combinations of drugs including α_1 blockers or minoxidil may be needed.

It has to be emphasised that these are only general principles. New drugs are constantly being introduced and views change about older drugs as experience accumulates. There are thus no hard and fast rules about the treatment of this common and serious disease.

Ischaemic heart disease

The coronary arteries supply the myocardium with oxygenated blood. Ischaemic heart disease is caused by atherosclerotic narrowing of the coronary arteries. The inadequate blood supply causes both atrophy of cardiac muscle with fibrous replacement and also damages the conducting tissues, causing unstable cardiac rhythm. Myocardial ischaemia can lead to either angina pectoris or myocardial infarction.

Angina pectoris and myocardial infarction

Angina pectoris is a pain in the chest, often substernal and radiating down the left arm. It is brought on by exercise, cold or emotion (Fig. 5.3). Angina due to effort is relieved by rest within a few minutes. The pain appears to be caused by transient oxygen deficiency in the myocardium, but is not severe enough to cause permanent structural damage.

Myocardial infarction causes prolonged severe chest pain which is not relieved by rest. The underlying myocardial oxygen deficiency is so severe that an irreversible necrotic injury is inflicted on the heart.

Management of angina. The mainstay of treatment is glyceryl trinitrate, but β blockers and calcium channel blockers are also valuable. Any predisposing causes, such as obesity, hypertension, hyperlipidaemia or anaemia, must also be treated. Violent effort and exposure to cold should be avoided.

1. *Glyceryl trinitrate* is a short-acting antianginal drug which is absorbed from a tablet put under the tongue. This avoids first-pass metabolism and allows rapid absorption into the systemic circulation without passage through the liver. Glyceryl trinitrate relaxes and dilates venules, but obstructed and rigid coronary arteries are not affected. Nevertheless, this drug is one of the most effective in treating anginal attacks because venous return and peripheral resistance are lessened and the work done by the heart is reduced. The tension in the ventricular wall in diastole is also lessened and this contributes to the reduced oxygen needs of the heart (Fig. 5.4). As an alternative, glyceryl trinitrate can be given transdermally via a self-adhesive plastic patch or as a spray given as a metered dose into the mouth. The long-acting nitrates may be useful in preventing angina or for acute attacks. They include isosorbide dinitrate and isosorbide 5-mononitrate.
2. *β blocking drugs.* Activation of the sympathetic nervous system by anger, fear, anxiety or effort may bring on an attack of angina. Blockade of the effects of the sympathetic nerves on the heart by β blockers such as propranolol and oxprenolol is often very effective in reducing the frequency and severity of anginal attacks. Whereas

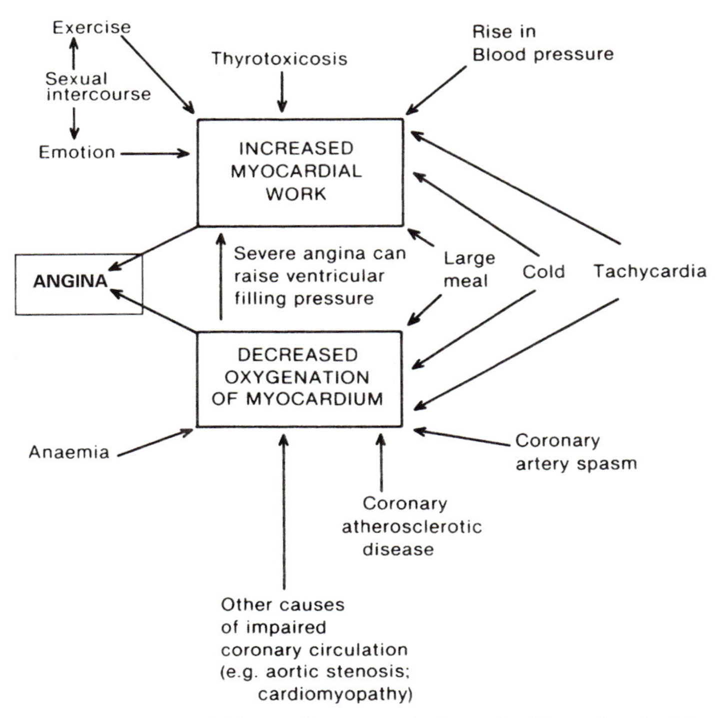

Fig. 5.3 Factors which contribute to anginal attacks. (Reproduced with permission from *Aids to Clinical Pharmacology and Therapeutics*.)

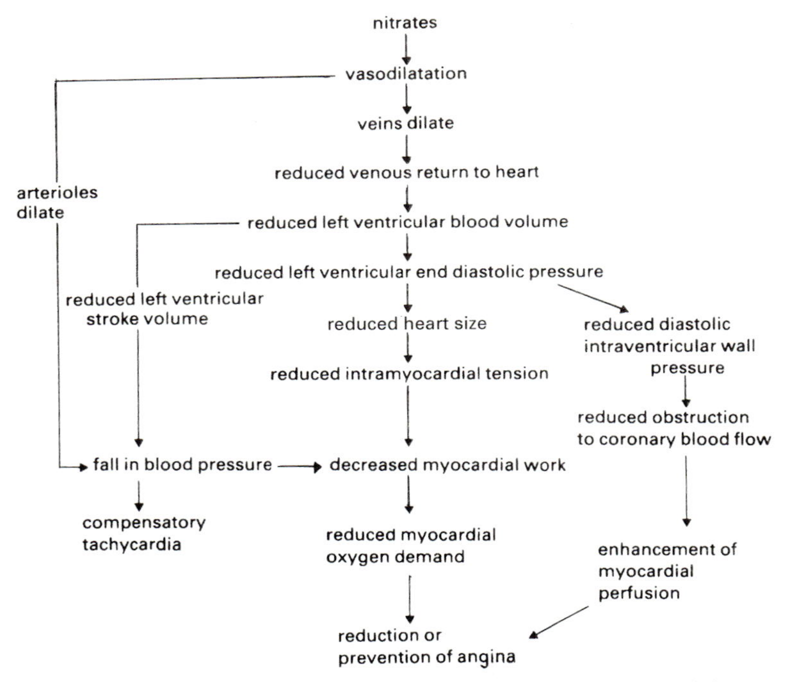

Fig. 5.4 Actions of nitrates in angina pectoris. (Reproduced with permission from *Aids to Pharmacology*.)

glyceryl trinitrate is taken when the anginal pain appears (or just before it is anticipated), β blockers are taken regularly several times a day. Although β blockers are often effective for the treatment of severe angina, a few patients are made worse. Bronchospasm may also be a problem.

3. *Calcium channel blockers*, such as *nifedipine* and *verapamil*, are of great benefit in angina and are increasingly widely used. Nifedipine is also an effective antihypertensive drug and verapamil is an antidysrhythmic.

4. *Aspirin* does not significantly affect the pain of angina but lowers the risk of myocardial infarction by its action of lessening the risk of thrombosis by inhibiting platelet aggregation.

Angina is not always persistent. In some, attacks stop completely after a time: in such cases drugs need only to be kept in reserve against the possibility of recurrence.

Myocardial infarction. This is usually characterised by agonisingly severe chest pain – often radiating into the neck or down the left arm. The pain persists for several hours and is not relieved by rest or by glyceryl trinitrate. *Myocardial infarction and angina can occasionally cause pain felt only in the left jaw. Rare though this is, the importance of accurate diagnosis and the avoidance of operative treatment for the pain will be obvious.* Characteristic electrocardiographic changes follow and indicate that part of the ventricular wall has suffered irreversible damage. There is no curative treatment but several measures may lower the mortality.

The underlying cause is severe restriction of the oxygen supply to the myocardium as a result of occlusion of a major coronary artery by thrombus. Although atherosclerosis is virtually invariably associated with myocardial infarction, the precipitating event is frequently a severe dysrhythmia.

The main treatment, to lower the mortality and effects of the acute attack, is to do everything possible to stop the development of cardiac arrhythmias and to limit spread of thrombosis in the coronary arteries. Survival from the acute attack almost invariably leaves the patient with an area of myocardial necrosis. The size of this infarct is an important factor affecting the prognosis.

The first consideration is to relieve pain and anxiety which can trigger catecholamine release and heighten the risk of dysrhythmias. Intravenous morphine is the drug of choice but nitrous oxide and oxygen are also effective. Administration of a β blocking agent can reduce the mortality of myocardial infarction by at least 30% and long-term β blockade should be continued after uncomplicated myocardial infarction.

Thrombolytic drugs such as streptokinase (Ch. 7), if given early, significantly lower mortality. Aspirin, in the acute attack, further reduces mortality and should be continued afterwards. The efficacy of thrombolytic drugs in lessening the risk of dying from a myocardial infarction suggests that they limit myocardial damage by preventing extension of thrombus in the coronary arteries.

Myocardial infarction is the chief cause of sudden death, but even this may sometimes be preventable if immediate cardiopulmonary resuscitation is given. Obviously this is not always successful but the more quickly it is started and the more efficiently it is done the better the results.

Prevention of atherosclerosis and coronary heart disease

Any measures that reduce the severity of atherosclerosis are likely also to lower the risk of coronary heart disease (CHD). The main risk factors for atherosclerosis are as follows:

1. Age
2. Hypertension
3. Cigarette smoking
4. High blood cholesterol levels
5. Insufficient exercise
6. Diabetes mellitus.

Substitution of animal fats by monosaturated and polyunsaturated vegetable fats in the diet lowers blood cholesterol levels, but the effect is small. Lowering total fat intake is more important. Greater consumption of antioxidants (β carotene, vitamins E and C) also appears to be associated with a lower incidence of coronary artery disease.

While epidemiological evidence for the beneficial effects of dietary manipulation may look impressive, their actual role remains unproven. Stopping smoking is certainly more important. Equally, better treatment of hypertension may also make a further impact on CHD statistics.

Management of thrombotic diseases

Thrombosis is a complex process involving both platelets and the clotting mechanism. On the venous side deposition of fibrin predominates, but in the fast-moving arterial blood, thrombi consist mainly of platelets with little fibrin. The nature of so-called 'coronary thrombosis' is more obscure, but platelet thrombi play a part in the production of most cases of myocardial infarction.

Early attempts to lower the mortality from myocardial infarction were directed towards prevention of fibrin thrombus formation with *anticoagulants*. More recently, and more logically, *antiplatelet drugs* such as aspirin have come into use for prevention of platelet thrombus formation or prevention of recurrence. *Fibrinolytic drugs* such as streptokinase are used for enzymatic breakdown of the fibrin component of thrombi.

Drugs used in the management of thrombotic disease are:

1. Anticoagulants
2. Fibrinolytic drugs
3. Antiplatelet drugs.

Anticoagulants

The main anticoagulants in use are *heparin* and *warfarin* (Ch. 7). Though at one time thought to be of value for myocardial infarction, their use has not lowered the mortality to any significant degree. Thrombus in arteries, such as the coronary arteries, is initiated by platelet aggregation and adhesion to the endothelium and it is impossible to give anticoagulants early enough to prevent fibrin deposition on the platelet thrombus. Anticoagulants may prevent extension of fibrin deposition but this has not been shown to be of significant benefit.

Uses of anticoagulants in cardiovascular disease

The main indications in heart disease are:

1. In atrial fibrillation to diminish fibrin thrombus formation and lessen the risk of detachment of fibrin emboli
2. During cardiac surgery to prevent fibrin deposition on the damaged endothelial surfaces
3. Prosthetic heart valves, to prevent fibrin deposition on these foreign surfaces and their attachments to the heart
4. In preparation for cardioversion (conversion to normal rhythm by a powerful DC shock) when minute emboli may be discharged when normal heart rhythm is established
5. For myocardial infarction, but their value is questionable.

The main indications for anticoagulation in other thromboembolic diseases include:

1. Prophylaxis of thromboembolic disease
2. In deep vein thrombosis to prevent extension of clot
3. For multiple cerebral emboli (little strokes) to prevent extension of fibrin deposition in the cerebral vessels
4. During renal dialysis to prevent fibrin deposition in the extracorporeal circulation
5. For pulmonary embolism to prevent further deposition of fibrin.

(For contraindications to and complications of anticoagulants see Chapter 7.)

Fibrinolytic (thrombolytic) drugs

Fibrinolytic drugs such as *streptokinase* activate circulating plasminogen to plasmin which breaks down fibrin thrombi. Given within the first 24 h after a myocardial infarction, fibrinolytic drugs can lower the mortality, but the earlier they are given the greater the benefit. Other fibrinolytic drugs of similar efficacy are *anistreplase* and *alteplase* (Ch. 7).

Antiplatelet drugs

Antiplatelet drugs interfere with platelet aggregation and adhesion. Aspirin is the only drug of proven efficacy for the prevention of recurrence of myocardial infarction. It may possibly also prevent myocardial infarction if taken long term by persons at risk, in a dose of 150 mg a day or 300 mg on alternate days. Aspirin, by blocking the enzyme cyclo-oxygenase (see Fig. 4.2) irreversibly prevents platelet thromboxane generation. Thromboxane production is affected more than prostacyclin production. Other drugs that interfere with platelet aggregation are dipyridamole, epoprostenol and ticlopidone, but these have not been shown to be any more effective than aspirin in lowering the mortality from myocardial infarction and may have more troublesome toxic effects.

Surgical treatment of ischaemic heart disease

In angina resistant to drugs, and in many patients who have had a myocardial infarction, the blood supply to the heart can be improved by a coronary aortic bypass graft.

Heart failure

Left ventricular failure

Left ventricular failure may be caused by hypertension, myocardial infarction or chronic valve disease (such as aortic stenosis or regurgitation). *Acute left ventricular failure* causes severe breathlessness due to interstitial and alveolar pulmonary oedema. The patient who is, in effect, drowning in his oedema fluid, must be placed in a sitting position to enable him to breathe and the following measures carried out.

1. To save life, oxygen must reach the alveolar capillaries. One-hundred per cent oxygen is given by face mask.
2. Oedema is removed as quickly as possible by using a powerful loop diuretic such as frusemide, ethacrynic acid or bumetanide. This not only removes fluid from the lungs but also causes vasodilatation which rapidly improves cardiac output.
3. If possible, the cause of the heart failure should be treated. If hypertension precipitated the heart failure, the blood pressure should be lowered with a fairly rapidly acting hypotensive drug such as diazoxide.
4. Morphine should be given to relieve the patient's fear and distress, and remove the compulsion to make excessive respiratory efforts. Diazepam is sometimes used instead of morphine.
5. Slow intravenous injection of glyceryl trinitrate may be given to lessen the work of the heart.

Right ventricular failure

This may be a secondary effect of left ventricular failure or may be a consequence of lung disease. Heart failure secondary to lung disease is known as *cor pulmonale* and is usually due to the common combination of longstanding chronic bronchitis and emphysema. An acute exacerbation of chronic bronchitis may precipitate respiratory failure, which in turn leads to right ventricular failure.

Management includes:

1. Oxygen (up to 30%) is given via a Venturi mask and the patient is encouraged to cough forcibly.
2. Sputum is sent for bacteriological examination and in the interim a broad-spectrum antibacterial such as co-trimoxazole or amoxycillin is given, but changed if necessary.
3. Sedatives, hypnotics or narcotic analgesics are absolutely contraindicated because of their depressant effect on respiration.
4. A bronchodilator such as salbutamol aerosol is given.
5. Digoxin and a diuretic such as chlorothiazide may be given in the acute stage, but there is usually no great urgency to start this aspect of treatment.

In the long term, heart failure is traditionally treated with a cardiac glycoside such as digoxin (see below) and a diuretic. However, vasodilators can substantially improve cardiac performance either by reducing peripheral resistance (hydralazine) or by dilating veins and reducing venous pressure (long-acting nitrates). Other drugs such as prazosin cause both arteriolar and venous dilatation and combinations of drugs can be tested until the optimal benefit is obtained. The ACE inhibitors are probably the most beneficial.

Cardiac glycosides have less effect on cardiac performance in long-term use and digoxin can often be withdrawn once the acute phase of failure has been controlled.

In treating heart failure, underlying diseases (thyrotoxicosis, valve defects, hypertension, etc.) must also be corrected. The sodium intake is lowered and drugs which cause sodium retention (NSAIDs and corticosteroids) should be avoided.

Diuretics

Diuretics increase the rate of urine production by the kidney and are used to eliminate oedema. The clinically useful diuretics are so powerful that they can induce a negative extracellular fluid balance – in other words they can dehydrate the patient. The most powerful (frusemide and ethacrynic acid) can induce an output of over 10 l of urine in a few hours. Most commonly, diuretics are given to eliminate oedema caused by heart failure, but they are often also effective in oedema due to kidney or liver failure. Another common use of diuretics is in the treatment of hypertension.

Diuretics are also useful to relieve localised oedema – as in the lungs or brain. The diuretics most often used are:

1. Thiazides (e.g. chlorothiazide, bendrofluazide)
2. Powerful short-acting ('loop') diuretics (e.g. frusemide, ethacrynic acid, bumetanide)
3. Aldosterone antagonists (spironolactone)
4. Potassium-retaining diuretics (e.g. triamterene, amiloride).

Thiazides. These are effective orally. They block sodium reabsorption in the distal renal tubule. Their action starts after 1 h and lasts about 6 h. The thiazides aggravate diabetes and cause loss of potassium, but in general are free from other serious side-effects. Occasionally, light-sensitivity dermatitis and gout may be precipitated.

Frusemide, bumetanide and ethacrynic acid. These can be given by mouth or injection. They act on the loop of Henle and distal tubule causing Na^+,Cl^- and K^+ loss. Diuresis begins 6 min after intravenous administration of frusemide and is completed after 4–6 h. These drugs induce massive loss of water, sodium and potassium from the body and can reduce the blood volume so severely as to precipitate hypovolaemic shock. More commonly, potassium loss develops and can enhance the toxicity of the cardiac glycosides. Uric acid excretion is inhibited and this can precipitate an attack of gout. Frusemide can interfere with glucose tolerance and in large doses can cause deafness.

Spironolactone. This causes diuresis only in those patients who have oedema and sodium retention due to hyperaldosteronism. Excessive amounts of aldosterone are secreted by patients suffering from renal or hepatic failure.

Potassium-retaining diuretics. The thiazides frusemide and ethacrynic acid can cause potassium deficiency. This may manifest itself as muscle weakness, atony of the gut, increased sensitivity of the heart to cardiac glycosides and cardiac arrest. This complication is countered by giving potassium salts or by using a potassium-retaining diuretic such as *amiloride* or *triamterene*. Triamterene does not lead to hypokalaemic states and in fact potentiates reabsorbing mechanisms in the kidney tubules. In the treatment of oedema due to congestive heart failure triamterene may be given with a potassium-losing diuretic, and thereby both potentiate the diuretic effect and avoid potassium loss.

Abnormalities of cardiac rhythm

The normal cardiac impulse arises in the sinoatrial node which consists of modified cardiac muscle. It repeatedly generates a wave of depolarisation which spreads in an orderly manner over the atria. The conducting tissue – the atrioventricular bundle (the bundle of His) – then carries depolarisation into the ventricles.

Depolarisation in the atria and ventricles results from a transient change in ionic permeability of the muscle cell membrane. These ionic changes activate the contraction mechanism of the muscle by increasing the amount of free intracellular calcium necessary for this process.

Abnormalities of rhythm of the heartbeat may consist of:

1. *Abnormal rate of discharge of the sinoatrial node.* Since the normal cardiac impulse arises in the sinoatrial node, abnormalities of rhythm originating in this nodal tissue are spoken of as sinus or supraventricular tachycardia (excessive rapidity), or sinus bradycardia (excessive slowing), of the heart rate.

2. *Ectopic impulses arising elsewhere in the heart than the sinoatrial node.* Extra beats may arise because of impulses firing sporadically from an abnormal focus in the atria or ventricles (atrial or ventricular exsystoles). Such an abnormal focus may repeatedly discharge and cause episodes of increased heart rate (paroxysmal atrial or ventricular tachycardia).

If many variable abnormal foci discharge in the atria, atrial contraction becomes uncoordinated and irregular. As a consequence, the ventricle is stimulated irregularly and, usually, rapidly. This is known as atrial fibrillation and causes the pulse to be irregular in both rhythm and volume.

Similarly, multiple varying ectopic foci in the ventricle cause uncoordinated contraction of the ventricle. This is ventricular fibrillation in which the myocardium is doing no more than twitching rapidly. When this happens, cardiac output immediately falls to zero and the patient becomes unconscious. Death follows within a few minutes.

3. *Abnormal conduction of the cardiac impulse.* Failure of the atrioventricular bundle to conduct the cardiac impulse from the atria to the ventricles is known as heart block. Conduction defects can also develop within the atria and impede the cardiac impulse from reaching the ventricles. In either event, extreme bradycardia may result; this causes a sudden lowering of cardiac output and attacks of unconsciousness.

Attacks of sinus tachycardia and atrial extrasystoles are not unusual in healthy persons. Atrial fibrillation can be the result of several diseases including rheumatic heart disease and thyrotoxicosis. Ventricular fibrillation may develop in the course of myocardial infarction or after cardiac surgery, or may be produced by drugs such as the cardiac glycosides, halothane and adrenergic stimulants, such as isoprenaline or adrenaline.

Arrhythmias arising in the atria do not usually immediately threaten life. By contrast, ventricular extrasystoles and ventricular tachycardia are dangerous because they may lead to ventricular fibrillation.

Sinus bradycardia and heart block may follow myocardial infarction or may be the result of an overdose of a cardiac glycoside.

Antiarrhythmic drugs

The following classification of antiarrhythmic agents is suggested for the non-specialist:

1. Cardiac glycosides
2. Quinidine-like drugs
3. β blockers
4. Drugs used for slow dysrhythmias; amiodarone and calcium blockers.

Cardiac glycosides. Of these, digoxin is the most commonly used. They have two therapeutic uses: in heart failure, and for rapid arrhythmias arising in the atria. Their main actions are:

1. To increase the force of cardiac contraction
2. To slow the heart by stimulating the vagus
3. To slow conduction down the atrioventricular bundle
4. To prolong the effective refractory period of the heart.

The beneficial effect of a cardiac glycoside on heart failure is by stimulating the force of contraction of the myocardium. The antiarrhythmic action is due to the other properties, of which the most important is to slow conduction down the atrioventricular bundle. The ventricles are thereby protected from excessively rapid stimulation coming from abnormal rhythms arising in the atria, such as atrial fibrillation.

The therapeutic dose of the cardiac glycosides is close to their toxic dose. Even when used at optimal levels they can cause side-effects such as nausea and vomiting. With increasing dosage there is severe slowing of the heart due to vagal stimulation. Heart block is another dose-dependent undesirable effect. In large doses, by contrast, the excitability of the myocardium is heightened and dangerous ventricular arrhythmias can result.

Because of these different toxic effects, the cardiac glycosides are contraindicated in sinus bradycardia and heart block, and in ventricular arrhythmias.

In the presence of a low blood potassium or a high blood calcium the toxic action of the cardiac glycosides may follow even modest doses.

Quinidine. Quinidine* is a drug which dampens the excitability of the myocardium, slows atrioventricular conduction and lessens the force of myocardial contraction. Practical disadvantages of quinidine are that it depresses the force of con-

*Quinidine is one of the few drugs discovered (in effect) by a patient. At the turn of the century the famous cardiologist Wenckebach was visited by a patient who complained that none of his doctors knew how to treat the irregular beating of his heart. Nevertheless he himself had found that it was ameliorated by taking quinine (quinine in those days was often taken as a tonic, hence 'tonic water'). Wenckebach was shrewd enough to take the information seriously and confirmed this effect of quinine, but found that its isomer, quinidine, was more effective. It is a pity patients' ideas about how their complaints are best treated are rarely so useful. Alternatively, it may be that patients should be listened to more carefully.

traction of the heart, lowers the cardiac output and can precipitate heart failure. It is now little used, but there are several drugs with qualitatively similar actions, in that they significantly inhibit myocardial excitability, but depress the force of contraction relatively little. They include *lignocaine*, *procainamide*, *mexiletine*, *flecainide*, *tocainide*, *lorcainide* and *disopyramide*. They are used mainly for the treatment and prevention of ventricular arrhythmias, such as ventricular extrasystoles and tachycardia. They may also be effective in rapid atrial arrhythmias, but are contraindicated in heart block and in heart failure.

Lignocaine is one of the safest and most useful agents for the control of fast arrhythmias in the early management of myocardial infarction. In order to get a quick but sustained effect, 50–100 mg of lignocaine is given intravenously. This can be followed, if necessary, by an infusion of 1.5–3 mg/min for up to 3 h.

Side-effects are uncommon but most often affect the nervous system. There may be confusion or excitability going on to convulsions. These effects are dose related.

β blockers. Blockers of the β actions of the sympathetic transmitter and of sympathomimetic drugs, include *propranolol*, *oxprenolol* and many others. As well as being used for the treatment of angina pectoris, hypertension and anxiety neurosis, these drugs are used to decrease the electrical excitability of the heart. The β blockers are used to treat ventricular arrhythmias, but are also effective in controlling atrial arrhythmias.

Propranolol has β_2 (bronchial) as well as β_1 (cardiac) blocking properties and can therefore cause bronchospasm. Propranolol also has some quinidine-like properties and lessens the force of cardiac contraction. *Metoprolol* and *atenolol* have partial β_1 selectivity, but can still produce bronchospasm in many asthmatics.

Miscellaneous. Isoprenaline is an agonist (stimulator) and therefore has all the actions on the heart of the catecholamines – including stimulation of rate of discharge of the sinoatrial pacemaker tissue and facilitating conduction in the bundle of His. Isoprenaline is used to treat excessive ventricular slowing due to failure of initiation or conduction of the cardiac impulse.

An excessively slow heart rate (sinus bradycardia) can be treated with *atropine*. This acts by blocking the parasympathetic supply to the heart (the vagus) which, when unopposed, has a slowing action on the rate of nodal discharge.

Amiodarone is an anti-arrhythmic drug which may be effective for abnormalities of cardiac rhythm that are resistant to other agents. In particular, it will usually control paroxysmal atrial fibrillation which has not responded to digoxin. Amiodarone is often effective in ventricular tachyarrhythmias, but is not indicated for heart block or bradycardia.

Verapamil and *diltiazem* act by impeding calcium flow across membranes. They are effective in angina as well as supraventricular tachycardia. Verapamil is now the drug of choice for rapid rhythms arising in the atria, particularly paroxysmal atrial tachycardia.

The main points regarding arrhythmias and their control by drugs can be summarised as follows, although it must be appreciated that this is a considerable oversimplification of the clinical and therapeutic problems.

1. Some atrial arrhythmias such as extrasystoles and mild overactivity of the nodal tissue (sinus tachycardia) are harmless and happen in normal subjects.

2. Rapid atrial arrhythmias may result in a fall in cardiac output, because of shortening of the time available for diastolic filling of the ventricles. It is often a feature of the failing heart, but is not an immediate threat to life. Atrial fibrillation and atrial flutter usually indicate underlying cardiac disease. The cardiac glycosides such as digoxin are particularly useful in rapid supraventricular tachycardias, because they protect the ventricle from excessive stimulation by slowing conduction down the atrioventricular bundle. β blockers are also used to treat atrial arrhythmias.

3. Extreme slowing of the heart (bradycardia) may be severe enough to cause loss of consciousness because of the fall in cardiac output. When this is due to a conduction defect (heart block), the situation may be improved by the use of isoprenaline or adrenaline.

Sinus bradycardia is treated with atropine, which blocks vagal activity. In heart block and sinus bradycardia the cardiac glycosides and β blockers are contraindicated.

4. Arrhythmias arising in the ventricle are always dangerous, as they can lead to ventricular fibrillation. Ventricular arrhythmias, which are a common consequence, and one of the main causes, of death after a myocardial infarction, may be treated with lignocaine followed by β blocking agents. The most reliable way of controlling ventricular arrhythmias due to ectopic foci is by giving a DC shock across the chest.

Cardiac pacemakers

In some disorders the sinus impulses reach the ventricle so slowly or irregularly that the patient can lose consciousness in the intervals between heartbeats (Stokes Adams attacks). Disorders such as this may be treated more satisfactorily by insertion of an electrical pacemaker than by drugs. Pacemakers act by delivering an electrical stimulus to the heart either at regular intervals or 'on demand' when the natural stimulus fails.

Treatment of ventricular fibrillation

This otherwise lethal condition is treated by electrical defibrillation. Electrodes and a conductive jelly are placed over the sternum, near the apex of the heart, and a brief high voltage shock given.

6. The respiratory system

Breathing is an apparently simple process by which oxygen is taken in and carbon dioxide eliminated by the lungs, but its control is complex. Drugs may affect the central nervous control of respiration or they may act on the lungs.

Drugs which depress respiration

Opioids

Opioid analgesics cause central depression of respiration. Thus, morphine, heroin and pethidine cause a considerable decline in the rate and depth of respiration and inhibition of the cough reflex. The respiratory effects of these drugs appear to be due to their action in diminishing the sensitivity of the respiratory centre to carbon dioxide. Normally, carbon dioxide is a potent physiological stimulus to breathing, but the opioids reduce its effectiveness at this site in the brain.

Methadone, pentazocine and phenazocine were initially thought to cause less respiratory depression, but doses equianalgesic to the older drugs cause a similar degree of respiratory inhibition. Depression of respiration caused by opioids is usually an undesirable side-effect. Nevertheless, this side-effect can be used to advantage when opioids are used to diminish respiratory effort in acute pulmonary oedema (due to left ventricular failure) or during assisted respiration with mechanical ventilators.

Severe respiratory depression due to morphine, pethidine, pentazocine and phenazocine is reversed by naloxone.

Hypnotics

Respiratory depression is caused by many hypnotic drugs, particularly barbiturates, which are not used for this purpose. Any central nervous depressant, including intravenous benzodiazepines, may lead to a dangerous degree of hypoxia in patients suffering from respiratory insufficiency due to chronic lung disease such as asthma or chronic bronchitis and emphysema. Intravenous midazolam is potentially more dangerous than diazepam because of its greater potency. Respiratory depression due to benzodiazepines can be quickly reversed with flumazenil.

Respiratory stimulants

Carbon dioxide is the most important respiratory stimulant, but occasionally drugs are used to stimulate breathing. If respiratory depression is due to opioid overdose, naloxone is usually effective. Respiratory depression due to overdose of hypnotic drugs or serious lung disease does not respond to, or is made worse by, opioid antagonists such as naloxone.

Respiratory stimulants such as doxapram should not be used for drug-induced respiratory depression as this can be dangerous and raise the mortality from hypnotic overdose. The main treatment of respiratory depression due to hypnotics and anaesthetics is positive-pressure artificial respiration.

BRONCHIAL ASTHMA

Asthma is characterised by attacks of reversible airway obstruction. Spasm of the bronchiolar smooth muscle contributes to the obstruction, but there is also a considerable degree of mucosal oedema and swelling together with plugging of bronchi by mucus.

Several factors can precipitate attacks of asthma in susceptible persons. These include allergy, infection, physical and chemical stimuli, and psychological influences. Their relative importance varies in different patients, but treatment may include elimination of allergens, antibiotic therapy and palliation of psychological stresses. But most important, asthmatic patients are treated with drugs that directly relieve the bronchial obstruction.

An important mechanism by which these factors cause airway obstruction is by release of mediators from sensitised mast cells in the lungs. When these cells are exposed to specific antigens or other harmful stimuli, they release a mixture of leukotrienes, particularly LTC_4 and LTD_4, histamine, 5-HT (5-hydroxytryptamine, serotonin) and some prostaglandins. These mediators induce bronchospasm, mucosal oedema, and increased leucocyte inflow and mucus secretion, all of which contribute to obstruction of the airways (Fig. 6.1).

Drugs currently used for asthma include:

1. Sympathomimetic drugs
2. Corticosteroids
3. Antimuscarinic drugs
4. Theophylline and other xanthines
5. Sodium cromoglycate and nedocromil.

Sympathomimetic drugs

Sympathomimetic drugs of the β agonist (stimulator) type such as adrenaline and isoprenaline, are effective in relaxing bronchial smooth muscle, reducing submucosal oedema and reducing the liberation of mediators from mast cells. However, they are obsolete for the treatment of asthma because of their cardiac effects. They have been replaced by drugs such as *salbutamol* and *terbutaline* which have selective β_2 stimulant (bronchodilator) actions and little effect on the heart.

Selective β_2 stimulant bronchodilators such as salbutamol and terbutaline are usually given as aerosols for the control of chronic asthma, but can also be given intravenously for severe attacks when their relatively slight β_1 effects on the heart are an advantage.

Salmeterol is also inhaled from an aerosol or *Diskinhaler*. It differs from other β agonists in that its action is prolonged and can protect against attacks for up to 12 h. It is useful for nocturnal asthma.

Corticosteroids

Local deposition of corticosteroids into the bronchial tree by inhalation of an aerosol reduces the severity of chronic asthma and greatly increases the responsiveness of the bronchi to β agonists. Very little of a steroid is absorbed from the lungs and their adverse systemic effects when they are used in this way are minimal.

Too much reliance may be placed on β_2 agonists the effectiveness of which may decline with prolonged use. In many cases they should be supplemented with inhaled corticosteroids because no other type of drug has such potent anti-inflammatory actions on the airways. *Beclomethasone dipropionate*, *budesonide* and *betamethasone valerate* from pressurised, metered aerosol sprays are used for this purpose.

Proliferation of *Candida* (thrush), in the oropharynx and upper airway may complicate such treatment, but rarely seems to be troublesome. Severe asthma unresponsive to other drugs should be treated with systemic steroids such as oral prednisolone. These may be given in large doses for a short period to terminate a severe, prolonged and refractory attack. In an emergency (*status asthmaticus*), intravenous hydrocortisone has to be given and may be life-saving. In other cases, corticosteroids may have to be given in smaller doses over a long period to reduce the frequency and severity of attacks. In these circumstances, systemic toxic effects (Ch. 10) have to be accepted.

There are about 2500 deaths a year from asthma in Britain, mainly as a result of undertreatment or failure to recognise and deal with worsening of the disease. A few of these deaths may be accounted for by cardiac complications resulting from combined treatment with theophylline and β agonists. If β agonists were more frequently combined with corticosteroids this death rate would be lowered.

Antimuscarinic drugs

Ipratropium (isopropyl atropine) and *oxitropium* are useful for patients who do not respond to

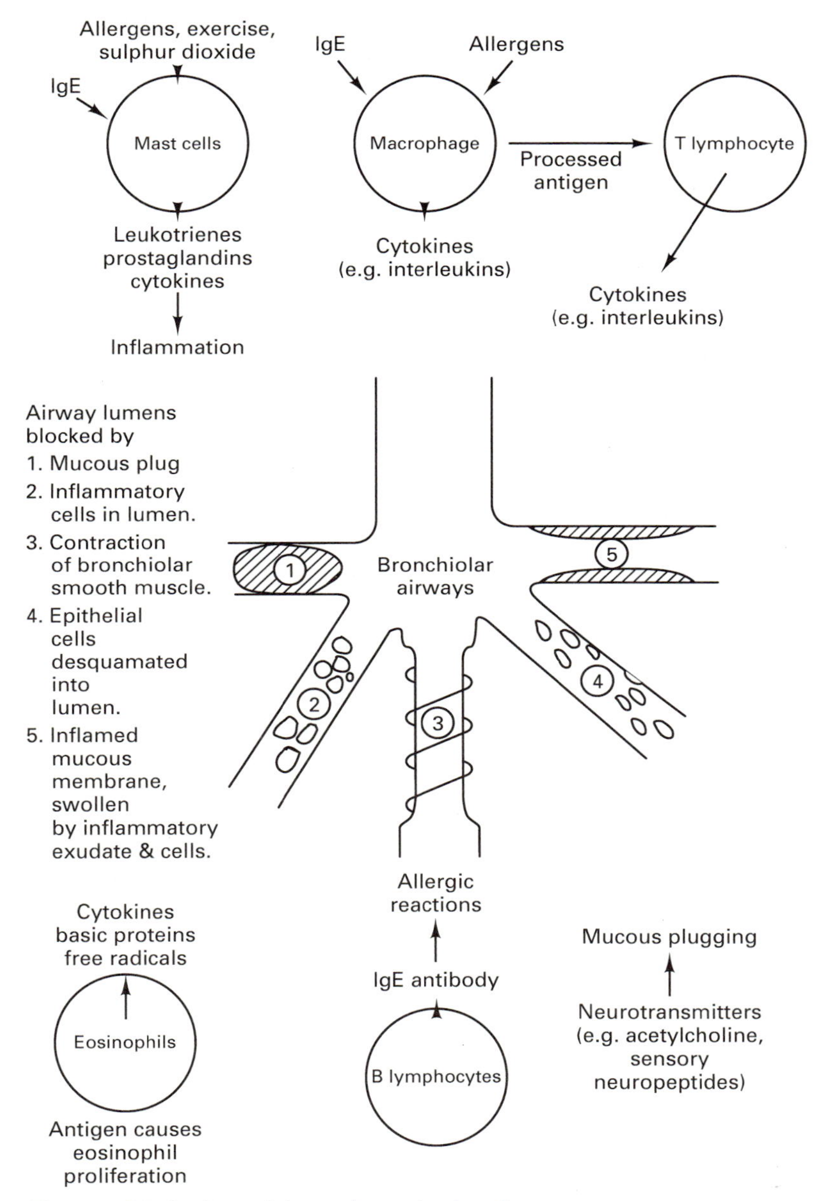

Fig. 6.1 Mechanisms of airway obstruction in asthma.

salbutamol and for asthma associated with chronic bronchitis, particularly in elderly patients.

Ipratropium is taken from an inhaler, but its onset of action is delayed for 30–60 min. The duration of action is 3–4 h and a dry mouth can be a troublesome side-effect. Oxitropium has a more prolonged action.

Theophylline and other xanthines

Theophylline is a xanthine, similar to caffeine. It is a mild diuretic, a central stimulant and a cardiac stimulant; it also relaxes smooth muscle. Theophylline is effective in terminating an attack of asthma when given by slow intravenous injection. Like the sympathomimetic drugs, theophylline relaxes smooth muscle and decreases mediator release from mast cells by raising their intracellular concentration of cyclic 3',5' - adenosine monophosphate (cAMP). The effects of theophylline on the heart are similar to those of adrenaline and when given rapidly can precipitate fatal ventricular fibrillation.

Theophylline is absorbed by mouth, but is a gastric irritant which causes vomiting. When combined with another molecule such as choline (as in choline theophyllinate) more theophylline can be given by mouth without causing nausea.

Theophylline itself is poorly soluble in water and is combined with ethylene diamine (aminophylline) for intravenous administration. Sustained-release oral preparations of aminophylline or theophylline are available and may be effective for controlling nocturnal asthma when sodium cromoglycate fails. However, aminophylline has no advantages over more selective drugs such as salbutamol for acute asthma, and is more dangerous.

Sodium cromoglycate and related drugs

Sodium cromoglycate is not used to terminate an attack of asthma but, taken prophylactically several times a day, may be effective in lessening the frequency and severity of attacks, particularly in children. It acts by blocking release of chemical mediators of asthma and preventing other bronchoconstrictor mechanisms by stabilising mast cell vesicles and by blocking irritant receptors in the respiratory mucosa. Thus, even when the patient is exposed to a specific allergen or to a chemical or physical irritant, histamine and leukotrienes are not released and parasympathetic outflow is not increased. The drug is inhaled as a powder or solution. Side-effects seem to be negligible, but not all patients respond.

Ketotifen is an antihistamine which has some sodium cromoglycate-like activity. It is taken orally and causes a dry mouth and sedation, and is little used now.

Nedocromil is another prophylactic which is currently only used for asthma in adults. It inhibits the release of chemical mediators from lung mast cells. It is given via a metered aerosol dispenser and is effective in preventing attacks due to allergy, exercise, cold or chemicals such as sulphur dioxide.

CHRONIC BRONCHITIS AND EMPHYSEMA

These two very common lung diseases frequently coexist. They are the most common cause of chronic obstructive pulmonary disease (COPD), a term which well describes their main effects. In effect, the patient suffers from chronic inflammation of the bronchi, varying degrees of airways obstruction due to progressive fibrosis, and loss of effective alveolar diffusing surface. Bronchospasm is typically associated. This chronically progressive picture is punctuated by acute exacerbations of lung infection.

Chronic bronchitis is not curable, but its progress can be slowed by stopping smoking, avoiding cold and damp environments and treating the infection and bronchospasm.

Acute infections of the lungs superimposed on chronic disease can precipitate right-sided heart failure (cor pulmonale) and respiratory failure.

Respiratory failure develops when lung function is so severely disturbed that the blood oxygen content falls, carbon dioxide content rises and blood pH falls. The patient is in danger of dying from lack of oxygen and yet, paradoxically, giving 100% oxygen may dangerously depress respiration. This is because hypoxia is the only remaining stimulus these patients have in order to breathe. Chronic intoxication with carbon dioxide, however, reduces the effectiveness of hypoxia as a respiratory stimulant. In practice, the patient is encouraged to breathe deeply and cough forcibly – using stimulants such as doxapram when necessary. Sedatives, hypnotics and opioids are absolutely contraindicated. Oxygen is given either intermittently or at a controlled concentration of 24–30% by using a Venturi mask.

The precipitating cause is usually an infection. Sputum should be taken for culture and in the interim a broad-spectrum antibacterial such as co-trimoxazole, ampicillin, amoxycillin or tetracycline is given.

If there is bronchospasm, salbutamol, ipratropium or prednisolone is given. Heart failure is an indication for giving a diuretic, such as chlorothiazide (Ch. 5).

It is important to encourage the patient to cough up sputum, and physiotherapy can help greatly. There is no clear evidence that expectorant drugs or mucolytics such as carbocisteine (carboxymethylcysteine) are of benefit.

Chronic obstructive pulmonary disease with its associated hypoxia is one of the few contraindications to the use of intravenous benzodiazepines because of their respiratory depressant effect.

Cardiac asthma

Cardiac asthma is mentioned only to differentiate it from bronchial asthma. It is an acute medical emergency because of the terrifying difficulty in breathing caused by waterlogging of the lungs (acute pulmonary oedema) which is the result of acute left ventricular failure. This in turn is often caused by a myocardial infarction, hypertension or valvular disease of the heart (Ch. 5). The patient can (as with bronchial asthma) often only manage to breathe when sitting upright, and any attempt to make a patient with cardiac asthma lie down is likely to be disastrous.

Cough suppressants

Antitussive drugs may be indicated when a cough is painful or unproductive, but suppression of coughing in patients with incipient respiratory failure or with excessive amounts of secretion in the lungs is harmful. The most commonly used drugs for this purpose are *codeine* and *pholcodine*. Codeine linctus is very widely used to control an irritating cough remaining after a respiratory infection has subsided. Morphine, diamorphine, methadone and pethidine are very powerful cough suppressants, but are not usually used for this purpose because of their high risk of dependence. Antihistamines, such as promethazine, are also cough suppressants and are present in many proprietary mixtures.

Expectorants are drugs which should facilitate the production and expectoration of sputum. Although ammonium salts, potassium iodide, ipecacuanha and squill increase bronchial secretion when given in near-emetic doses, they probably play no useful role in lung disease apart from a placebo effect.

7. The blood

Blood formation

The main factors required for blood formation are:

1. Iron
2. Vitamin B_{12}
3. Folic acid.

Deficient intake, failure of absorption or excessive blood loss can lead to anaemia (deficiency of haemoglobin). Many symptoms result from impaired oxygen-carrying capacity of the blood, but deficiency of haematinic factors can also cause oral mucosal disorders.

Erythropoiesis is regulated by the growth factor *erythropoietin*, which is mainly secreted by the kidney. Anaemia in chronic renal failure is a result of depressed erythropoietin production.

Iron

Sources and absorption

The Western daily diet contains 10–20 mg of iron, of which about 10% is absorbed. Absorption is from the small intestine and enhanced by:

1. Low intestinal pH
2. Ascorbic acid
3. High protein diet.

Iron deficiency

The main cause is chronic blood loss from such causes as menstrual bleeding, excessive loss during parturition and gastrointestinal bleeding (peptic ulcer, piles or tumours).

Dietary deficiency of iron is uncommon, but may be relative as a result of making up for large demands due to pregnancy or menstrual or other loss. Alternatively, the diet may have a low iron content in the elderly, for example, who may largely depend on tea and biscuits. Absorption is depressed by:

1. Gastric achlorhydria
2. Phytates
3. Tetracyclines
4. Phosphates
5. Bulky, high fibre diets.

Treatment of iron deficiency

The underlying cause must first be found and treated. Iron is usually given by mouth as ferrous sulphate, gluconate or fumarate. Ferric salts are less well absorbed. Oral iron (100–200 mg per day) should be continued for 6 months to restore normal reserves.

In emergency, or if the response to oral iron is poor, parenteral iron (iron dextran, iron sorbitol citric acid or saccharated iron oxide) can be given, but this can sometimes cause fever, urticaria, headache, joint pains or vomiting.

Vitamin B_{12}

Vitamin B_{12} consists of a nucleotide with four pyrrol rings combined with cobalt. There are several interconvertible forms such as hydroxycobalamin, cyancobalamin and methylcobalamin in which cobalt is attached to hydroxy, cyanide or methyl group, respectively.

Mode of action

Vitamin B_{12} is required for the synthesis of methionine thymidinic acid and conversion of methylmalonic acid to succinic acid. Deficiency blocks methylation of methyltetrahydrofolate. As a consequence folate fails to enter cells and DNA formation is impaired.

Sources

Vitamin B_{12} is present in meat and offal, particularly liver. The daily requirement is 1–2 μg. A vegetarian diet contains 0.5 μg/day derived from milk and bacterial contamination of food. Normal body stores of vitamin B_{12} last for 3–5 years before becoming signicantly depleted. It is absorbed from the lower ileum, but only in conjunction with intrinsic factor. Intrinsic factor is a glycoprotein secreted by normal gastric parietal cells. It forms a stable acid complex with vitamin B_{12}.

Vitamin B_{12} deficiency

Vitamin B_{12} deficiency is mainly due to pernicious anaemia and defective absorption. A totally vegetarian (vegan) diet gives rise to vitamin B_{12} deficiency exceptionally rarely. Possible causes of deficiency include:

1. Failure of absorption due to absence of intrinsic factor secretion, as in pernicious anaemia (the most common cause) or after gastrectomy
2. Intestinal disease (e.g. Crohn's disease or jejunal diverticulosis)
3. Absence of vitamin B_{12} in a vegan diet.

Effects of vitamin B_{12} deficiency. Vitamin B_{12} deficiency causes a megaloblastic anaemia and some deficiency of granulocytes. It also causes subacute combined degeneration of the spinal cord with neurological or psychiatric effects, or both. A sore tongue is sometimes the first symptom. Neurological and oral signs can antecede any fall in haemoglobin levels, but the haematological disorder is shown by abnormally large erythrocytes (macrocytosis) with a high mean corpuscular volume (MCV).

Treatment. Vitamin B_{12} is given by injection in the form of hydroxycobalamin. Its effect is shown by reticulocytosis which starts within a few days and reaches a peak within a week. The exceptionally rare dietary deficiency should be treated by modification of the diet.

Folic acid

Folic acid is pteroylglutamic acid which is responsible for several steps in purine and pyrimidine synthesis. Folate deficiency results in megaloblastic changes in the bone marrow and macrocytic anaemia.

Sources and absorption

Folic acid is present in green leaves (*folium*, Latin for leaf) and the daily requirement of 100–150 μg is supplied by a conventional diet. Folic acid is absorbed in the duodenum and upper ileum. Normal body stores last for about 4 months.

Folic acid deficiency

Possible causes include:

1. Malabsorption
2. Excessive demands (pregnancy, chronic haemolytic anaemia) or loss (long-term dialysis)
3. Drugs (alcohol, methotrexate and other folic acid antagonists, phenytoin, primidone, phenobarbitone, nitrofurantoin)
4. Dietary deficiency.

The effects are megaloblastic bone marrow changes and macrocytic anaemia. Macrocytosis is an early sign of alcohol dependence.

Treatment. Folic acid worsens the neurological effects of vitamin B_{12} deficiency which must therefore be excluded. The cause of folic acid deficiency must be remedied if possible. Oral folic acid is then given at a dose of 5 mg/day.

Oral manifestations of impaired blood formation

Possible oral effects include glossitis, recurrent aphthae, susceptibility to candidosis and angular stomatitis. 5–10% of patients with recurrent aphthae, particularly those in whom ulcers start or worsen late in life, are found to have iron, vitamin B_{12} or folic acid deficiency. Oral effects can sometimes precede the fall in haemoglobin level.

HAEMOSTASIS

Haemostasis after injury depends first on formation of platelet thrombi followed by clotting. The clotting cascade is shown in Figure 7.1. Platelet thrombi are sufficient to plug puncture wounds but, since they also form on damaged areas of endothelium, they contribute to blockage of coronary arteries. In the slow-moving venous blood, extensive fibrin thrombi may be deposited, particularly in immobile limbs. Fragments may break off to form emboli which can, for example, block the pulmonary arteries.

Drugs are used to improve haemostasis in haemorrhagic diseases such as haemophilia. Antiplatelet drugs are used to counteract platelet aggregation on atheromatous plaques in those at risk from myocardial infarction, or on prosthetic heart valves. Anticoagulants are used particularly to lessen the risks of deep vein thrombosis and other types of thromboembolic disease. Other drugs acting on the haemostatic mechanisms are thrombolytic agents and inhibitors of fibrinolysis.

HAEMORRHAGIC DISORDERS

HAEMOPHILIA

The most common major haemorrhagic disorder is haemophilia A which affects about 5 in 100 000 of the population: it is approximately 10 times as common as haemophilia B. It is a sex-linked genetic trait causing deficiency of procoagulant factor VIII. Haemophilia B is due to deficiency of factor IX. It is inherited in the same way as, and is clinically indistinguishable from, haemophilia A.

Treatment of bleeding in the haemophilias or preparation for surgery is by giving the deficient factors, which are derived from normal human blood. The antifibrinolytic agent tranexamic acid is usually also given to stabilise clot formation and may be sufficient alone for minor operative procedures on patients with mild haemophilia.

Preventive treatment

Ideally, regular prophylactic replacement of factor VIII (AHF) is provided. However, this necessitates daily injections of AHF which is in short supply and expensive. Its use may also lead to antibody formation or transmission of viruses. Many haemophiliacs have developed hepatitis or AIDS

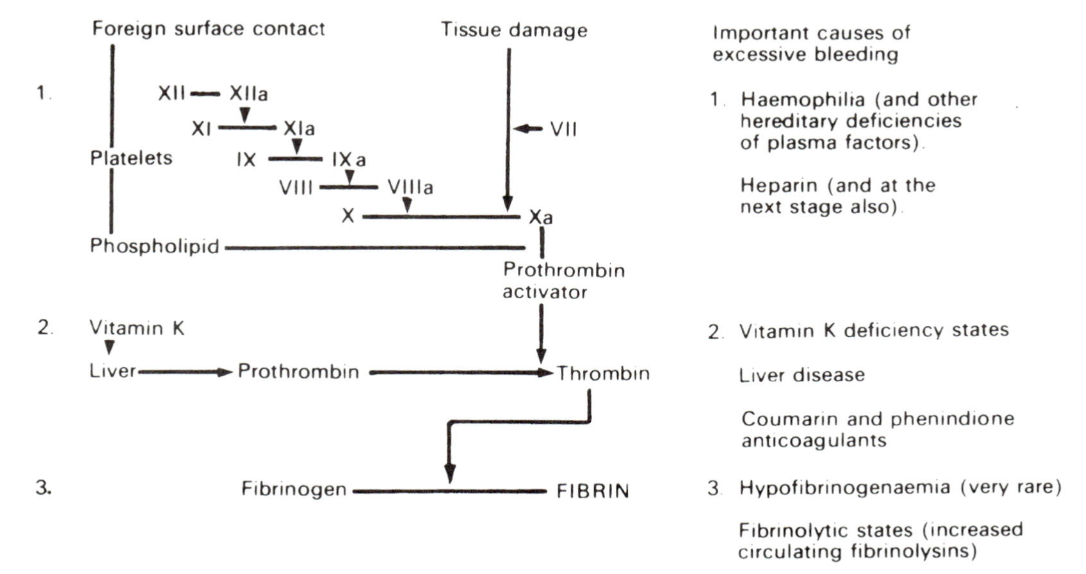

Fig. 7.1 The clotting mechanism and areas of action of some hereditary and acquired haemorrhagic diseases. The complexity of the sequence of events leading up to clotting is shown, demonstrating in particular the main areas where deficiencies or drugs may interfere with the process. (The precise sequence of interaction of the individual plasma factors is of little importance in the present context.)

from factor VIII products. Blood donors are therefore screened for HIV and hepatitis B antibodies and the factor VIII is heat treated. Increasing reliance is therefore placed on desmopressin and tranexamic acid. As in other haemorrhagic disease, aspirin is contraindicated at all times.

Replacement therapy

Human freeze-dried factor VIII concentrate (factor VIII fraction, dried) is used when the deficiency is sufficiently severe. This preparation is stable for a year at 40°C, but once reconstituted should be used without delay. In milder cases (factor VIII levels within 5–25% of normal) desmopressin (see below) may be satisfactory, and is increasingly used.

Dental management

Dental extractions can be lethal unless managed correctly. Dental care must be planned from an early age to reduce dental disease and operative intervention to a minimum. For dental surgery, haemophiliacs require the care of specialists in several disciplines and should be treated in Haemophilia Reference Centres, or associated units.

The dose of factor VIII given before operation depends both on the severity of haemophilia and the amount of trauma involved. Factor VIII is effective only for about 12 h and must be given regularly at least twice daily postoperatively for major surgery. A factor VIII level of 50–75% is needed for dental extractions. Factor VIII may also need to be given postoperatively, but many patients can be managed with the antifibrinolytic tranexamic acid, which is given for the following 10 days.

Antifibrinolytic drugs in haemophilia

Natural fibrinolysis is brought about by activation of plasminogen to plasmin (Fig. 7.2). It prevents propagation of thrombi formed at minute areas of endothelial damage. Tranexamic acid is given (30 mg/kg) orally, four times a day starting 24 h preoperatively. It significantly reduces factor VIII requirements by preserving the stability of the clot as it forms.

Topical tranexamic acid also helps to reduce bleeding: 10 ml of a 5% solution used as a mouthrinse for 2 min, four times daily for 7 days is recommended.

Desmopressin

Desmopressin, an analogue of posterior pituitary extract, temporarily corrects the haemostatic defect in mild haemophilia by releasing factor VIII C (endogenous procoagulant) and von Willebrand factor into the blood. It is given as an intravenous infusion (0.5 μg/kg, repeated 12 hourly if necessary). It may be useful for patients with factor VIII inhibitors and is increasingly widely used for the management of mild haemophilia for such purposes as dental extractions. As desmopressin also causes release of plasminogen activator, tranexamic acid should also be given to counteract the enhanced fibrinolytic activity.

Desmopressin may cause facial flushing and slight tachycardia, but the chief adverse effect is tachyphylaxis (declining response to repeated administration).

Haemophilia B

The principles of management of haemophilia B are the same as those for haemophilia A, except

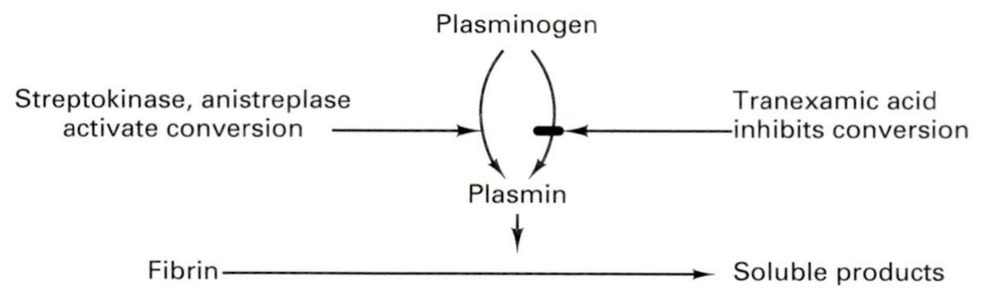

Fig. 7.2 The process of plasminogen activation and the opposing effects of thrombolytic (left) and antithrombolytic (right) drugs on it.

that factor IX replacement is needed before surgery. Human dried factor IX concentrate is available as a powder to be reconstituted with distilled water for intravenous injection. It is given (20 units/kg) 1 h preoperatively. The standard preparation may also contain factors II, VII and X. Factor IX is more stable than factor VIII. Its half-life is often up to 2 days, so that replacement therapy can sometimes be given at longer intervals than for haemophilia A.

Von Willebrand's Disease

Von Willebrand's disease (pseudohaemophilia) is characterised by deficiency of von Willebrand factor and factor VIII. It is usually inherited as an autosomal dominant trait, but a severe form of the disease may be inherited as a sex-linked recessive trait, like true haemophilia. Von Willebrand's disease affects from 1 to 45 per 100 000 of the population and is at least as common as haemophilia A. Von Willebrand's disease not only affects females as well as males but, unlike haemophilia, usually causes purpura of mucous membranes and the skin rather than a clotting defect. It is then less difficult to manage. Gingival haemorrhage is more common than in haemophilia and haemarthroses are rare. Although the disorder is usually less severe than haemophilia A, postoperative haemorrhage can be troublesome. Only a minority have factor VIII levels low enough to cause severe clotting defects as well as a prolonged bleeding time. However, the severity does not correlate well with the factor VIII level.

Typical findings in von Willebrand's disease are a prolonged bleeding time, usually a prolonged activated partial thromboplastin time (APTT), low levels of von Willebrand factor (factor VIII R: Ag), and low factor VIII C and VIII R: RCo (ristocetin cofactor) levels. The low level of factor VIII R results in poor platelet adhesion after trauma. Platelets usually fail to aggregate in the presence of ristocetin, thus causing purpura as a typical sign of the disease.

Management

Aspirin is contraindicated, as in haemophilia, but most cases can be managed with desmopressin. However, the severe subgroups of von Willebrand's disease have to be managed in a similar way to haemophilia A except that factor VIII has a prolonged half-life and less frequent infusions may be required.

ACQUIRED COAGULATION DEFECTS

Acquired haemorrhagic disorders are considerably more common than the congenital diseases but, except for liver disease, are usually less severe. Important causes include:

1. Anticoagulant therapy
2. Vitamin K deficiency or malabsorption
3. Liver disease
4. Disseminated intravascular coagulation (DIC)
5. Fibrinolytic states.

Aspirin and other non-steroidal anti-inflammatory analgesics can worsen any bleeding tendencies by interfering with platelet aggregation.

Anticoagulants

The commonly used anticoagulants are heparin for short-term treatment and coumarins for long-term treatment.

Heparin

Heparin is given by injection and acts immediately. It is a mixture of sulphated polysaccharides and greatly accelerates the action of antithrombin III which reduces the action of thrombin and factors IX, X, XI and XII. It thus inhibits the thrombin – fibrinogen reaction. It prolongs prothrombin, activated partial thromboplastin and thrombin times. These indices have to be monitored to control prolonged treatment.

Pharmacokinetics. Heparin is precipitated by gastric acid. It is usually given by intravenous or subcutaneous injection (intramuscular injection commonly causes haematomas) and acts immediately. Its effect is usually lost within less than 6 h of the last injection ($t_{\frac{1}{2}}$ = 60 to 90 min).

Uses of heparin. These include:

1. Deep vein thrombosis
2. Pulmonary embolism
3. For haemodialysis and other artificial circulation techniques

4. Acute obstruction of a limb artery
5. Disseminated intravascular coagulation in selected cases only
6. Anticoagulation during pregnancy (it does not cross the placenta).

Heparin is usually given for the first 36 h of anticoagulation and the process is prolonged as necessary with an oral anticoagulant which is given at the same time to allow it time to act.

Toxic effects. These include:

1. Spontaneous bleeding
2. Allergy occasionally
3. Osteoporosis (with chronic daily administration of very high doses).

Spontaneous bleeding affects up to 5% of patients and is countered with protamine sulphate.

Dental management of patients on heparin anticoagulation. Since heparin acts for only 4–6 h, surgery can safely be carried out after 6–8 h, when its effects have ceased. In renal dialysis patients, surgery is best carried out on the day after dialysis as the effects of heparinization have then ceased and there is maximum benefit from dialysis. In emergency situations, intravenous protamine sulphate can be used to reverse the effect of heparin.

Oral anticoagulants

Coumarins, of which *warfarin* is the drug of choice, antagonise the action of vitamin K (Fig. 7.3). They thus prolong the prothrombin and activated partial thromboplastin times. The action of vitamin K is antagonised by inhibition of vitamin K epoxide reductase. This blocks the conversion of vitamin K epoxide to the reduced form (vitamin KH_2). Vitamin KH_2 is the cofactor in the carboxylation of glutamate residues in the inactive proenzyme forms of factors II, VII, IX and X, as well as anticoagulant proteins C and S. The effects of oral anticoagulants are therefore delayed until these vitamin K products have been used up.

Pharmacokinetics. Warfarin is completely absorbed from the gut and is 97% bound to plasma albumin. It has a half-life of 44 h, but there is a 12-fold variation. Like all oral anticoagulants, warfarin enters the fetus; oral anticoagulants are therefore contraindicated in pregnancy.

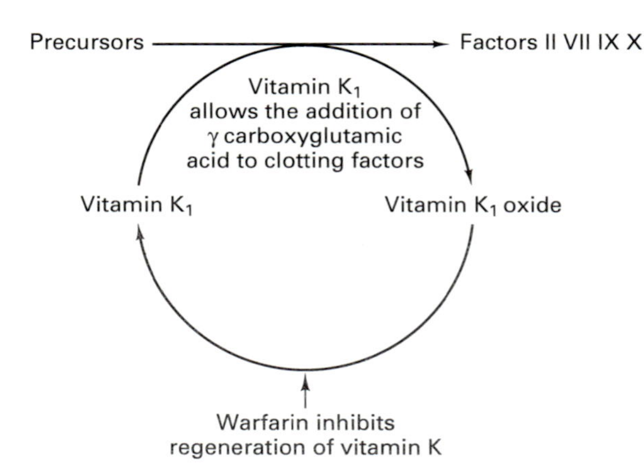

Fig. 7.3 Outline of the mechanism of production of clotting factors by vitamin K from precursors and the site of action of the coumarin anticoagulant warfarin. (Reproduced with permission from *Aids to Pharmacology*.)

The full effects are delayed for 48–72 h. For an immediate effect, heparin is given at the same time. Warfarin treatment should maintain a prothrombin time of 2–2.5 times the control (control 11–15 s), or a thrombotest of 5–20%. Prothrombin times are recorded as the international normalised ratio (INR), a ratio of 2–3 being the usual therapeutic range.

Uses of warfarin. These include:

Limited duration administration

1. Prophylaxis of thromboembolic disease
2. Deep vein thrombosis
3. Pulmonary embolism
4. Preparatory to cardioversion.

Long-term or life-long administration

1. Atrial fibrillation
2. Prosthetic heart valves.

Contraindications. These include:

1. Active or potential bleeding lesions
2. Haemorrhagic diseases
3. Head injuries
4. Diabetic retinopathy.

Interactions. The effects of oral anticoagulants are enhanced by:

1. Protein-binding drugs (e.g. aspirin, phenylbutazone, sulphonamides (including co-

trimoxazole and metronidazole) which displace the anticoagulant from plasma proteins.
2. Withdrawal of barbiturates causing cessation of enzyme induction
3. Amiodarone which inhibits metabolism.

Effects are decreased by:

1. Reduced absorption by cholestyramine
2. Enhanced metabolism, e.g. barbiturates, rifampicin, carbamazepine, griseofulvin.

The risk from haemorrhage during anticoagulant treatment is also enhanced under the following circumstances:

1. Irregular tablet taking
2. Concurrent liver disease or obstructive jaundice, which impair vitamin K metabolism or absorption
3. Prolonged broad-spectrum antibiotic (tetracycline) therapy, which reduces vitamin K synthesis in the gut (theoretically)
4. Liquid paraffin, which leads to loss of vitamin K (theoretically)
5. Use of aspirin and other non-steroidal anti-inflammatory agents which can cause gastric bleeding and also interfere with platelet function.

Under such circumstances as these, the thrombotest should be repeated within 24 h of surgery. If anticoagulant therapy is being given for a prosthetic heart valve, prophylaxis against infective endocarditis should also be given.

Precautions for dental surgery during anticoagulant therapy

Stopping or reducing the dose of anticoagulants can lead to rebound thrombosis. This has led to thrombosis of prosthetic cardiac valves and even thrombotic deaths after dental surgery. There should be no interference with anticoagulant treatment until an acceptable level of activity has been agreed. The INR (prothrombin time) or the thrombotest are the main laboratory tests used for monitoring oral anticoagulant activity. Blood (citrated) for the thrombotest must be collected in siliconised containers and tested within a few hours of venepuncture.

In practice, minor surgery (simple extractions of a few teeth) may be carried out safely with no change in anticoagulant treatment if the prothrombin time is within the normal therapeutic range (INR 2–3 times normal) and thrombotest 15% or higher). However, regional blocks should not be used and surgical trauma should be kept to a minimum. After extractions a little haemostatic material (e.g. oxidised cellulose) may be sutured over the socket, but is not essential.

More major oral surgery should be carried out in hospital, with the cooperation of the physician. Anticoagulation may need to be modified, but if anticoagulation is to be continued vitamin K for arrest of bleeding should preferably be avoided as it makes subsequent anticoagulation difficult. For minor bleeding, administration of tranexamic acid may be adequate. Life-threatening haemorrhage is controlled by stopping the anticoagulant and giving prothrombin complex concentrate (PCC). If this is unobtainable, fresh frozen plasma can be given, but is less effective.

Vitamin K deficiency and malabsorption

Vitamin K is absorbed from the diet and also synthesised by the gut flora. It is a fat-soluble vitamin and its absorption in the small gut depends on the presence of bile salts. After transport to the liver, vitamin K is used for the synthesis of factors II (prothrombin), VII, IX and X.

Haemorrhagic disease may result from inadequate amounts of vitamin K reaching the liver, particularly as a result of obstructive jaundice or malabsorption. Alternatively, vitamin K metabolism can be impaired by anticoagulants or severe liver disease. In the latter, many haemostatic factors cannot be formed from vitamin K, which becomes of little or no value.

Dental aspects. Dental management in vitamin K deficiency may be complicated both by the clotting defect and the underlying disorder, particularly obstructive jaundice.

The underlying disease should be corrected in possible, but vitamin K can be given for emergency surgery. *Phytomenadione* (5–25 mg) is the most potent and rapidly acting form and should be given by slow intravenous injection. The INR (prothrombin time) should be monitored after 48 h and, if still prolonged, parenchymal liver disease should be suspected.

Liver disease

Liver disease is an important cause of bleeding disorders. The haemostatic defects in liver failure include impaired vitamin K metabolism with failure of production of many clotting factors, enhanced fibrinolysis, and thrombocytopenia. As a consequence, haemorrhage can be severe and difficult to manage. An early sign of liver damage due to paracetamol overdose is prolongation of the INR, so that bleeding is a complication. Antifibrinolytic treatment and fresh frozen plasma may sometimes be effective. If there is an obstructive element to the disease and if parenchymal disease is mild, vitamin K may be effective.

Disseminated intravascular coagulation

Disseminated intravascular coagulation (DIC), also known as consumption coagulopathy or defibrination syndrome, is an uncommon, complex and not fully understood process in which the main effect is probably activation of haemostasis-related mechanisms within the circulation. Possible precipitating causes include incompatible blood transfusions, severe sepsis, obstetric complications, severe trauma or burns, and cancers in various sites. In head injuries, some degree of DIC may be found in over 50% of cases.

Possible effects of disseminated intravascular coagulation include:

1. *Haemorrhagic tendencies*. These result from consumption of platelets and clotting factors internally and from activation of the fibrinolytic system.
2. *Thrombotic phenomena*. Clotting in capillaries can cause vascular occlusion and can damage any organ. The kidneys, liver, adrenals and brain are particularly vulnerable.
3. *Haemolysis*. Red cells become damaged as a result of the changes in the capillaries (microangiopathic haemolysis).
4. *Shock*. Shock may be caused by adrenal damage or obstruction of the pulmonary circulation by fibrin deposition and other factors.

The overall mortality may be 50% and is mainly due to the underlying disease.

Management. The management of disseminated intravascular coagulation is difficult. The main principles include:

1. Correction of the primary disease, if possible
2. Treatment of shock, blood loss, hypoxia and pH disturbances
3. Administration of intravenous heparin if there is limb thrombosis, pulmonary embolism or peripheral gangrene
4. Replacement of coagulation factors with whole blood if there is haemorrhage
5. Administration of an antifibrinolytic drug (aprotinin) if there is excessive fibrinolysis.

Fibrinolytic states

Thrombolytic (fibrinolytic) drugs, such as streptokinase and urokinase, and local activation of plasmin by infection, for example, may cause abnormal bleeding. Dental surgery should be deferred where possible in patients on fibrinolytic therapy.

THROMBOLYTIC DRUGS

Thrombolytic drugs activate the conversion of plasminogen to plasmin which breaks down fibrin into soluble products (Fig. 7.2). The physiological effect of plasmin is the removal of small fibrin thrombi which may form at sites of endothelial damage and so maintain vascular patency.

The main use of thrombolytic drugs is in the early treatment of myocardial infarction.

Streptokinase

If given within a few hours of the attack, streptokinase lessens the mortality from myocardial infarction, but still confers some benefit if given within 24 h. Its effects are additive with those of aspirin and the drugs should usually be given concomittantly.

Streptokinase is given by slow intravenous infusion. It causes vasodilatation and so may cause hypotension.

Adverse effects. Bleeding and allergy are the main adverse effects.

Contraindications. These include haemorrhagic diatheses or active bleeding, a recent stroke, severe uncontrolled hypertension and recent streptococcal infection.

Other thrombolytic agents

Antistreplase and alteplase are as effective as streptokinase, but vary in their immunogenicity and tendency to cause bleeding. Urokinase is of no proven benefit in myocardial infarction.

ANTIFIBRINOLYTIC DRUGS

Tranexamic acid.

This inhibits plasminogen activation and enhances clot stabilisation. It is useful in a variety of haemorrhagic conditions including haemophilia, as described earlier, and for overdose of streptokinase.

Aprotinin

This inhibitor of plasminogen is proteolytic enzyme used for: patients at risk from major blood loss from, for example, major heart surgery; some haemorrhagic states, such as disseminated intravascular coagulation; and controlling bleeding secondary to thrombolytic treatment.

ANTIPLATELET DRUGS

Platelet aggregation plays a major role in the initiation of thrombus formation. Antiplatelet drugs may inhibit thrombus formation in fast-moving arterial blood where anticoagulants are ineffective, but may be used in conjunction with anticoagulants under certain circumstances.

Aspirin

Aspirin inhibits the release of platelet products and platelet aggregation by irreversibly inhibiting cyclo-oxygenase. This blocks production of labile endoperoxides and thromboxane A_2 and this is longer lasting than inhibition of prostacyclin.

Aspirin (300 mg daily) is effective for the secondary prevention of myocardial infarction. Evidence that lower doses (300 mg on alternate days, or 75 mg per day) are as effective, or possibly more effective, has yet to be confirmed. Aspirin may also be effective for the primary prevention of myocardial infarction in high-risk patients. It also reduces mortality if given (150 mg/day) for a month after myocardial infarction. Low doses of aspirin (75–100 mg/day) are also given after coronary artery bypass surgery to lessen the risk of graft occlusion and reinfarction.

Dipyridamole

Dipyridamole inhibits adenosine uptake. It inhibits platelet phosphodiesterase and raises platelet cAMP levels. It is sometimes used with aspirin after coronary artery bypass surgery or with warfarin in patients with prosthetic heart valves. However, its effectiveness is uncertain.

8. Allergic reactions and the immune response

Inflammation is a major component of many immunologically mediated diseases, and in such conditions is harmful rather than protective. Common examples are the inflamed and swollen bronchial linings in asthma and the inflamed joints of rheumatoid arthritis.

Immunologically mediated diseases fall into two main groups, namely:

1. *Reactions to exogenous allergens.* These give rise to the common allergies such as asthma, urticaria and hay fever, collectively known as atopic disease, as well as acute anaphylaxis. They are type I reactions mediated by IgE and release of mediators from mast cells.
2. *Autoimmune diseases.* These less common diseases are characterised by formation of autoantibodies to host cell components. Rheumatoid arthritis and thyroiditis are the most common examples; others are lupus erythematosus, Addison's disease and pemphigus vulgaris.

Generally speaking, there are considerable differences between the management of these two groups of diseases, even though inflammation plays a major role in both groups.

Inflammation is the response to a variety of mediators. Drugs may antagonise these mediators by inhibiting their synthesis or release, or by blocking receptors and thus lessen inflammation. Other drugs can modulate immune reactions by affecting lymphocyte function.

CHEMICAL MEDIATORS OF INFLAMMATION

Eicosanoids

Eicosanoids (*eekosi*, Greek for 20) are mediators derived from 20C essential fatty acids, mainly from membrane arachidonic acid from all types of cells. Eicosanoids include prostaglandins D, E and F, prostacyclins, thromboxanes and leukotrienes LTB_4, LTC_4 and LTD_4.

Arachidonic acid is liberated from membrane phospholipids by phospholipase A_2 which has been activated by calcium ions and calmodulin. Phospholipase is inhibited by drugs which lessen the availability of calcium ions, while glucocorticoids induce the synthesis of lipocortin, a protein which blocks phospholipase activity.

Physical stimuli activate the entire system (Fig. 8.1) by causing inflow of calcium ions which accelerate arachidonic acid formation.

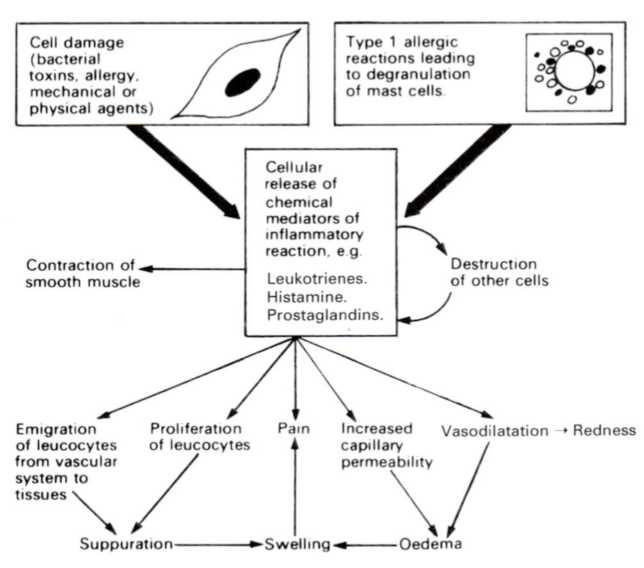

Fig. 8.1 Diagrammatic representation of the mechanisms and interactions involved in allergic and other inflammatory reactions.

Prostaglandins (PG), prostacyclins (PGI), leukotrienes (LT) and thromboxanes (TX)

Vascular effects

PGE_2 is a potent vasodilator of arterioles, precapillaries and postcapillary venules. It thus lowers blood pressure and enhances blood flow to viscera.

PGD_2 in low concentration is a vasodilator, but in high concentrations it is a vasoconstrictor. PGD_2 and PGF_2 constrict pulmonary arteries and veins.

TXA_2 is a potent vasoconstrictor and platelet aggregator.

The prostacyclin, PGI lowers blood pressure by vasodilatation and causes reflex tachycardia. Endothelial PGI_2 inhibits platelet aggregation.

LTC_4 and LTD_4 cause vasodilatation, hypotension and exudation of plasma from postcapillary venules with 1000 times the potency of histamine.

Leucocyte effects

LTB_4 causes positive chemotaxis of neutrophils, eosinophils and monocytes. In high concentrations it causes aggregation and degranulation of neutrophils, and superoxide formation.

PGE_2 inhibits the differentiation of B lymphocytes and, as a consequence, formation of plasma cells.

Effects on smooth muscle

PGF and PGD_2 constrict bronchial and tracheal smooth muscle. Asthmatics are particularly sensitive to the action of $PGF_2\alpha$, but PGE relaxes bronchial smooth muscle.

PGE and PGF contract intestinal longitudinal muscle and can cause diarrhoea and bile reflux.

Pain

Injected prostaglandins cause pain which is delayed in onset but persistent. PGE, PGI_2 and LTB_4 sensitise afferent nerve endings to chemical and physical stimuli and induce hyperalgesia. In this way they enhance the pain caused by the release of bradykinin in inflamed tissue.

Effects on gastrointestinal secretion

PGE and PGI_2 inhibit gastric acid and pepsin secretion. Prostaglandins also increase secretion of mucus which protects the gastric mucosa.

Platelet activating factor (PAF)

Platelet activating factor is a lipid product from membrane phospholipids of leucocytes, platelets, endothelial and other cells.

Its synthesis is triggered by antigen–antibody complexes, chemotactic peptides, thrombin, exposed collagen and PAF itself. Synthesis depends on phospholipase, acetyltransferase and calcium ions: it is inhibited by corticosteroids.

Actions of PAF include:

1. Contraction of smooth muscle such as that of the bronchioles
2. Vasodilatation (but reduction of renal blood flow) and enhanced vascular permeability
3. Stimulation of platelet and neutrophil aggregation, causing liberation of LTB_4
4. Stimulation of monocyte and eosinophil aggregation and chemotactic for eosinophils
5. Gastric ulceration
6. Hyperalgesia.

Histamine

Unlike the mediators described above, histamine is synthesised and stored particularly in mast cells, but also in basophils and neurones. It is distributed throughout the body, but is in greatest concentration in skin, lungs and alimentary mucosa.

Antigen and IgE cause release of histamine, PGD_2 and LTC_4 from mast cells. Antigen–antibody complexes activate a membrane G protein which causes phospholipase C to form phosphatidyl choline and lysophosphatidic acid.

Histamine is one of several mediators of acute inflammation and immediate type hypersensitivity reactions. It is also involved in gastric secretion and transmission in the CNS. The effects of histamine depend on which of at least two groups of histamine receptors (H_1 and H_2) are stimulated (Table 8.1).

H_1 actions are blocked by antihistamines such

Table 8.1 Actions of histamine on H_1 and H_2 receptors

H_1 only	H_2 only	H_1 and H_2
Enhanced permeability of postcapillary venules	Gastric acid and pepsin secretion	Dilatation of limb arterioles
Constriction of coronary and basilar arterioles	Dilatation of gastric mucosal arterioles	Pain and itching
Dilatation of facial arterioles	Increased rate, force and automaticity of heart	
Broncho-constriction	Inhibition of IgE dependent degranulation of mast cells	

as chlorpheniramine or terfenadine which are used for urticaria and hay fever, as discussed later. H_2 blockers such as cimetidine have little or no effect on allergic diseases, but diminish gastric acid secretion and are used for peptic ulceration (Ch. 12).

5-Hydroxytryptamine (5-HT, serotonin)

5-HT is also a mediator of inflammation. It is stored in platelets but not human mast cells. Its effects depend on which of the many receptors is involved.

Among its other effects, 5-HT initially relaxes then constricts vascular smooth muscle. 5-HT agonists or antagonists may be given for migraine (Ch. 4), but none are currently used for management of inflammatory disease.

Cytokines (lymphokines)

Cytokines are soluble products of lymphocytes and have a great variety of actions affecting immune responses among others. Cytokines produced by T lymphocytes include δ-interferon (δ-IFN) and interleukin 2 (IL-2). IL-2 is a T-cell growth factor secreted by helper (CD4) cells. IL-3 is a multipotential colony-stimulating factor, one form of which stimulates granulocytes and monocytes. B-cell growth factor, B-cell diffusion factor, macrophage activating factor, suppressor and helper factors, transfer factor and lymphotoxin are some of many other cytokines.

Neutrophil products

Neutrophils and their products play a major role in inflammatory reactions. Neutrophil cationic proteins enhance vascular permeability, neutrophil immobilisation, histamine release and monocyte chemotaxis.

Neutrophil acid proteases act on kininogen to form kinin.

Neutral proteases degrade collagen, basement membrane and fibrin. They also cleave the complement components C3 and C5 to form active products, catalyse kinin formation from kininogen and enhance vascular permeability.

The complement system

Activation of the complement system leads to formation of many active products. The latter include anaphylotoxins $C3_a$ and $C5_a$ which can trigger release of histamine from mast cells. $C5_a$ and activated C567 complex are potent chemotactic factors.

One activator of C3 to form $C3_a$ is plasmin, which also converts kininogen to kinin and prekallikreinin to kallikreinin.

Kinins

Kinins are peptides which contract smooth muscle. Bradykinin, by contrast, is a non-peptide which is 10 times more active as a vasodilator than histamine. It also induces pain and enhances vascular permeability.

The action of kinins is terminated by kininases such as angiotensin 1 converting enzyme.

DRUGS WHICH MODULATE INFLAMMATORY AND IMMUNE REACTIONS

Antihistamines

H_1 receptor blocker antihistamines, such as *cyclizine*, are mainly effective for allergic rhinitis, and urticaria, but not asthma. They are also effective for motion sickness and have antimuscarinic effects which may contribute to their antiemetic properties. Most are also sedating apart from those such as *astemizole* and *terfenadine* which do not penetrate the CNS.

Inhibitors of histamine release

Sodium cromoglycate and its analogues appear to inhibit mediator release by stabilising the mast cell membrane. Sodium cromoglycate sometimes effectively prevents asthmatic attacks, but is generally more effective in children than adults. It may control exercise-induced as well as allergic asthma in some patients.

Sodium cromoglycate is remarkably non-toxic but may cause irritation and coughing on inhalation.

Nedocromil has similar actions to cromoglycate but, after inhalation, is absorbed into the circulation and, as a consequence, has a more widespread action on mast cells. It also appears to be more effective than cromoglycate for adults, but may cause transient headache or nausea.

Ketotifen has actions like those of sodium cromoglycate, but is predominantly an H_1 antihistamine and causes drowsiness. It has little value in the treatment of asthma.

β Sympathetic agonists

Adrenaline and selective β agonists combat allergic inflammatory reactions mainly by physiological antagonism of mediator activity on the target organs themselves. This is achieved by their action on different cell receptors from those which bind mediators (Fig. 8.2). Sympathetic agonists relax bronchial smooth muscle by raising the intracellular concentration of cyclic adenosine monophosphate (cAMP).

Adrenaline will also suppress the histamine-induced triple response and histamine release from the lungs of sensitised animals. Adrenaline and other sympathetic agonists also suppress mediator release from IgE-sensitised mast cells.

Adrenaline combats the effects of inflammatory mediators mainly because of its ability to induce:

1. Bronchial muscle relaxation (β_2 effect)

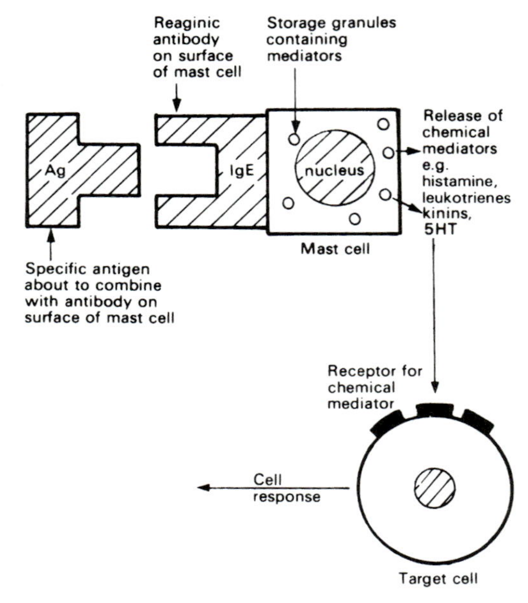

Fig. 8.2 Diagrammatic representation of the specific way in which antigen binds to antibody, triggering the release of chemical mediators which act in turn on the target cell.

2. Vasconstriction particularly in mucosae, skin and viscera (α effect) and decreased capillary permeability
3. Lessening mucosal oedema partly by diminishing mediator release.

Adrenaline is the first line of treatment in acute anaphylaxis and other acute life-threatening allergic reactions. It acts within minutes of injection and can be given by the subcutaneous, intramuscular or intravenous routes according to the severity of the reaction. The tendency of adrenaline to cause arrhythmias by its direct β effects on the heart is a possible hazard particularly when given intravenously, but the risk is small in comparison with the immediate threat to life from circulatory collapse.

The action of adrenaline is brief (up to 30 min) and may have to be given again. β agonists such as salbutamol which are longer acting and more selective in their action are, therefore, more appropriate for combatting asthma (Ch. 6).

Immunosuppressive drugs

Drugs which have major immunosuppressive effects fall into two main groups, namely:

1. Non-cytotoxic agents – corticosteroids and cyclosporin
2. Cytotoxic agents – azathioprine, methotrexate and others.

The immune response, whether humoral (antibody) or cell mediated, depends on division and differentiation of lymphoid cells, and protein synthesis. The anticancer drugs which act by interfering with cell division, growth and protein synthesis have immunosuppressive actions. In practice, these same drugs are called 'immunosuppressive' when they are used for such purposes as the prevention of rejection of a graft or transplant, and 'cytotoxic' when they are used in cancer chemotherapy.

For prevention of graft rejection, adrenal glucocorticoids, particularly semisynthetic analogues such as prednisolone, are used in large doses.

Cytotoxic drugs, used to suppress or prevent rejection reactions, include:

1. *Alkylating agents*, e.g. cyclophosphamide and chlorambucil
2. *Antimetabolites*:
   a. Antipurines, e.g. mercaptopurine, azathioprine and thioguanine
   b. Antifolates, e.g. methotrexate.

Azathioprine is frequently used with prednisolone for immunosuppression.

An arbitrary and misleading distinction is often made between corticosteroids and immunosuppressive agents (cytotoxic drugs). Both are immunosuppressive and enhance susceptibility to infection. However, corticosteroids differ from cytotoxic agents in their wide range of other actions (Ch. 10) unrelated to immunosuppression. Cytotoxic drugs, by contrast, can induce severe bone marrow depression and may lead to tumour formation. However, the adverse effects of cytotoxic drugs have to be accepted for achieving the deep immunosuppression necessary to prevent organ graft rejection or severe autoimmune disease. Azathioprine, methotrexate and cyclophosphamide are examples of drugs used for these purposes.

A major action of such drugs is to inhibit nucleic acid synthesis and thus block protein production and cell division. The result is that antibody production may be depressed or that lymphokines, which are normally formed by sensitised lymphocytes and which may contribute to target cell damage, are also not synthesised.

Cytotoxic drugs have serious toxic effects, particularly bone marrow suppression, promotion of tumour formation and abnormal susceptibility to infection (Ch. 9).

As a result of depression of cell-mediated immunity, viral and fungal infections are common complications of longer term use and are a major hazard for organ transplant patients and any others receiving immunosuppressive treatment.

Corticosteroids

Several mechanisms are involved in the immunosuppressive and anti-inflammatory actions of corticosteroids and effects vary with dosage.

1. Intracellular receptor binding leads to synthesis or activation of *lipocortin*. Lipocortin inhibits phospholipase A_2 and release of arachidonic acid from phospholipids. Synthesis of leukotrienes, prostaglandins, thromboxane and prostacyclin is thus blocked.
2. Production of IL-2 is depressed by blocking the activation of IL-1 and IL-6 genes. T lymphocyte proliferation is thus depressed as is the function of T cells.
3. Lymphokine release and the response to lymphokines are diminished.
4. In high doses, corticosteroids are cytotoxic to immature T lymphocytes and some of their mature counterparts.

The overall effects of corticosteroids are predominantly depression of cell-mediated immune responses and anti-inflammatory action. Antibody production and antigen–antibody interactions are not inhibited, except insofar as they are dependent on T-cell activity.

In the case of asthma or anaphylaxis, it is probable that the benefits of corticosteroids are mainly:

1. To lessen the output of mediators
2. To protect target cells from such mediators.

The integrity of cell membranes is stabilised and capillary permeability is reduced. Oedema and cellular exudate are thus reduced in inflamed areas (the bronchi in asthma), and in anaphylactic reactions leakage of fluid from the circulation is diminished.

Like other immunosuppressive drugs, corticosteroids enhance susceptibility to infection. Fungal infection (oropharyngeal thrush), for example, is a common consequence even of local deposition of corticosteroids from inhalers for asthma.

Cyclosporin

Action. Cyclosporin blocks T-cell proliferation by inhibiting activation of IL-2 and other lymphokine genes. The mechanism is probably by inactivating an isomerase called *cyclophilin*.

Uses. Cyclosporin is absorbed when given by mouth and can also be given intravenously. Its main use has been in organ transplantation and for prevention and treatment of graft-versus-host disease. Cyclosporin may be effective for some autoimmune diseases, lichen planus and psoriasis. Its advantages over cytotoxic drugs are that there is less susceptibility to opportunistic infections unless immunosuppression is excessive, and less risk of lymphoma promotion.

Toxic effects. Cyclosporin is nephrotoxic, but the effect is reversible if treatment is stopped early. Other toxic effects are gingival hyperplasia, hypertrichosis, hepatic impairment and metabolic hyperkalaemia.

Azathioprine

Actions. Azathioprine is metabolised in the liver to 6-mercaptopurine, then to its active metabolite 6-thioinosinic acid. DNA and RNA synthesis is blocked by inhibition of synthesis of adenylic and guanylic acids from inosinic acid. T-cell proliferation is thus blocked. The action of azathioprine is at a late stage in the process of T-cell action; thus it is usually given with prednisolone or other immunosuppressive drugs.

Uses. Azathioprine is used in organ transplantation typically in combination with prednisolone and cyclosporin. It is also used for autoimmune diseases such as pemphigus vulgaris to lessen the dose of corticosteroids and their toxic effects, or as an alternative if toxic effects are intolerable.

Toxic effects. Marrow suppression is the main short-term effect and with it there is enhanced susceptibility to infection. Later there is a risk of lymphoma.

9. Antitumour drugs and cytotoxic chemotherapy

Basic principles

Many anticancer drugs interfere with cell replication by blocking nucleotide synthesis. Hence they act preferentially on dividing cells. As a result, rapidly proliferating normal tissues as well as tumour cells tend to be damaged. The most vulnerable normal tissues are therefore:

1. Bone marrow (haemopoietic cells)
2. Gonads
3. Gastrointestinal tract lining
4. Hair follicles.

Some anticancer drugs, such as alkylating agents, are cycle specific and act at all phases of the cell cycle. Others, such as methotrexate, 6-mercaptopurine and vinca alkaloids, act only at a particular phase of the cell cycle (Fig. 9.1). A few act equally on resting (G_0) phase and dividing cells.

The proportion of tumour to normal cells that are killed (the therapeutic index), varies with each drug. Non-cycle-specific drugs are highly toxic since they tend to damage normal and tumour cells equally. Cycle-specific drugs may kill a higher proportion of tumour cells if the dose is high enough, but this may lead to unacceptable toxic effects. The effect of phase-specific drugs, by acting only on cells in the sensitive phase of the cycle, reaches a plateau and further increase in the dose does not increase cell killing (Fig. 9.2). Cycle- and phase-specific drugs are unlikely to be

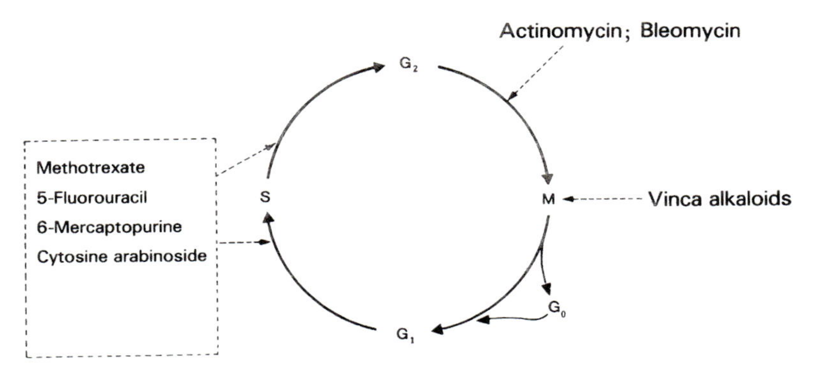

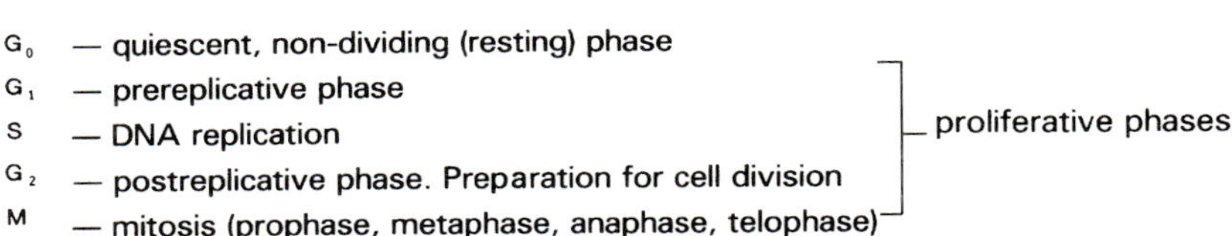

Fig. 9.1 Diagram to show the sites of action of important cytotoxic drugs on the cell cycle. (Reproduced with permission from *Aids to Pharmacology*.)

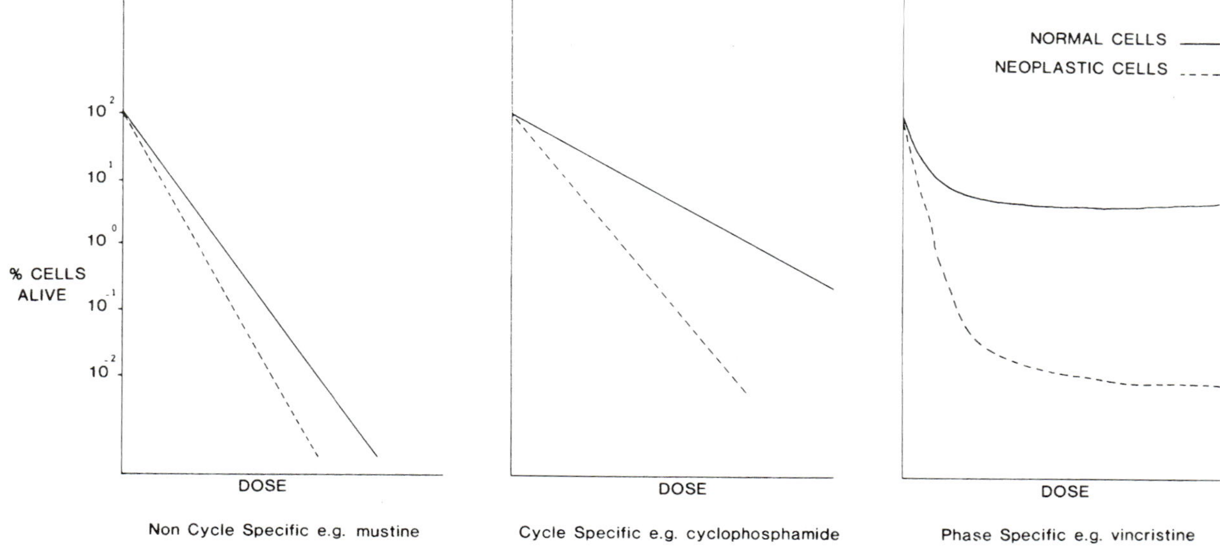

Fig. 9.2 The relative effects on survival of normal and of cancer cells of non-cycle-specific, cycle-specific and phase-specific anticancer drugs. (Reproduced with permission from *Aids to Pharmacology*.)

effective against slow-growing tumours with many cells in G_0 phase.

Tumour cells typically proliferate more rapidly than normal cells, but their growth rate is not uniform. Their variable growth rate tends, therefore, to overlap that of normal tissues, with consequent difficulties in obtaining maximum tumour cell killing without excessive toxicity. Small tumours often consist of a higher proportion of rapidly dividing cells than large ones and tend to be more susceptible to chemotherapy. Surgical reduction of the bulk of large tumours may therefore make chemotherapy more effective.

General principles of cancer chemotherapy

1. Cure probably depends on elimination of all tumour cells or reducing them to such small numbers that body defences can destroy the remainder.

2. An antitumour drug cannot be given in a single dose sufficient to kill all the tumour cells because its toxic effects are likely to kill the patient. Two strategies are to give smaller doses at intervals or to use several drugs at the same time so that their efficacy is enhanced, but their toxicity is not correspondingly greater.

3. A given dose of drug kills a corresponding proportion of tumour cells in unit time. The number of cancer cells before treatment therefore determines the number that survive and the smaller the tumour the better the result. Nevertheless, many cancers in the oral and perioral regions that can be detected while still very small have a poor prognosis.

4. Clinical manifestations of cancers in many sites appear only after they have reached a considerable size. Treatment has therefore to be prolonged if there is any chance of cure.

5. Cancer chemotherapy generally causes severe toxic effects and treatment depends on trying to achieve a balance between toxicity and efficacy.

6. Repeated sessions of drug treatment (intermittent pulsed chemotherapy) (Fig. 9.3) may be successful by allowing more rapid recovery of normal body cells than tumour tissue.

7. Cytotoxic treatment is frequently given after surgery or radiotherapy of cancer (adjuvant chemotherapy). Its aim is to eradicate or prevent seeding of metastases. It is effective in some patients with breast cancer.

8. Cytotoxic chemotherapy alone is rarely curative. Its chief therapeutic successes have been

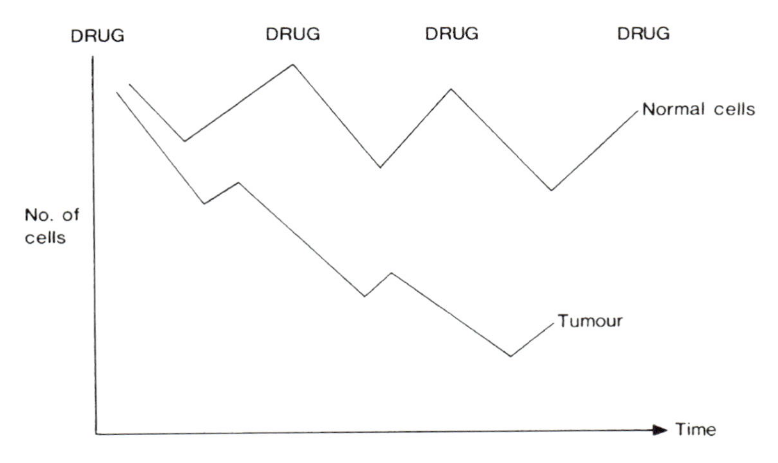

Fig. 9.3 (Reproduced with permission from *Aids to Pharmacology*.)

in childhood (lymphocytic) leukaemia, some lymphomas (particularly Hodgkin's disease and African Burkitt's lymphoma), testicular tumours, choriocarcinoma and embryonal childhood tumours. Other cancers such as small cell lung cancer, ovarian cancer and myeloma show an initial response, i.e. are chemoresponsive, but are not usually chemocurable.

ANTICANCER DRUGS

These include:

1. Alkylating agents
2. Antimetabolites
3. Plant alkaloids
4. Antitumour antibiotics
5. Other antineoplastics
6. Hormones
7. Biological response modifiers.

Alkylating agents

Mode of action. These drugs inhibit cell replication by forming covalent bonds with bases in nuclear DNA and bind bases in opposite strands of the DNA double helix. Strand separation before DNA replication is thereby blocked. They also alkylate proteins, including enzymes, causing cellular dysfunction.

Uses. Examples are mustine, ifosfamide, busulphan, lomustine (CCNU), carmustine, chlorambucil, melphelan and cyclophosphamide. They are mainly used for lymphomas, chronic lymphocytic leukaemia and myeloma.

Alkylating agents suppress cell division in the marrow and in this way cause leucopenia (particularly granulocytopenia), anaemia and thrombocytopenia. They also damage DNA and inhibit gametogenesis. They are themselves, carcinogenic and prolonged administration raises the risk of developing leukaemia.

Alkylating agents are also immunosuppressive due to their inhibition of lymphoid cell division and their destructive action on circulating lymphocytes. Some, such as cyclophosphamide, are used for this purpose (Ch. 8).

Antimetabolites

Antimetabolites have several actions such as blocking metabolic steps in the synthesis of purines and pyrimidines from folic acid. Antimetabolites are structurally similar to a natural component in the synthetic pathway and thus combine with the enzyme responsible for synthesising the natural substance. The important action of antimetabolites used in tumour therapy is to block synthesis of nucleic acids. The result is that nuclei cannot divide, cytoplasm cannot grow and cell division is blocked.

An important antifolate antimetabolite is *methotrexate*. It is used in the treatment of Hodgkin's disease and acute leukaemia. The antipurine substance *6-mercaptopurine* is also used to treat acute leukaemia. Other antimetabolites are 5-fluorouracil, cytosine arabinoside and 6-thioguanine.

Bone marrow suppression is the main dose-limiting action of these drugs.

Plant alkaloids

Vinca alkaloids (from periwinkle) include *vincristine*, *vinblastine* and *vindesine*. They block mitosis by binding to tubulin to prevent microtubule formation. As a consequence the mitotic spindle cannot form. These drugs are used for acute leukaemias, lymphomas and embryonal tumours.

Etoposide and *teniposide* are alkaloids derived from mandrake root. Like the vinca alkaloid they are mitotic spindle poisons. They are active in small cell carcinoma of the lung.

Antitumour antibiotics

These are antibiotics but too toxic for antibacterial use. They block synthesis of DNA and messenger RNA by intercalating with the DNA helix. They thus block protein synthesis and cell growth. Examples are *doxorubicin*, *daunorubicin*, *epirubicin* and *bleomycin*.

Other antineoplastics

Cisplatin and *carboplatin* are platinum coordination compounds. They selectively inhibit DNA synthesis and may be effective for testicular and ovarian cancers and, possibly, for bladder and some head and neck cancers. Cisplatin in particular is ototoxic and nephrotoxic, and causes severe vomiting and diarrhoea. It can also cause a blue line in the gingivae by deposition of platinum compounds.

Hormones and hormone antagonists

Oestrogens. The growth of some tumours such as those of the breast and prostate is hormone dependent. Oestrogens such as stilboestrol may delay the extension of carcinoma of the prostate.

Before the menopause, oestrogens may accelerate the growth of breast carcinoma, but after the menopause the same hormones sometimes slow down proliferation of this tumour.

Corticosteroids. Very high doses of glucocorticoids, such as hydrocortisone and prednisolone, are lymphocytoxic and are often given with the antimetabolite azathioprine for lymphomas and lymphocytic leukaemia.

Tamoxifen is a hormone antagonist which blocks oestrogen receptors in target organs and is currently the drug of choice for breast cancer with metastases in postmenopausal women. In some patients it will cause metastases to resolve with remarkable success. It is also being increasingly used as the first line of treatment for breast cancer in younger women.

Biological response modifiers

Interferons have activity against hairy cell leukaemia and some other tumours. *Interleukin-2* can cause regression of some tumours such as renal cell carcinoma.

RADIOTHERAPY

X-rays and other forms of radiation used in the treatment of tumours have a complex action on dividing cells. Amongst the observable effects are chromosomal breakages and abnormalities in cell division.

Radiotherapy is used in the treatment of some skin tumours, Hodgkin's disease, lymphomas, and a wide variety of carcinomas, and has largely displaced surgery in certain sites such as the mouth.

COMPLICATIONS OF CYTOTOXIC CHEMOTHERAPY

The main problems are the result of the non-specific cytotoxic action of these drugs upon the marrow and other rapidly proliferating normal cells, particularly the following:

1. *Gastrointestinal tract.* Anorexia, distressingly severe nausea, vomiting or diarrhoea are common. The cells lining the gastrointestinal tract are vulnerable since they are constantly replaced and hence are rapidly dividing.

2. *The bone marrow.* Anaemia and leucopenia are common. The latter contributes to an abnormal susceptibility to infection.

3. *Immunosuppression.* The corticosteroids and azathioprine are frequently used in combination and together suppress lymphocyte production, are lymphocytotoxic and depress lymphocyte function in other ways. Cell-mediated immunity is greatly impaired or abolished. Viral and fungal infections are a common consequence and infection is the chief cause of death during cytotoxic or immunosuppressive treatment. Many infections are due to organisms that are harmless to healthy persons (opportunistic infections). The susceptibility to infective complications is compounded in patients with leukaemia or lymphomas – diseases for which cytotoxic agents are usually used. Both the disease itself and the cytotoxic agents impair resistance to infection. The mouth is often the first or main site of these infections. Periodontal bacteria, for example, can become pathogenic in these circumstances to cause oral ulceration or septicaemias.

4. *Teratogenic effects.* Cytotoxic agents are among the few drugs in clinical use with proven capability of damaging the developing fetus.

5. *Carcinogenic effects.* The development of new tumours, particularly lymphomas and leukaemia after cytotoxic chemotherapy, is a significant hazard. Several cytotoxic drugs are mutagenic and under experimental conditions, some of them have been shown to be carcinogenic.

Irradiation is also potentially carcinogenic and second neoplasms can follow such treatment. Cancers of various types have been a long-term effect on the immediate survivors of the atomic bombs dropped on Japan at the end of the Second World War.

6. *Sterility.*

7. *Hair loss.* The rapidly dividing cells of hair follicles are vulnerable to cytotoxic drugs such as cyclophosphamide. Complete baldness can result and is distressing, particularly for women. However, the hair eventually grows again.

Antiemetics to combat cytoxic-associated nausea

Nausea and vomiting caused by cytotoxic drugs can be distressingly severe and difficult to control. The main antiemetics used for this purpose are domperidone, phenothiazines such as prochlorperazine, dexamethasone, and the 5-HT_3 antagonists, granisetron or ondansetron. Antihistamines are of little value.

Oral complications of cytotoxic treatment

1. *Ulceration.* Methotrexate in particular causes oral ulceration, as do other cytotoxic drugs such as 5-fluorouracil, daunorubicin and bleomycin to a somewhat lesser degree. Oral ulceration may be the first sign of toxicity and may be so severe as to prevent continuation of chemotherapy.

2. *Infections.* Cytotoxic drugs promote oral infections, particularly by *Candida albicans* and also by unusual organisms such as staphylococci and Gram-negative bacilli.

3. *Bleeding.* Drug-induced thrombocytopenia can cause excessive gingival bleeding or other signs such as mucosal purpura.

4. *Neoplasms,* particularly lymphomas, associated with the use of cytotoxic agents for immunosuppression may develop in the mouth.

Oral infections can be controlled with varying degrees of success by meticulous oral hygiene and by frequent rinses with a 0.2% solution of chlorhexidine. If an identifiable pathogen can be isolated, specific antimicrobial treatment should be given. Oral candidosis, for example, is common and should be treated with topical nystatin or miconazole (Ch. 16).

10. Hormones and the skeleton

Hormones and their modes of action

The anterior pituitory gland, influenced by releasing and release-inhibiting factors from the hypothalamus, produces both hormones which act on target organs and others which control the secretions of other endocrine glands (Fig. 10.1). Hormones, in turn, affect target cells by different mechanisms, as summarised in Figure 10.2.

Sex hormones

In both sexes, the adrenal cortex produces oestrogens, progestogens and androgens. The testes are the main site of androgen production, while the ovaries produce oestrogens and progestogens.

Androgens, such as *testosterone propionate, methyltestosterone* and *testosterone,* are used for hypogonadism in the male. Androgens are also used as anabolic agents in wasting diseases and in chronic renal failure.

Oestrogenic drugs include *stilboestrol, ethinyl oestradiol* and *mestranol.* Some of the progestogens are given to prevent osteoporosis: others have been used to suppress lactation. Oestrogen–progestogen mixtures are effective in a wide range of gynaecological disorders, particularly of the menstrual cycle.

Destruction of the pituitary leads to gonadal hypofunction because of failure of production of luteinising hormone and follicle stimulating hor-

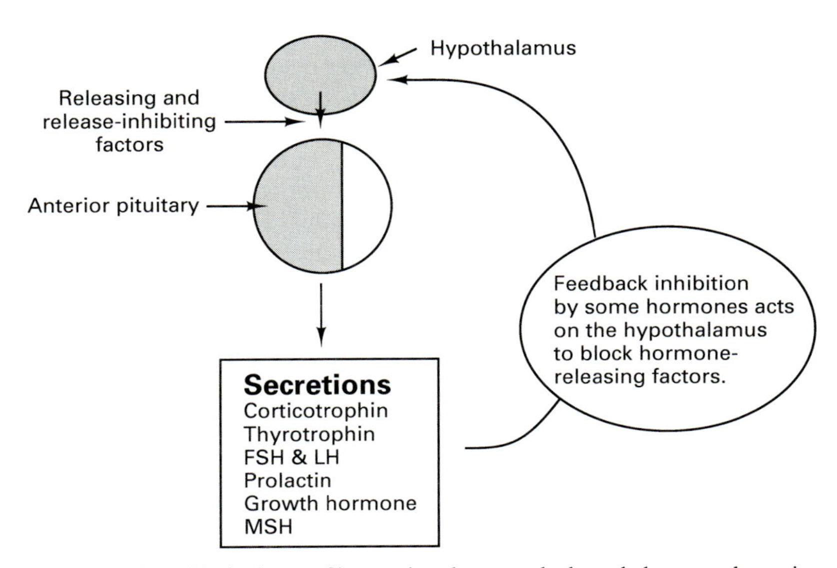

Fig. 10.1 Simplified scheme of interactions between the hypothalamus and anterior pituitary and of feedback mechanism of anterior pituitary secretions. FSH, follicle stimulating hormone; LH, luteinising hormone.

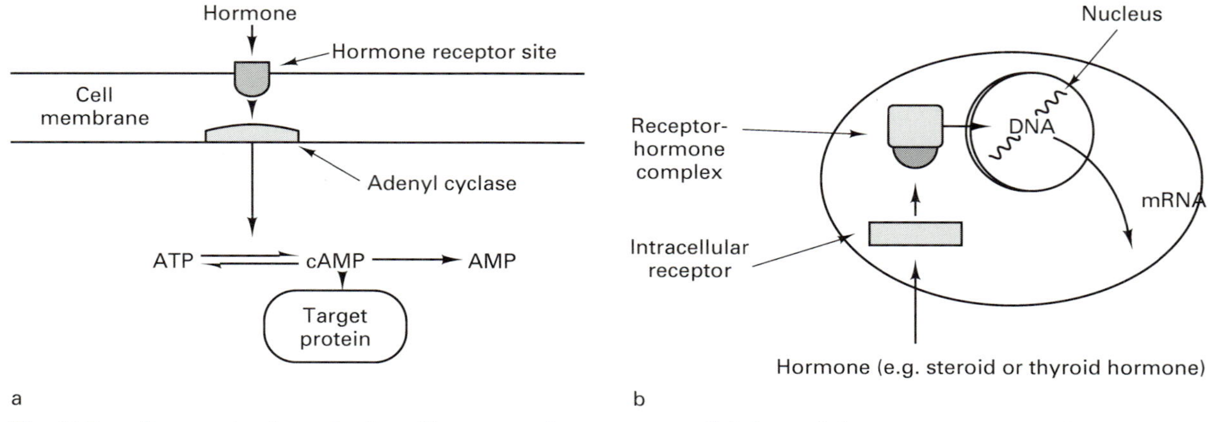

Fig. 10.2 **a** An example of a mechanism of hormone action on a target cell. **b** Intracellular receptors are targets for some hormones. The hormone - receptor complex enters the nucleus and stimulates formation of specific messenger RNA (mRNA).

mone. This may be treated with gonadal steroid replacement or by administration of gonadotrophins such as human menopausal gonadotrophin. This has both luteinising and follicle stimulating properties.

Partial destruction of the pituitary may lead to overproduction of prolactin. This results in galactorrhoea, amenorrhoea, impotence and infertility. Treatment can be with the ergot alkaloid, bromocriptine, which inhibits the release of prolactin and is the drug of choice to stop normal lactation.

Important uses of sex hormones are as follows:

1. Replacement treatment of gonadal failure
2. Menstrual disorders
3. Oral contraception
4. Treatment of hormone-dependent cancers (see Ch. 9).

ORAL CONTRACEPTIVES

The most effective oral contraceptive is an oestrogen–progestogen combination. It acts mainly by inhibiting ovulation due to suppression of pituitary gonadotrophin release. Additional mechanisms which contribute to their high contraceptive effectiveness are by increasing the viscosity of the cervical mucus, and by depressing tubular motility and endometrial development.

The patient takes the combined pill for 20 or 21 days, leaves a 7-day gap and then starts to take the pill again for a further 20 or 21 days. During the 7-day gap there is usually uterine haemorrhage.

Adverse effects

Serious side-effects are rare with steroidal contraceptive agents, but minor toxic effects are common. These include nausea, breast discomfort, headache or migraine, aggravation of diabetes, ankle swelling, weight gain, bleeding in midcycle and failure to bleed during the 7-day gap. The progestogen appears to be mainly responsible for changes such as lethargy and depression. However, the range of possible toxic effects from oral contraceptives is wide (Table 10.1).

The mortality from cardiovascular disease due to myocardial infarction is about three to five times greater than in non-users of the pill. The risk increases with age, pre-existing hypertension and cigarette smoking. The use of oral contraceptives after the age of 35 years may, therefore, be inadvisable. After stopping oral contraceptives, fertility may be subnormal for several cycles in a minority of women.

The benefits of oral contraceptives have to be balanced against the risks, and it is generally agreed that their level is acceptable, bearing in mind that the hazards of pregnancy and labour may be higher. But in women who continue to take these agents for 20 or more years, the effects are uncertain.

Table 10.1 Effects of oestrogen and progestogen components of oral contraceptives

Oestrogen effects	Progestogen effects	Combined effects
Breakthrough bleeding	Acne	Hypertension
Carbohydrate intolerance	Depression	Irregular bleeding
Cerebral arterial thrombosis	Hirsutism	Myocardial infarction
Cervical erosions	Lessened libido	Post-pill amenorrhoea
Cloasma	Vaginal dryness	
Depression		
Menstrual cramps		
Migraine		
Oedema		
Vaginal discharge		
Vaginal candidosis		
Venous thrombosis		

Associations between oral contraceptives and cancer

There appears to be a greater risk of cervical carcinoma among users of contraceptive drugs compared with those who use intrauterine contraceptive devices. Prolonged use of the pill is also associated with a greater risk of endometrial cancer.

Neither of these findings establishes a cause-and-effect relationship between use of the pill and cancer. Nevertheless, oral contraceptive agents with low oestrogen and low progestogen content are probably preferable for long-term use.

Dental aspects of oral contraceptive use

Mild deterioration of gingivitis with increased gingival oedema, and possibly also of periodontitis, may result from use of oral contraceptives. The greater risks associated with hypertension and ischaemic heart disease, particularly in older women who are smokers and use oral contraceptives, also need to be considered if a general anaesthetic has to be given.

Broad-spectrum antibiotics such as amoxycillin are said to diminish the action of combined oral contraceptives by interfering with the absorption of the oestrogenic component. However, this is a largely theoretical consideration, particularly after a single dose used for prophylaxis of infective endocarditis. Moreover, with prolonged courses of broad-spectrum antibiotics (more than 2 weeks) resistance to this interference develops and the oestrogen is absorbed normally.

Note: those with a passion for accuracy may have noticed that *the* pill is not *a* pill. Pills consist of the drug made up in a pasty mixture that sets hard: they are now obsolete because of the variability of dissolution and absorption. The pill is, in fact, a tablet, i.e. highly compressed powder.

THYROID HORMONES

The thyroid gland secretes thyroxin (T4) and tri-iodothyronine (T3). These hormones stimulate the metabolism of tissues and raise their rate of utilisation of glucose and oxygen. The metabolic rate partly depends on the thyroid hormones so that in hypothyroidism (myxoedema) the basal metabolic rate (BMR) is abnormally low, whilst in hyperthyroidism (thyrotoxicosis) the BMR is high.

Hypothyroidism

The thyroid hormones are needed during development for growth of the skeleton and for normal brain maturation. Congenital absence or hypofunction of the thyroid, due for instance to iodine deficiency, leads to dwarfing, mental deficiency and other consequences due to the low BMR. This clinical entity is known as cretinism.

In adults or children, hypothyroidism is treated by oral administration of T4. In the adult the smallest dose of thyroxin which will raise the metabolic rate to normal is used. Cretinism is treated by giving the largest tolerable dose of thyroxin as soon as the disorder is recognised, to prevent mental deficiency and dwarfing.

Patients suffering from severe myxoedema may have such a low metabolic rate that they become comatose, particularly after taking sedative drugs. T4 takes about 48 h before it starts to raise the metabolic rate and, therefore, may not be suitable for such an emergency. Under these circumstances T3 is often given. Not only is it about five times more active than T4, but it raises the metabolic rate within 6 h.

Hyperthyroidism

In addition to the raised metabolic rate, increased secretion of T3 and T4 enhances responsiveness of the tissues to sympathetic activity. As a consequence, severely thyrotoxic patients often have cardiac arrhythmias and may be more sensitive to adrenaline. A β blocker such as propranolol is often effective in treating fast arrhythmias in hyperthyroidism. There is, however, *no* clinical evidence to support the suggestion that the use of adrenaline in dental local anaesthetics is contra-indicated in patients with hyperthyroidism.

The treatment of thyrotoxicosis may be by operation (partial thyroidectomy) or by destruction of some of the thyroid cells by radioactive iodine (iodine-131). Alternatively, drugs, namely *carbimazole* or *propylthiouracil*, may be given. Both of these drugs block the synthesis of T3 and T4 by preventing incorporation of iodine into their organic precursors. Side-effects of these drugs include rashes (common) and neutropenia (rare).

Calcitonin

Calcitonin (thyrocalcitonin) is secreted by the C cells in the parafollicular regions of the thyroid gland and also by the thymus and parathyroids. It is concerned with calcium homeostasis, as discussed below.

DIABETES AND ANTIDIABETIC AGENTS

Insulin is the antidiabetic peptide secreted by the β cells of the pancreatic islets of Langerhans. If insufficient insulin is produced, diabetes mellitus develops. Glucose cannot then be fully used by cells so that there is excessive breakdown of the glycogen and fats within them. Fats are not completely oxidised but are broken down to acetoacetate, acetone and β-hydroxybutyrate (so-called acetone or ketone bodies). When these substances enter the circulation they are excreted on the breath and in the urine, and ketosis is said to be present.

In diabetes the blood glucose is raised. Large amounts of glucose therefore enter the renal tubules by way of the glomerular filtrate to cause an osmotic diuresis. Polyuria leads to dehydration and thirst.

Diabetic patients are also excessively susceptible to infection – particularly by staphylococci or *Candida albicans*. Serious arterial disease frequently leads to retinopathy, renal disease, occlusive coronary artery disease and occlusion of peripheral limb vessels. Acute episodes of ketosis, acidosis and loss of consciousness (diabetic coma) may punctuate the course of this chronic illness.

There are two major types of diabetes: insulin-dependent diabetes mellitus (IDDM), which is typically of early onset; and non-insulin-dependent diabetes mellitus (NIDDM), which is typically late in onset. Juvenile-onset diabetes starts in adolescence or early adult life and is characterised by weight loss, ketosis and the inability of the pancreas to produce insulin. In maturity-onset diabetes the patient is usually obese and has raised levels of circulating insulin. However, lack of exercise, obesity and age lead to insulin resistance in the tissues and thus to a relative lack of insulin.

Young, thin diabetics with ketosis usually need insulin to correct their metabolic abnormalities. Maturity-onset diabetes may be corrected by dietary measures and weight loss only, but many elderly diabetics require, in addition to dieting, oral hypoglycaemic agents such as sulphonylureas

Table 10.2 Actions of insulin

1. Enhances glucose uptake by muscle and fat
2. Inhibits gluconeogenesis
3. Promotes conversion of glucose to glycogen and fatty acids
4. Promotes conversion of fatty acids to triglycerides and inhibits reverse reaction; thus deposition of fat is enhanced
5. Promotes conversion of aminoacids to proteins and inhibits reverse reaction

or biguanides. Any diabetic who develops ketosis, acidosis or hyperglycaemic coma needs insulin.

Insulin

Insulin is a peptide which is traditionally crystallised out from acid extracts of beef or pig pancreas, but human insulin is now also synthesised using recombinant DNA techniques. Insulin is destroyed by proteolytic digestive enzymes and is therefore given by injection, usually subcutaneously.

The action of insulin is to lower the blood sugar by several mechanisms (Table 10.2).

In diabetic coma, insulin may be injected intramuscularly or intravenously and when rapid action is needed soluble insulin is used. For a more prolonged effect, protamine zinc insulin slowly releases insulin from the protein–insulin complex. Insulin zinc suspension is in the form of crystals, the size of which determines the duration of effect.

A diabetic often needs a combination of insulins in an attempt to keep the blood sugar at a steady level in the face of varying demand.

Monocomponent and human insulins. Allergy to insulin can develop against such substances as insulin precursors remaining in the solution or to insulin from a particular animal – usually bovine insulin. These reactions can often be avoided by the use of newer, highly purified insulins obtained from a single species of animal and monocomponent insulins from which allergenic substances such as proinsulin have been removed. Alternatively, human (recombinant DNA) insulin can be given.

Toxic effects of insulin

These are summarised in Table 10.3.

Table 10.3 Toxic effects of insulin

1. Hypoglycaemia
2. Local and systemic allergy (uncommon)
3. Insulin resistance due to insulin antibodies
4. Acquired enhanced susceptibility to insulin
5. Lipodystrophy (localised fat atrophy at the site of injection), particularly with older, less pure insulins

Hypoglycaemia. If too much insulin is given either by accidental overdose or relative to inadequate carbohydrate intake, hypoglycaemia can result. Hypoglycaemia may develop, for example, in a dental patient who is prevented by treatment from eating at the expected time. Mild hypoglycaemia causes excessive hunger. More severe hypoglycaemia may produce signs similar to fainting or drunkenness. The patient may become confused, ataxic, or argumentative, and eventually develops convulsions and coma.

If recognised early, hypoglycaemia can be reversed by giving sugar by mouth. Once consciousness is lost, glucose must be given intravenously and is usually quickly effective. Hypoglycaemia which does not respond adequately to glucose alone may be reversed temporarily with injections of *glucagon*. This is another peptide hormone secreted by the α cells of the islets of Langerhans of the pancreas. It has a hyperglycaemic action by accelerating hepatic breakdown of glycogen.

Diabetic patients who need a general anaesthetic must have carefully arranged doses of insulin and glucose to tide them over the period of starvation and unconsciousness and to prevent either hypoglycaemia or ketosis (see below). Prolonged hypoglycaemia can lead to death or permanent brain damage.

Allergy. Allergic reactions to insulin can cause localised itching and swelling at the site of injection, or generalised urticaria. In general, pig insulin is less allergenic than beef. Another type of immune reaction to insulin is insulin resistance. Allergy to monocomponent or even to human insulin can occasionally develop. Nevertheless, newly diagnosed diabetics are usually given human insulin.

Localised fat atrophy. This reaction at the site of repeated subcutaneous injections, appears as localised depression of the skin.

Management of insulin-dependent diabetics requiring surgery

The main measures include:

1. Admit to hospital 48 h preoperatively.
2. Change to soluble insulin three times daily.
3. During surgery infuse insulin 3 units/h plus 6 g of glucose per hour. Blood glucose should be monitored hourly and these infusion rates may need to be modified to achieve levels of 6–8 mmol/l.
4. Continue with above regimen until oral feeding and intermittent insulin injections can be resumed.
5. Patients with mild diabetes not requiring insulin should have blood glucose levels monitored hourly into the postoperative period.

Non-insulin-dependent diabetes should have their blood glucose levels monitored during the operation and the postoperative period.

Oral hypoglycaemic drugs

These agents are principally used for maturity onset, non-ketotic diabetes which cannot be adequately controlled by diet alone. There are two main groups of orally active hypoglycaemic drugs:

1. Sulphonylureas
2. Biguanides.

Sulphonylureas act by increasing the release of insulin from the pancreas. Thus they are only effective in the presence of functioning islet tissue. Two commonly used members of this group are *tolbutamide* and *chlorpropamide*. Tolbutamide is rapidly destroyed in the liver and has to be taken two or three times a day. Its action is greatly enhanced and prolonged by severe liver disease. Chlorpropamide is not metabolised, but is excreted unchanged via the kidney. It can be effective for over 24 h when given only once daily. Its action is potentiated by renal failure. *Glibenclamide* has an action intermediate in duration between tolbutamide and chlorpropamide, but like the latter can be taken once daily. Tolbutamide is preferable for use by the elderly in whom chlorpropamide and glibenclamide can cause prolonged hypoglycaemia. These drugs can cause hypoglycaemia, but this is usually easily managed by giving glucose or sugar by mouth. Another disadvantage of the sulphonylureas is that they tend to increase appetite. This may be troublesome, in that it may add to the patient's difficulties in keeping to their carbohydrate- and calorie-restricted diets.

Biguanides such as *metformin* have similar uses to the sulphonylureas, but have the advantage for obese diabetics that they tend to diminish appetite. Biguanides appear to act at tissue level by enhancing the action of circulating insulin. Unlike the sulphonylureas they have no hypoglycaemic action in the total absence of functioning islet cells.

The biguanides and sulphonylureas have a synergistic action and the two types of drug may be given together. Both phenformin and metformin are rapidly absorbed from the gut and rapidly excreted unchanged by the kidneys. They are given twice or three times daily.

ADRENAL CORTICAL HORMONES: CORTICOSTEROIDS

The adrenal cortex secretes cortisol (hydrocortisone), aldosterone and some of the sex hormones. Cortisol is a *glucocorticoid*, and raises the blood glucose by accelerating the breakdown of tissue glycogen. Aldosterone is a *mineralocorticoid* which controls sodium and water excretion.

The glucocorticoids have powerful anti-inflammatory and antiallergic actions. As a result, drugs such as hydrocortisone and prednisolone can be life-saving in severe refractory asthma and anaphylaxis. The mechanism of this effect is via a mediator substance, *lipocortin*. The steroid enters many types of cell, binds to cytoplasmic receptors and the combination enters the nucleus which is stimulated to produce the specific mRNA for lipocortin synthesis. Lipocortin mediates several actions, which include:

1. Inhibition of phospholipase and thus inhibiting synthesis of prostaglandins and leucotrienes. The prostaglandins cause the pain, oedema and vasodilatation of acute inflammation. Leukotrienes mediate cellular infiltration, mucosal

secretion and bronchoconstriction in more prolonged inflammation (Ch. 8).

2. Inhibition of production of interleukin 2. This substance, secreted by lymphocytes, also stimulates proliferation of T lymphocytes. Because steroids block proliferation of T cells in this way, cell-mediated immunity is depressed.

3. Inhibition of release of and the response to lymphokines. Lymphokines are proteins released from lymphocytes in severe inflammation (such as rejection of a foreign tissue graft or necrosis in a granuloma) which destroys tissue cells.

Clinical uses of glucocorticoids

There are two main applications for glucocorticoids, namely:

1. As replacement of the steroid in patients with adrenal insufficiency due to adrenal or pituitary disease
2. For suppression of inflammatory and immunologically mediated diseases such as rheumatoid arthritis, eczema and asthma.

Corticosteroids enter the general circulation when given orally or by injection. Alternatively, the drug may be applied locally to skin or mucous membranes. This gives a high concentration at the site of inflammation with relatively little systemic absorption.

Cortisol (hydrocortisone) has mineralocorticoid activity as well as glucocorticoid and anti-inflammatory effects. Mineralocorticoids promote retention of sodium and water, and loss of potassium by the kidney. These actions help to restore blood pressure, and fluid and electrolyte balance in cases of adrenal insufficiency but play no part in anti-inflammatory effects. Cortisone, a synthetic drug, is also inactive until converted in the liver to cortisol. Hydrocortisone is therefore given when a rapid response is required.

Corticosteroids are used in physiological amounts in replacement therapy and successfully reverse the tendency to hypoglycaemia, dehydration and hypotension due to adrenal insufficiency in such conditions as Addison's disease.

When anti-inflammatory activity is required, a steroid with predominantly glucocorticoid (anti-inflammatory) actions should be used to avoid the oedema and hypertension which hydrocortisone may cause. Synthetic steroids include *prednisolone, triamcinolone, betamethasone* and *dexamethasone*. Prednisone is inactive until converted in the body to prednisolone. The latter is used instead of prednisone.

The relative potencies of the different corticosteroids are shown in Table 10.4.

Table 10.4 Equivalent anti-inflammatory doses of glucocorticoids

	Dose (mg)
Bethamethasone	2.5
Cortisone acetate	100
Dexamethasone	2.5
Hydrocortisone	80
Methylprednisolone	16
Prednisolone	20
Triamcinolone	16

Adverse effects

When used as anti-inflammatory agents, very large doses of glucocorticoids are given. If given briefly for acute reactions such as anaphylaxis this has no adverse effects, but long-term use of even small doses causes a variety of toxic effects (Table 10.5).

Table 10.5 Major toxic effects of corticosteroids

1. Feedback inhibition of the pituitary-adrenal system
2. Glucocorticoid actions
3. Mineralocorticoid actions

Pituitary-adrenal inhibition. Prolonged steroid therapy in childhood can arrest growth by inhibiting pituitary growth hormone release, depressing protein synthesis and probably by other actions also.

Another important consequence of prolonged steroid treatment is adrenal cortical suppression. During corticosteroid treatment and for up to 2 years after cessation of steroid administration, the adrenal cortex cannot produce its normal outpouring of cortisone in response to stress. Under these circumstances, for example if the patient breaks a leg, develops a severe infection, undergoes an operation under general anaesthesia or goes into status asthmaticus, acute adrenal insufficiency with severe hypotension may develop. This can be prevented by giving large doses of steroids (Ch. 19).

Glucocorticoid actions. The toxic effects of glucocorticoids include aggravation of pre-existing diabetes or development of diabetes in a prediabetic individual. This is due to enhanced gluconeogenesis. Peripheral utilisation of glucose may also be depressed.

Depression of the inflammatory response and of cell-mediated immunity can allow infection to progress unchecked. Infection is the chief cause of death of patients on prolonged corticosteroid treatment.

Anabolism (conversion of amino acids to proteins) is depressed but catabolism is not. Thus there is muscle wasting and loss of bone matrix, causing osteoporosis. Increased capillary fragility and loss collagen in the skin, causes purpura. Healing and fibrosis are also inhibited.

Peptic ulceration and gastric haemorrhage can result from concurrent use of corticosteroids and nonsteroidal inflammatory drugs.

Fat is deposited in particular sites, notably face, shoulders and abdomen. The face becomes moon-shaped – one of the characteristic signs of prolonged corticosteroid therapy.

Mood changes. A feeling of well-being is not uncommon, but may go on to euphoria or, rarely, psychotic states.

Anti-vitamin-D action. Absorption of calcium from the gut is impaired and hypercalcaemia in diseases such as sarcoidosis (but not hyperparathyroidism) is reversed.

Mineralocorticoid actions. Sodium and water retention lead to oedema and hypertension. Potassium loss causes muscular weakness.

Treatment of adrenal insufficiency

Both the glucocorticoid and mineralocorticoid properties of corticosteroids are needed. The glucocorticoid action is provided by hydrocortisone. To combat hyponatraemia, dehydration and hypotension, a pure mineralocorticoid steroid is also given. Aldosterone is the natural mineralocorticoid secreted by the adrenal cortex, but a synthetic steroid (*fludrocortisone*) has very powerful mineralocorticoid activity, but negligible glucocorticoid and anti-inflammatory effects and is an effective substitute.

In the body cortisone is converted to cortisol (hydrocortisone). When a rapid action is needed as in hypotensive and Addisonian shock, anaphylactic shock or status asthmaticus, hydrocortisone in large doses is injected intravenously. Hydrocortisone is also preferred in chronic illness because of individual variation in the ability of the liver to convert cortisone to cortisol.

The actions of corticosteroids have been considered from the viewpoint of their pharmacological actions. Their clinical usefulness and also their adverse effects are summarised in Table 10.6.

A moon-face appearance often passes for healthy plumpness and the complexion is often of very good colour. These, with the subjective feelings of well-being, often effectively mask serious disease with a spurious and dangerously misleading appearance of good health. It is important to bear this in mind when assessing a patient for surgery and general anaesthesia.

Uses of corticosteroids in oral disease

Corticosteroids are used for non-infective, inflammatory conditions, such as recurrent aphthae and lichen planus, where there is no identifiable cause that can be removed.

Table 10.6 Actions of corticosteroids

1. Carbohydrate metabolism (raised blood sugar)
2. Anti-inflammatory and antiallergic
3. Lowered resistance to infection
4. Mineral metabolism – sodium and water retention can raise the bood pressure
5. Depression of protein synthesis leading to delayed wound healing
6. Fat deposition, particularly in the face, shoulders and abdomen
7. Anti-vitamin-D action – impaired calcium absorption from the gut can cause osteoporosis
8. Adrenocortical suppression
9. Growth arrest in children
10. Mood changes

The actions of corticosteroids under these circumstances are probably mainly anti-inflammatory.

The preparations available are hydrocortisone lozenges (hydrocortisone hemisuccinate 2.5 mg) and triamcinolone dental paste.

Recurrent aphthae

For this disease hydrocortisone lozenges can be allowed to dissolve as slowly as possible in the mouth. Two or three a day are taken every day if ulceration is very frequent (a week or so between the healing of one crop and the outbreak of another). There is no evidence that this level of dosage (up to 7.5 mg of hydrocortisone a day) has any adrenal suppressive effect. Since the disease is subject to natural remissions and the effectiveness of treatment difficult to assess, this treatment should be continued for no more than 2 months, then stopped for a month to assess progress. If ulcers recur, a further course of treatment can be given.

Triamcinolone dental paste is triamcinolone acetonide (0.1%) in a vehicle consisting of gelatin, pectin and methyl cellulose. This imbibes water to form a gel which adheres firmly to the oral mucosa. This protective layer keeps the corticosteroid in contact with the lesion, but is difficult for patients to apply.

The usefulness of corticosteroids for aphthous stomatitis is limited. Only a minority of patients respond well; stronger corticosteroids or systemic administration achieve no better results.

Lichen planus

Hydrocortisone lozenges and triamcinolone paste can also be used for atrophic or erosive lesions of lichen planus, but with limited effect. The more potent anti-inflammatory corticosteroids are more effective, but preparations for topical oral use are not generally available. For severe oral lichen planus unresponsive to topical steroids, systemic corticosteroids are effective. Triamcinolone paste is sometimes helpful in the management of gingival lichen planus (so-called desquamative gingivitis).

Bullous stomatitis

Mucous membrane pemphigoid can often be treated with topical corticosteroids while lesions remain localised to the mouth. The more potent corticosteroids such as beclomethasone dipropionate or betamethasone valerate are more effective, but the only available preparations of these that can be conveniently used in the mouth are the sprays used for the treatment of asthma. Such sprays deliver a metered dose of 100 μg per puff, but this can be repeated until enough corticosteroid is deposited on the lesion. If ocular bullae develop, systemic corticosteroids become necessary.

Pemphigus vulgaris is an autoimmune disease. Epithelial cells lose their normal adherence to one another causing oral ulceration and disintegration of the skin surface with fatal effects if untreated. The disease responds well to immunosuppressive treatment but very large doses of corticosteroids (100 mg of prednisolone a day) are needed to control the disease. To lower this dose, azathioprine is given in addition, but even so, a typical regimen would be prednisolone 40–60 mg/day plus azathioprine 100–150 mg/day. Prolonged treatment such as this may lead to a sustained remission.

Management of dental surgery in patients on systemic corticosteroids

When patients have been on long-term corticosteroid therapy, and possibly for up to 2 years after withdrawal, adrenocortical function is depressed. A stressful situation such as an injury or operation under general anaesthesia can then precipitate acute hypotension and circulatory failure. This may be fatal. Protection must therefore be provided by giving full doses of hydrocortisone as it is less difficult to prevent such a crisis than to treat it.

Short-term prophylactic use of corticosteroids has no significant ill-effects and it is safer to err on the side of giving too much rather than too little for this dangerous condition.

A general guide to the management of patients under long-term corticosteroid treatment is as follows:

1. Major oral surgery must be carried out in hospital.

2. Minor operations including extractions should preferably be carried out under local anaesthesia, but intravenous hydrocortisone should be given prophylactically.

3. If even a brief general anaesthetic is unavoidable, then a corticosteroid must be given prophylactically. At least 100 mg of hydrocortisone succinate should be given intravenously just before the operation and the patient's condition carefully watched throughout. If there is any sign of a falling blood pressure, immediate hydrocortisone supplementation (100–500 mg intravenously) must be given.

4. For extractions under local anaesthesia 100 mg of hydrocortisone should be given intravenously and repeated if there is the least doubt as to the patient's condition.

5. Patients should be kept under observation for at least an hour after the operation. If the blood pressure starts to fall at least 200 mg of hydrocortisone should be given intravenously and the patient transferred to hospital.

6. Restorative dentistry under local anaesthesia is probably not dangerous. There is probably no need for corticosteroid supplementation but, on the other hand, there should be no hesitation in giving large amounts intravenously if circulatory collapse seems imminent.

The suggestion of doubling the patient's normal dose of corticosteroid the day before and on the day of treatment is probably ineffective, as relatively enormous doses (hundreds of milligrams) are needed to prevent or manage circulatory collapse.

Steroid antagonists

A few drugs block steroid synthesis. The main example is *metapyrone*, which controls the symptoms of and is used for the preoperative management of Cushing's disease. *Aminoglutethimide* inhibits steroid production in the adrenals and also blocks conversion of androgens to oestrogens in the tissues. It is used as a hormone antagonist in the treatment of breast cancer.

PARATHYROID HORMONE AND CALCITONIN

The control of body calcium

Calcium plays several essential roles in the body. These include formation and maintenance of the skeleton, the control of secretory processes and the functioning of excitable tissues such as nerve and muscle. Calcium in trace quantities is also essential for blood clotting and various other enzymic reactions. The amounts needed for these latter processes are, however, so small that they are not affected by the blood calcium level. If the blood calcium level fell sufficiently low, death due to cardiac arrhythmia would come long before clotting or other enzymic processes were impaired.

The concentration of calcium in the plasma and other body fluids is dependent on:

1. The amount of calcium absorbed from the intestine
2. The amount of calcium excreted in the urine
3. The equilibrium between mobilisation from, and deposition of calcium into bone.

The skeleton forms the main bulk of calcium salts in the body and acts as their reservoir.

Several factors influence these basic processes. These include vitamin D, parathyroid hormone and calcitonin (Fig. 10.3).

Vitamin D

Vitamin D exists in several forms. The natural fat-soluble vitamin is *cholecalciferol* (vitamin D_3). *Calciferol* (vitamin D_2) is a semisynthetic product which is used therapeutically. When ultraviolet light acts on the skin it converts an inactive precursor, *7-dehydrocholesterol*, into vitamin D_3.

Vitamin D_3 is absorbed from the gut. Cholecalciferol is then converted by the liver and kidney into a metabolite (*1,25–dihydroxycholecalciferol*) which enhances intestinal absorption of calcium and promotes calcification of skeletal tissue. There is a minor effect on the kidney enhancing calcium reabsorption. Thus, the active vitamin enhances calcium absorption from dietary sources by potentiating intestinal transport of the

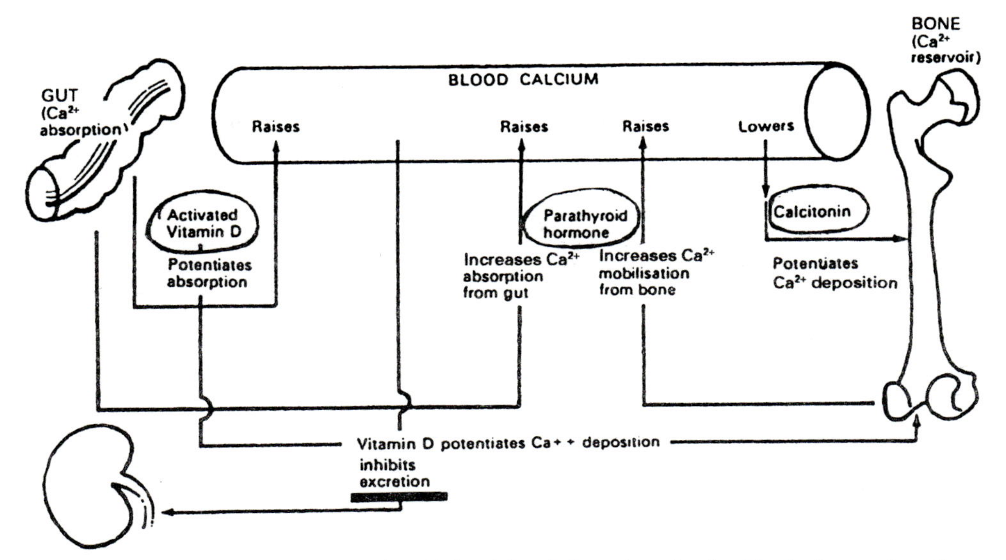

Fig. 10.3 Diagram indicating the way in which calcium balance is maintained by the interaction of three main agents (vitamin D, parathyroid hormone and calcitonin) on calcium absorption and deposition or resorption from bone.

ion. Calcium and phosphate enter the kidney in the glomerular filtrate. Vitamin D increases re-absorption of renal tubular calcium into the circulation and decreases the reabsorption of phosphate (Fig. 10.4).

If there is relative or absolute lack of vitamin D there is failure of calcification of the organic matrix of replacement bone. In adults, this results in osteomalacia, in which the bones are greatly weakened. In children, vitamin D deficiency causes rickets. The mechanism of the disease process is similar but in developing bones, rickets causes disorganisation of the zone of provisional calcification of the epiphyseal cartilage

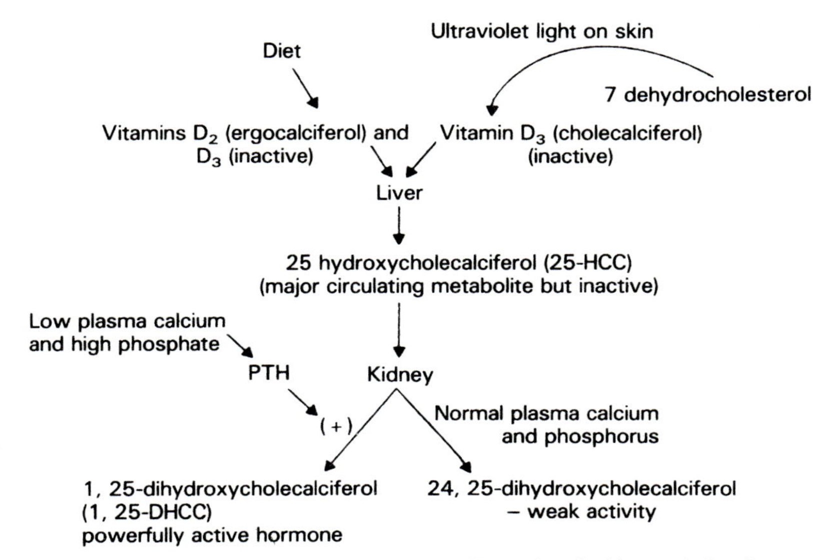

Fig. 10.4 Metabolic activation of vitamin D. (Reproduced with permission from *Aids to Pharmacology*.)

and the epiphyseal plates become thickened, wide and uneven.

Malabsorption syndromes are also potential causes of vitamin D deficiency, while chronic renal disease (either genetic or inflammatory) can also cause excessive bone mineral loss. The latter condition, known as renal rickets, is relatively resistant to vitamin D.

An important consequence of vitamin D deficiency is hypocalcaemia which may be severe enough to result in tetany or convulsions.

Parathormone

The parathyroid gland secretes the peptide hormone, parathormone (PTH). A fall in blood calcium triggers release of PTH, while a raised blood calcium inhibits its release.

PTH acts on bone, intestine and excretory mechanisms. PTH mobilises calcium from bone and thus raises plasma calcium at the expense of bone calcium. This is its most important action. Overactivity of the parathyroid glands due to hyperplasia or a PTH-producing tumour causes bone resorption, osteoclastic activity and disappearance of bone matrix. Advanced disease is characterised by so-called *osteitis fibrosa cystica*, but this is now rare.

Osteitis fibrosa cystica consists of areas of bone destruction which resemble cysts in radiographs, but are solid aggregations of soft tissue consisting mainly of osteoclasts.

PTH potentiates the action of vitamin D by mediating absorption of calcium by the intestine. PTH decreases excretion of calcium into the urine, faeces, sweat and milk.

Hypofunction of the parathyroid causes a lowering of blood calcium, which may lead to tetany.

Calcitonin

As noted earlier, calcitonin is secreted by the thyroid gland, but its physiological function is not understood. Calcitonin given as a drug depresses blood calcium levels, and its actions are, in general, opposite to those of PTH. Osteoclastic bone resorption is slowed and injection of calcitonin causes an immediate fall in blood calcium. It acts principally by increasing uptake of calcium by bones. However, overproduction of calcitonin by a thyroid tumour does not have this effect.

Clinical applications of calcitonin. Porcine and synthetic salmon calcitonin (*salcatonin*) are available. Prolonged use of porcine calcitonin can provoke production of neutralising antibodies. Salcatonin is less immunogenic.

The main uses of calcitonin are for treatment of hypercalcaemia and severe Paget's disease. In the latter it relieves pain and some of the neurological complications such as deafness.

Hypercalcaemia. Causes include immobilisation, vitamin D intoxication, sarcoidosis, multiple myeloma, malignancy of bone and some other cancers, and hyperparathyroidism. Calcitonin acts rapidly and can reverse severe hypercalcaemia which might otherwise be fatal due to renal failure or cardiac arrhythmias.

Paget's disease

Paget's disease is characterised by anarchic bone deposition and resorption causing the bones to become much thickened but weaker. In the early stages especially, osteoclastic activity predominates and may cause hypercalcaemia and severe bone pain. Both can be corrected by calcitonin but there is usually antibody production after a time.

For long-term treatment, bisphosphonates such as *disodium etidronate* are used. Disodium etidronate is absorbed onto hydroxyapatite crystals and slows both their rate of growth and resorption. This slows the high rate of bone turnover typical of Paget's disease and etidronate is currently the treatment of choice since it can be given in repeated courses without diminished activity.

The main factors controlling blood calcium are summarised in Table 10.7.

Table 10.7 Major factors affecting blood calcium levels

1. Dietary intake of vitamin D and calcium
2. Parathormone secretion. Raises blood calcium, mobilising calcium from bones and enhancing absorption by potentiating the action of vitamin D
3. Injected calcitonin opposes the action of parathormone and lowers blood calcium mainly by increasing deposition of calcium in the bones
4. Absorption of calcium may be depressed in intestinal diseases causing malabsorption as in steatorrhoea
5. Excretion of calcium is enhanced in some chronic renal diseases
6. Demands for calcium rise during pregnancy and lactation and may not be balanced by intake
7. Ionisable calcium is depressed when there is alkalosis (overbreathing with loss of CO_2 or vomiting with loss of gastric acid) and can lead to tetany

11. Nutrition: vitamins

Vitamins catalyse metabolic processes and are essential for normal health. Vitamins (apart from synthesis of vitamin K in the gut) are supplied by a conventional diet and, despite widespread belief to the contrary, vitamin supplementation is rarely needed. Those who habitually take vitamin tablets benefit the multimillion pound 'health food' industry, rather than themselves. However, there is suggestive evidence that some vitamins in higher doses than needed to prevent deficiencies may lessen the risk from diseases such as myocardial infarction or cancer.

Vitamin deficiencies result from:

1. Malnutrition
2. Abnormal diets
3. Malabsorption diseases.

Vitamin deficiencies produce well-defined diseases, but it is very rare for deficiency of a single vitamin to develop. Vitamin deficiencies are usually multiple and associated with general malnutrition. As a consequence, vitamin deficiencies are seen in Britain and the rest of the Western world only in particular groups of people. These include food faddists (vegans, those who eat a pure vegetable diet with no meat or dairy products of any sort) and chronic alcoholics. In the past, scurvy developed among the crews of sailing ships who, on journeys lasting many months, were completely deprived of fruit or green vegetables. Some vitamin deficiencies are due to failure of absorption rather than dietary deficiencies. The main examples are vitamins B_{12} and K deficiencies which affect blood formation (Ch. 7).

Fat-soluble vitamins (A, D, E and K)

Vitamin A

Vitamin A (retinol) is present in fish, milk, egg yolk and liver. Its precursor or provitamin (β carotene) is present in carrots and green vegetables. Vitamin A is essential for formation of retinal pigment (visual purple). Deficiency of vitamin A leads to impaired vision in poor light (night-blindness). Severe vitamin A deficiency is one of the most common causes of blindness in developing countries by causing corneal softening, infection and scarring.

Vitamin A also affects the behaviour of epithelium; deficiency causes glandular epithelium to undergo squamous metaplasia, while squamous epithelium tends to become hyperkeratinised. Analogues of vitamin A (retinoids) such as etretinate are available for treatment of severe congenital disorders of keratinisation and intractable psoriasis. Adverse effects are frequent and most patients develop dryness and cracking of the lips and many develop a dry mouth or nose. Etretinate is also teratogenic. Isotretinoin is another retinoid used in dermatology for severe acne. As well as being teratogenic, oral isotretinoin can cause hyperostosis, corneal opacities and premature fusion of the epiphyses.

The suggestion that vitamin A may possibly have a protective action against tumour formation is currently under investigation. Low dose β carotene and isotretinoin have been reported to lessen the risk of malignant change in oral leukoplakia. There is also some evidence that men with cancer of the head and neck region have a lower than average vitamin A intake. In marginally malnourished children with no overt signs of vitamin deficiency, administration of vitamin A raises their resistance to infection such as the pulmonary complications of measles. β carotene and other antioxidants such as vitamin E and ascorbic acid may possibly have some protective effect against myocardial infarction. However, overindulgence in vitamin A can be toxic.

Toxic effects. Chronic hypervitaminosis A can cause dry itching skin, gingivitis, mouth fissures and muscle pains. Intracranial pressure may be raised. It may also be teratogenic so that pregnant women are warned to avoid eating liver (a rich source of vitamin A) and taking vitamin A supplements.

Vitamin D

The main source of vitamin D is in fish liver oils but small amounts are present in eggs and butter. In strong sunlight vitamin D is synthesised in the skin. In Britain margarine is fortified with vitamins A and D, but requirements are small except during periods of bone growth and pregnancy.

Deficiency of vitamin D in the growing child causes rickets. This was said to have disappeared from Britain but cases may still be seen, especially among immigrants, particularly in Scotland and the north of England where lack of sunlight, a high carbohydrate diet and possibly also the use of wholemeal flour, containing phytates which impair the absorption of calcium, appear to be contributory.

Another factor likely to contribute to rickets among those who use wholemeal flour is that the latter is the only form of flour to which calcium is not added as a legal requirement.*

There is no basis for the idea that dental caries is due to vitamin D deficiency and poor calcification of the teeth. Countries where malnutrition is rife show a lower incidence of dental caries than in the West where the diet is often excessive, particularly in respect of sugar. Giving vitamin D and calcium for the prevention or reduction of dental caries is valueless. There are also dangers associated with raising children's intake of vitamin D since they are likely to be having foods such as milk and cereals fortified with this vitamin. Some children are sensitive to the action of this potent drug and hypervitaminosis D causes hypercalcaemia and renal calcinosis.

The role of vitamin D in calcium homeostasis has been discussed in Chapter 10.

Vitamin K

Vitamin K is present in green leaves and fruit and also synthesised by gut microorganisms which probably provide the main source. True vitamin K deficiency is seen only in the newborn who lack a gut flora to synthesise vitamin K and are certainly not eating green vegetables. Otherwise, deficiency results from malabsorption due to such diseases as obstructive jaundice.

Vitamin K is a precursor of prothrombin, an essential clotting factor (Ch.7). Hypothrombinaemia caused by deficiency of vitamin K is treated by giving acetomenaphthone by injection. However, this is ineffective when there is severe liver disease since prothrombin cannot then be synthesised. Vitamin K is of no value as a non-specific haemostatic agent when there is no deficiency.

Vitamin E

Vitamin E, an antioxidant, was for a long time thought to be of no medical importance. However, in the USA in particular, vitamin E has been consumed on a considerable scale because of a pathetic and misplaced belief that, since it is necessary for normal reproductive activity of rats, it enhances sexual vigour in humans. The effect of vitamin E in humans is quite different, but it has been difficult to establish whether vitamin E deficiency can genuinely affect humans, largely because of the very long time it takes to deplete the normal body stores.

However, vitamin E deficiency can result from syndromes such as abetalipoproteinaemia where fat absorption is defective, and can lead to degenerative neurological disorders and retinal

*This is due to pressure from the health food lobby. Rickets may therefore be one of the benefits of an additive-free diet.

lesions in children. High doses of vitamin E can considerably improve neurological function in this condition, especially if treatment is started early, but even affected adults may benefit. This rare neurological disorder is the only known effect of vitamin E deficiency in humans, though in doses above normal dietary needs it is thought to give some protection against myocardial infarction.

Water-soluble vitamins (B group and C)

B group vitamins

Vitamin B_1 (thiamin, aneurin). The main sources are the husks of grain and peas, beans and eggs. Deficiency of thiamin causes the disease known as beriberi which is virtually only seen in the Far East, but a similar deficiency state may develop in chronic alcoholics. Polyneuritis, cardiac failure and mental disorder are the main features.

Vitamin B_2 (riboflavin). This is widely distributed in yeast products, meat, offal, milk and green vegetables. Riboflavin deficiency is exceedingly rare but causes cracking of the lips (cheilitis), stomatitis, a sore tongue with a pebbly surface, and dermatitis. As a consequence vitamin B (usually as a mixture of B vitamins) is often given for a sore tongue, but is unlikely to be effective since the causes are elsewhere.

Vitamin B_6 (pyridoxine). This is also widely distributed and the sources are similar to those of riboflavin. Pyridoxine acts as a coenzyme in many metabolic processes but it is uncertain whether pyridoxine deficiency is a definable disease in man and no clinical syndrome has so far been ascribed to it apart from peripheral neuropathy due to isoniazid treatment.

Nicotinamide. The main sources of nicotinamide are also meat, offal and whole grains. Severe deficiency of nicotinamide produces pellagra (literally 'rough skin') with glossitis, dermatitis, diarrhoea and dementia as its classical features. Pellagra is usually a multiple deficiency state associated with malnutrition and rarely, if ever, a pure nicotinamide deficiency.

Folic acid. Folic acid is necessary for normal blood formation (Ch. 7). It may also prevent neural tube defects (spina bifida) and mothers at risk are currently advised to raise their intake of this vitamin.

Ascorbic acid (vitamin C)

The main sources are fresh green vegetables and fresh fruit. The vitamin is easily oxidised and destroyed by cooking. If sources of vitamin C are cut off, deficiency takes several months to develop. Scurvy is exceedingly rare in Britain, though it is a possible hazard for the isolated elderly living on a restricted diet (tea and buns).

Vitamin C is concerned with collagen formation and deficiency also affects platelet function. Vitamin C deficiency (scurvy) is characterised by a rash, purpura and mental changes. Purpura may be severe and contributes to the production of spongy, swollen and bleeding gums which are seen in advanced disease. Vitamin C has no beneficial effect on common, plaque-related gingivitis.

There is an enhanced risk of gastric cancer in those who consume large amounts of salt-preserved foods such as salt cod and some oriental pickles. Vitamin C is thought to have a protective effect in such populations.

Lest it be thought that scurvy is of historical interest only, a 24-year-old engineer was reported in 1983 to have the disease in classical form including swollen, bleeding gums. He had lived largely on peanut butter sandwiches, recalled having eaten an apple 4 years previously but could not recall ever having eaten an orange.

It has been suggested that massive doses of ascorbic acid prevent or ameliorate the common cold. This is unproven and the effect, if any, is marginal.* Moreover, cessation of megadose intake of ascorbic acid can lead to rebound deficiency and scurvy.

*In one bizarre case, intravenous injection of no less than 80 g of ascorbic acid proved to be lethal. This really does seem to be carrying prevention too far.

12. The alimentary system

Indigestion (dyspepsia)

Indigestion is not a disease but a variety of symptoms such as a feeling of distension (flatulence), abdominal discomfort or pain, acid reflux (heartburn), intolerance of some foods, and nausea. These symptoms frequently have no organic cause, but can result from acid reflux into the oesophagus, peptic ulcer, cancer of the stomach and many other gastrointestinal diseases. Features strongly suggestive of functional dyspepsia are that the patient often has anxiety traits and, despite persistence of symptoms for long periods, remains well and does not lose weight. However, organic disease must be excluded before dyspepsia is treated symptomatically.

The treatment of functional indigestion is important because: (1) it is one of the most common complaints in medicine, (2) the cost of treatment runs into many millions of pounds annually, and (3) patients need to be reassured of the absence of serious organic disease.

Management of dyspepsia. Organic disease must first be excluded by appropriate investigation. Non-drug treatment includes reassurance, stopping smoking, reducing alcohol intake, and exclusion of provocative foods such as fried foods. The main drugs effective for dyspepsia are antacids and H_2 receptor antagonists (see below).

Antacids. The most satisfactory preparation of antacids for indigestion or peptic ulcer pain is the combination of aluminium glycinate or hydroxide and magnesium trisilicate or hydroxide. These are effective buffers but do not cause alkalosis, and are long-acting. The mildly constipating effect of aluminium compounds is also counteracted by the mildly purgative action of the magnesium hydroxide. Liquid mixtures are more effective than tablets – the latter are simply more convenient to carry around.

Hiatus hernia and gastro-oesophageal reflux. These conditions can be due to displacement of the oesophagogastric junction and part of the stomach into the thorax. Because the pinching action of the diaphragm has been lost, gastric contents repeatedly reflux into the oesophagus. This process causes heartburn and other symptoms. In many patients the oesophagogastric sphincter mechanism is incompetent without the junction being displaced. Thus there seems to be little relation between the physical changes and the symptoms, many of which are probably functional.

Frequent and regular administration of antacids suppresses symptoms by reducing the irritant action of gastric acid on the oesophageal mucosa. Local anaesthetics with antacids are sometimes used to diminish oesophageal pain. An alternative approach is to increase the viscosity and solidity of the gastric contents in order to reduce reflux. Alginic acid is used in this way.

Metoclopramide increases the tone of the oesophagogastric sphincter and the magnitude of peristaltic waves down the oesophagus. Further benefit in hiatus hernia is provided by the action of the drug in hastening gastric emptying through the pylorus. Metoclopramide is often also used as an antiemetic. *Cimetidine* and *ranitidine* (see below) are frequently effective in relieving the symptoms of gastro-oesophageal reflux, but *omeprazole*, a *proton pump inhibitor*, suppresses gastric acid production and is the most effective drug for otherwise intractable reflux oesophagitis.

Achalasia. This disorder of oesophageal motility is due to deficiency in the autonomic nerve supply and causes difficulty in swallowing. Amyl nitrite helps the condition by relaxing the oesophagogastric sphincter. Parasympathomimetic drugs such as methacholine may also help.

Antiemetic drugs

Several drugs antagonise the vomiting response. These may act on the vomiting centre in the brain or on its nervous connections (Fig. 12.1). Alternatively, drugs may have a direct action on the alimentary tract.

1. *Hyoscine* and most of the antihistamines (such as *cyclizine* and *diphenhydramine*) have a central antiemetic action and are useful for preventing motion sickness and vomiting associated with vertigo. They act on muscarinic receptors in the vomiting centre and histamine (H_1) receptors in the vestibular nuclei.

2. *Chlorpromazine* and *trifluoperazine* are antipsychotic drugs but are also powerfully antiemetic. They are not effective against travel sickness, but are active against vomiting due to toxic and metabolic causes. They act by inhibiting dopamine receptors in the chemoreceptor trigger zone in the brain stem.

3. *Metoclopramide* has both peripheral and central antiemetic actions. It is not effective against travel sickness, but prevents vomiting due to many

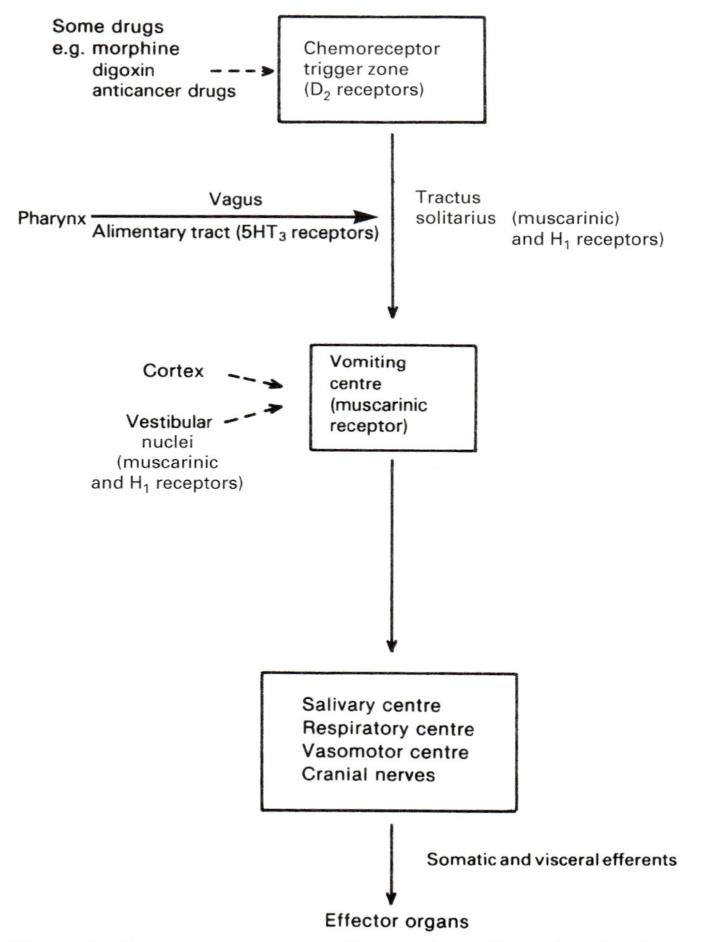

Fig. 12.1 Receptor centres controlling vomiting. (Reproduced with permission from *Aids to Pharmacology*.)

toxic and metabolic causes. Metoclopramide increases oesophageal and gastric motility. It also accelerates peristalsis in the small intestine. Like the phenothiazine drugs, metoclopramide has a central inhibitory action on the chemoreceptor trigger zone in the brain. This normally has a stimulatory effect on the vomiting centre when activated.

As mentioned earlier, the action of metoclopramide on the chemoreceptor trigger zone of the vomiting centre is because it is a dopamine receptor blocker. It can thus cause involuntary movements, particularly in young persons, and especially trismus.

4. *Domperidone* has a similar action to metoclopropamide but is less likely to cause the involuntary movement and muscular spasm that may result from metoclopropamide. However, domperidone also has a powerful inhibitory effect on the chemoreceptor trigger zone.

5. The specific 5-HT_3 antagonists, *ondansetron* and *granisetron* are potent antiemetics given for nausea following irradiation or cytotoxic drug treatment.

6. *Steroids*, such as dexamethasone, are useful antiemetics in anticancer treatment or terminal illness.

Vomiting or retching during dental procedures (such as impression taking) is mainly caused by anxiety and can often be prevented by sedation.

Gastric secretion and peptic ulceration

Acid and pepsin are secreted by the gastric mucosal cells. The parasympathetic nerve to the stomach is the vagus. When this is activated gastric secretion is increased. When food enters the stomach, gastrin is secreted and further stimulates acid production.

Cholecystokinin-pancreozymin and secretin, released by the small intestine, depress gastric acid production. Gastrin acts by stimulating histaminocytes which, by releasing histamine from the stomach wall, stimulates acid secretion (Fig. 12.2).

Peptic ulceration is a localised area of inflammation and loss of epithelium in the alimentary tract. A peptic ulcer will only form at a site where acid and pepsin come in contact with the mucosa. The most common sites are the lower end of the oesophagus, stomach and duodenum. The condition may present as pain or as a complication of the ulcer such as perforation or haemorrhage. The gastric mucosa is protected from acid and pepsin by the intrinsic resistance of its epithelium and by mucus (the mucosal barrier). The mediator of these protective mechanisms is gastric prostaglandin which acts physiologically to modulate gastric acid secretion, promote epithelial resistance and increase mucus secretion.

Inhibition of gastric prostaglandin production by non-steroidal anti-inflammatory drugs (NSAIDs) such as aspirin can thus cause or aggravate peptic ulceration. *Misoprostol*, a synthetic prostaglandin analogue, successfully antagonises the irritant effect of NSAIDs on the stomach.

The following are some of the medical approaches to the treatment of peptic ulceration:

1. *Bed rest* not only diminishes peptic ulcer symptoms, but accelerates healing. It is not known why this is so effective, but complete rest may lessen autonomic nervous stimulation of secretion.

2. *Stopping smoking* is also a surprisingly effective means of accelerating ulcer healing.

3. *H_2 receptor blocking drugs.* Histamine has several actions. H_1 effects include vasodilatation, increased capillary permeability and bronchoconstriction; H_2 effects are stimulation of acid and pepsin secretion by the stomach, contraction of the uterus and stimulation of the heart. H_2 blocking drugs therefore inhibit acid and pepsin secretion by the stomach and are very effective in accelerating the healing of peptic ulcers. *Cimetidine*, *ranitidine*, *famotidine* and *nizatidine* are H_2 blockers in current use.

Cimetidine rarely causes significant side-effects, but there may occasionally be confusion or dizziness in the elderly, and drugs such as oral anticoagulants, phenytoin and benzodiazepines may be potentiated by inhibition of their metabolism in the liver. Mild gynaecomastia and nephritis have also been reported. Ranitidine appears to be remarkably free from side-effects. However, they should not be given for indefinite periods. Courses of 1–2 months are preferable. Needless to say, it should also be established that a gastric ulcer is not malignant before starting treatment with these drugs.

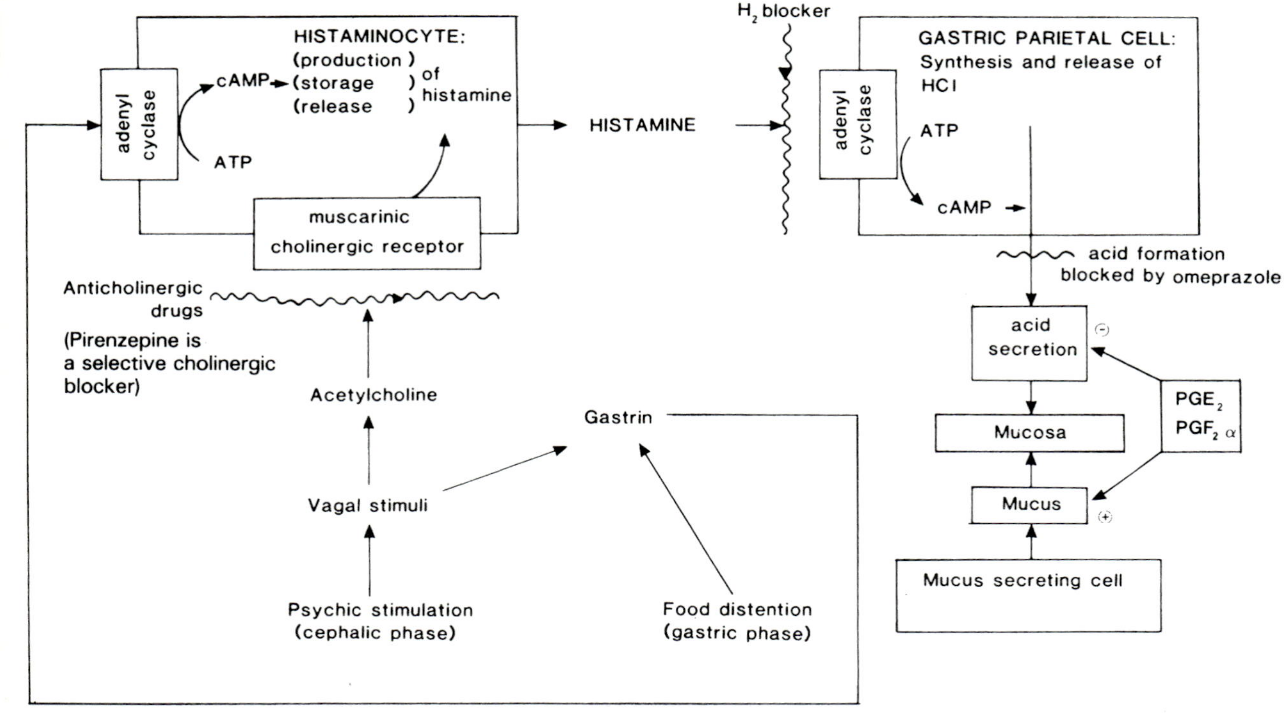

Fig. 12.2 Diagrammatic representation of the relationship between histaminocytes (enterochromaffin-like cells) and parietal cells in the gastric mucosa. (Reproduced with permission from *Aids to Pharmacology*.)

H_2 blockers are particularly effective in accelerating the healing of the majority of duodenal ulcers and are also valuable for reducing acid secretion in such conditions as severe reflux oesophagitis with ulceration or bleeding from erosive gastritis. Although these drugs are frequently highly effective in promoting the healing of peptic ulceration, the relapse rate after cessation of treatment is high.

4. *Omeprazole* induces complete and prolonged inhibition of acid secretion by blocking the proton pump (H^+/K^+-ATPase) system in the gastric parietal cells. It is used for the Zollinger–Ellison syndrome and when other antiulcer treatments have failed.

Drugs such as H_2 blockers and, particularly, omeprazole, which inhibit gastric acid production, may allow bacterial colonisation and excessive nitrosamine production. These substances are potentially carcinogenic and, although gastric cancer has not been shown to complicate treatment with H_2 blockers or omeprazole, these drugs should not be given for indefinite periods.

5. *Bismuth chelate.* Bismuth compounds are weak antacids. Nevertheless, tripotassium dicitratobismuthate rapidly heals duodenal ulcers. Although enhanced prostaglandin and depressed acid production may contribute, an important effect is its antibacterial action on *Helicobacter pylori*, an organism that is associated with peptic ulceration. Antibiotics such as amoxycillin or metronidazole given with bismuth compounds accelerate the healing of peptic ulcers.

6. *Antimuscarinic drugs.* Atropine and related drugs such as propantheline and poldine may help some forms of dyspepsia, but rarely benefit patients with peptic ulcer. By contrast, the selective M_1 antimuscarinic drug *pirenzepine* selectively blocks gastric muscarinic receptors which drive acid secretion and accelerates the healing of peptic ulcers.

7. *Sucralfate* is a salt of sucrose sulphate. It binds to the ulcer crater and exerts a local antacid and antipepsin action. It is as effective as H_2 blockers in promoting the healing of peptic ulcers.

8. *Antacids* such as sodium bicarbonate and

aluminium hydroxide reduce gastric acidity and thus diminish the activity of gastric pepsin. Although antacids may relieve the pain of peptic ulceration, they do not accelerate healing unless large doses are given frequently for an impractically long period. In general, antacids are not toxic, but excessive consumption can lead to side-effects. Large doses of sodium bicarbonate produce alkalosis, whilst calcium carbonate in excess can induce hypercalcaemia. Magnesium and aluminium compounds are therefore preferred.

Small frequent meals have antacid properties, due to the repeated exposure of the gastric contents to the amphoteric groups in dietary protein.

9. *Carbenoxolone sodium* is a derivative of liquorice root. It prolongs gastric epithelial cell life-span and increases mucus secretion, but water retention, hypertension, cardiac failure and pulmonary oedema can complicate treatment. Carbenoxolone accelerates the heating of gastric ulcers, but has largely been replaced by H_2 blockers or omeprazole.

10. *Metoclopramide* reduces peptic ulcer symptoms, but does not affect healing.

11. *Prostaglandins*, such as *misoprostol*, a synthetic analogue of PGE_1, accelerate the healing of peptic ulcers. As mentioned earlier they act physiologically to modulate acid secretion, promote epithelial resistance and increase mucus production. By contrast, NSAIDs aggravate peptic ulceration because they inhibit prostaglandin synthesis.

Drugs used to control diarrhoea

Mild infections should not be treated with antibiotics, but symptomatic relief may be provided by drugs that decrease intestinal motility or reduce the fluid content of the stools. In more severe diarrhoea the first line of treatment is to replace water and electrolytes.

1. Drugs which reduce peristalsis include atropine, *diphenoxylate* and *mebeverine*. Morphine and codeine reduce propulsive gut activity by inducing static spasm of the smooth muscle of the intestinal wall.

2. Greater viscosity of the gut contents may be achieved by agar, kaolin, methyl cellulose or bran.

3. Infective diarrhoea, the bugbear of tourists to hot countries, is caused by strains of *Escherichia coli*, *Salmonella*, *Campylobacter*, *Clostridia*, *Shigella* and *Staphylococcus aureus* as well as protozoa and viruses. Many of these organisms produce enterotoxins which accelerate transport of water and salt through the bowel wall to cause rapid distension of the gut. Some strains of *E. coli* and some other bacteria also invade the intestinal mucosa.

The main measure is to repair fluid loss. Drugs which reduce intestinal mobility are contraindicated. Severe bacterial diarrhoea should be treated by giving *trimethoprim* or *ciprofloxacin*. Erythromycin or ciprofloxacin are given for *Campylobacter* infection, a common cause of diarrhoea.

Other treatments for diarrhoea due to specific illnesses include steroids and sulphasalazine for ulcerative colitis and Crohn's disease.

Enteric fever (typhoid and paratyphoid)

Enteric fever is a rare disease, is common in underdeveloped countries and occasional cases or minor epidemics from a variety of sources can break out elsewhere. It is one of the few important infections where chloramphenicol may need to be given, but ciprofloxacin is an alternative.

Purgatives

The use of purgatives has diminished greatly over the years because of changed beliefs about the causes and consequences of constipation. At the same time the hazards of the regular use of laxatives have become known. Laxatives comprise four main groups:

1. Bulking agents
2. Faecal softeners
3. Stimulant laxatives
4. Osmotic laxatives.

Bulk purgatives. These promote peristalsis by increasing the volume of the intestinal contents. This induces reflex stimulation of the intestinal musculature. Bran, agar and methyl cellulose act in this way.

Guar gum is another fibrous product which produces a bulky gel when mixed with water.

This not only shortens intestinal transit time, but reduces the absorption of glucose and lipids from the intestine. It may thus help in the management of diabetic patients as well as acting as a purgative.

Faecal softeners. These mainly act in the last few feet of intestine and include liquid paraffin and *docusate sodium.* Liquid paraffin is not recommended because it can cause lipid pneumonia, paraffin granulomas in the abdominal lymph nodes and pruritus ani.

Stimulant laxatives. These stimulate activity of the gut wall. Senna contains an anthroquinone (emodin) which acts in this way. *Bisacodyl* is another irritant purgative which undergoes enterohepatic recirculation. *Docusate* acts as a stimulant as well as a faecal softener.

Osmotic laxatives. These act by retaining in the intestine, water which by its bulk effect stimulates peristalsis. *Magnesium sulphate* is used when a rapid bowel evacuation is needed. *Lactulose* is a non-absorbed carbohydrate which acidifies the contents of the intestine and causes an osmotic diarrhoea. Lactulose is used in the treatment of hepatic encephalopathy, a serious complication of liver failure in which nitrogen-containing compounds are absorbed and cause neurological disorders and coma. Commonly used drugs which can cause liver failure are overdose of paracetamol and aspirin in children if it precipitates Reye's syndrome.

13. Toxic effects of drugs

Drugs are usually given for a single therapeutic purpose, but no drug has a single action. The undesired actions of drugs are called toxic effects or side-effects, whether or not they have a substantially harmful effect on the patient. Iatrogenic disease is a somewhat pretentious name for disease caused by drugs or any other kind of medical treatment. It is supposed to mean 'disease produced by doctors', but 'disease which produces doctors' is probably a more correct literal translation.

Toxic effects of drugs fall into the following categories:

1. Dose-independent actions
2. Dose-dependent effects
3. Drug interactions
4. Idiosyncrasy.

Dose-independent toxic actions of drugs

Dose-independent reactions are mainly allergic. There is frequently no way of predicting whether a patient is going to develop such a reaction. The first exposure to a drug may have no adverse effects, but subsequent exposures cause allergic responses. A previous history of asthma, infantile eczema, hay fever or urticaria usually indicates a greater risk of drug allergy.

Allergy to drugs ranges from mild local itching to fatal anaphylactic shock. In general, the shorter the interval between drug administration and the onset of clinical signs of allergy, the more serious the reaction. A general guide is that reactions which begin within half an hour may be life-threatening, while those which start on the following day are usually relatively mild.

Anaphylaxis is a dangerous early allergic response and may lead to fatal cardiovascular collapse and bronchospasm or laryngeal oedema. A serious reaction of this sort can follow an injection or, rarely, oral administration of penicillin in susceptible persons. Drug treatment of this complication may be life-saving. Intramuscular adrenaline and intravenous chlorpheniramine (Ch. 19) reduce oedema of the respiratory passages, relax bronchiolar smooth muscle and raise the blood pressure.

Urticaria, a generalised acute allergic reaction affecting the skin, consists of widespread areas of redness, itching and swelling. It can follow administration of a specific allergen. Local application of a cooling lotion such as calamine may relieve the irritation. Itching and swelling may also be lessened by giving an antihistamine such as chlorpheniramine by mouth. Antihistamines should not be applied to the skin because they themselves can cause sensitisation.

Local allergy (contact dermatitis) can be caused by a wide range of drugs. Repeated handling of antibiotics such as streptomycin, for example, can cause contact dermatitis. Similarly, an area of itching and swelling may appear over the site of repeated insulin injections.

Specific allergic sensitisation is frequently a result of skin medication, particularly the use of creams containing antihistamines, antibiotics or local anaesthetics. Once an eczematous reaction has been induced it is important to avoid contact with the sensitising drug even after the lesion has healed.

It is highly questionable whether contact allergy can affect the oral mucosa. Authenticated examples are so rare as to defy credence.

Delayed reactions

Allergic reactions do not always quickly follow the first administration of the drug. Toxic effects with an immunological basis can develop suddenly after prolonged exposure to a drug. A delayed reaction of this sort to penicillin may take the form of arthritis and fever (serum sickness reaction). Similarly, a delayed reaction to the antituberculous drug isoniazid can cause fever.

Immune responses to some drugs (such as the hypotensive agent hydralazine) can cause an illness similar to acute disseminated lupus erythematosus. The effects include fever, raised erythrocyte sedimentation rate, arthritis, pleural effusion, rashes and, rarely, kidney damage.

The antimalarial and antirheumatic drug chloroquine can have a toxic effect on the retina months after first exposure.

Dose-dependent effects of drugs

These may either be exaggerations of their therapeutic actions or side-effects unrelated to the therapeutic action.

Cytotoxic drugs such as methotrexate, cyclophosphamide and 6-mercaptopurine act as anticancer drugs or immunosuppressive agents by inhibiting division of tumour and immunologically active cells. However, normal body tissues that undergo continuous cell division are also damaged. Thus, large doses of this kind of drug will inevitably lead to marrow suppression (anaemia, leucopenia and thrombocytopenia), inhibition of gonadal activity (temporary or permanent sterility), intestinal effects (haemorrhage and diarrhoea) and suppression of hair follicle activity (baldness).

An example of dose-dependent toxic effects which are not part of the therapeutic action of a drug are the side-effects of the cardiac glycosides. Digoxin (used for treatment of heart failure or rapid supraventricular arrhythmias), can cause loss of appetite, nausea, vomiting, and (in the elderly) mental changes such as confusion and excitement if given in large doses.

Drug interactions

The main types of drug interaction are:

1. Interactions outside the body
2. Chemical interactions in the intestine
3. Pharmacological interactions
   a. Potentiation
   b. Antagonism
   c. Enzyme induction
   d. Enzyme inhibition
   e. Drug binding to plasma proteins.

Interactions outside the body. Mixing the bronchodilator drug theophylline with a wide range of other substances (including some antibiotics and antihistamines) produces precipitation in vitro. Such mixtures should not be injected.

Chemical interactions in the intestine. An example is the binding of calcium or iron salts to tetracycline if given at the same time. Absorption of both is prevented as a consequence.

Potentiation. Cerebral depressants such as the barbiturates, antihistamines or benzodiazepines have an additive effect on each other if more than one is given. Ethyl alcohol has the same effect, and when given in addition to hypnotics can lead to dangerous respiratory depression.

Antagonism. An example of a drug terminating the therapeutic action of another drug is the abolition of the hypotensive effect of guanethidine or clonidine (both largely obsolete) by the simultaneous administration of the tricyclic antidepressives imipramine or amitriptyline.

Enzyme induction. Some drugs enhance the ability of the body to metabolise drugs. This process of enzyme enhancement is termed *induction.* The antiepileptics, phenytoin and carbamazepine are inducers of drug metabolising enzymes. One consequence is that some other drugs are metabolised rapidly and their actions are weaker and briefer. Examples of drugs which are less effective if given after an inducing agent include:

1. Coumarin anticoagulants
2. Oral contraceptives, androgens and oestrogens
3. Hydrocortisone and synthetic glucocorticoids
4. Tricyclic antidepressants
5. Phenothiazine antipsychotics
6. Vitamin D_3 and folic acid.

Thus, while a patient is taking carbamazepine, oral contraceptives may become less effective, and pregnancy has occasionally followed. By contrast, when treatment with the enzyme-inducing drug is stopped, metabolism of many drugs slows down and an anticoagulant (for example) could cause abnormal bleeding.

Prolonged phenytoin treatment causes relative deficiency of vitamin D_3 and this in turn can lead to osteomalacia. The antibiotic, rifampicin is also an inducing agent which can interfere with the activity of the contraceptive pill and warfarin.

Enzyme inhibition. The monoamine oxidase inhibitors (MAOIs) block the activity of several oxidase enzymes. When a patient is being treated with a MAOI, drugs normally removed by oxidation may have undesirably prolonged and intense actions. The most severe reactions are with pethidine – they usually lead to respiratory depression, hypotension and coma, and have occasionally been fatal.

Drug binding to plasma proteins. Many drugs travel in the blood partly in a free form and partly bound to plasma proteins – particularly albumin. The active form of the drug is free and unbound. A decline in the proportion of bound drug will therefore potentiate drug activity. Such a change may be caused by drugs competing for binding to plasma proteins. An example is the administration of amiodarone to a patient who is being maintained on an anticoagulant dose of warfarin. Amiodarone binds preferentially to the plasma albumin and displaces the warfarin from the protein binding sites. Thus the concentration of unbound (active) warfarin rises, with a parallel increase in its anticoagulant action. The overall result is that amiodarone given to a patient maintained on warfarin may lead to haemorrhage, unless the dose of warfarin is correspondingly lowered.

Patients with a low plasma albumin level bind drugs to an abnormally small extent – a larger amount remains unbound and therefore in the active form. Thus patients with hypoalbuminaemia show greater steroid toxic effects when given prednisolone.

Idiosyncrasy

This term, which has been argued about for generations, means no more than its common usage suggests, i.e. behaviour peculiar to an individual. In pharmacological terms, it means an unusual and unexplained type of adverse reaction to a drug. It is to be hoped that with growing knowledge of factors affecting drug metabolism, disposition and excretion, the term will disappear.

Susceptibility to adverse reactions

Some patients appear to be particularly prone to toxic reactions due to certain drugs. This may be due to:

1. Genetic predisposition
2. An acquired characteristic or disease.

Genetic factors. These can change the effectiveness of drugs in either direction. The antituberculous drug isoniazid is metabolised, and consequently inactivated, by acetylation. About one-third of the population possess the capacity to metabolise isoniazid rapidly. These individuals are known as 'rapid acetylators', and in such cases standard doses of isoniazid, for example, will not maintain adequate antituberculous blood concentrations of the drug. On the other hand, they may be less prone to develop the toxic effects of isoniazid, even with high doses.

Suxamethonium is a short-acting muscle relaxant. Its effect usually lasts about 4 min since the action of the drug is terminated by the hydrolytic action of the plasma enzyme pseudocholinesterase. About 1 in 4000 of the population lack normal plasma pseudocholinesterase. These people appear normal in every other respect but, if given suxamethonium, may remain paralysed for many hours and need artificial respiration.

Patients who suffer from inherited deficiency of the red cell enzyme glucose-6-phosphate dehydrogenase can develop acute haemolytic anaemia when given drugs such as the antimalarial pamaquine and the antibacterial nitrofurantoin, or in some cases aspirin. The enzyme deficiency may otherwise produce no clinical effects apart from a greater susceptibility to haemolytic jaundice.

Acquired factors. These can change drug responses in many ways and drug interactions form one type of example. For example, previous treatment with barbiturates results in enhanced metabolism and, therefore, a weaker effect of tricyclic antidepressants and phenothiazine antipsychotics. By contrast, patients who are treated with monoamine oxidase inhibitors have excessive sensitivity to the sedative actions of opioids.

Diseases may also change drug responses. Two important examples are liver and kidney disorders.

1. *Liver disorders.* Patients with liver disease can suffer delays in drug detoxification, abnormal brain sensitivity and coagulation defects.

Morphine and other opioids, tricyclic antidepressants and hypnotics may have excessive effects because detoxification by the liver is delayed. The response to cerebral depressants in general is also exaggerated because of abnormalities in brain function which accompany liver failure.

The liver is the main site of synthesis of the plasma clotting factors. In hepatocellular disease factors V, IX and X and prothrombin are deficient, so that even small doses of anticoagulants can lead to uncontrollable haemorrhage.

2. *Kidney disorders.* In renal failure, drugs which are principally excreted by the kidneys can accumulate in the body and reach toxic levels. Thus, concentrations of penicillin can rise so high as to cause neurological damage. Streptomycin, kanamycin, neomycin and gentamicin also have to be administered less frequently (every 24–48 h instead of twice daily), otherwise deafness may develop due to VIIIth nerve damage.

Similarly, digoxin and chlorpropamide, which are mainly excreted by the kidneys, must be given in smaller doses (or alternative drugs found) in the presence of renal failure.

Effects on fetal development (teratogenic effects)

Unlike the toxic effects described above, some drugs affect the development of the fetus and do not necessarily have any adverse action on the mother. The most striking example is the thalidomide tragedy which resulted in the birth of many hundreds of children with appalling abnormalities, of which the absence of limbs was the most obvious. By contrast, thalidomide appears to be relatively safe for adults and is used, for example, by specialists for disablingly severe major oral ulcers and leprosy.

A few other drugs, notably antitumour agents and the vitamin A derivatives such as isotretinoin, have been shown clinically to be teratogenic. Tretinion or isotretinoin should not be taken by pregnant women, but despite the warnings it has been estimated that in the USA several hundred babies with congenital deformities have been born to mothers who have been taking this drug for skin disease.

In contrast to the few drugs with proven teratogenic effects on humans, virtually any drug can have this effect experimentally if given in a suitable dose at a critical stage in fetal development to some animal. Different species in fact differ widely in their vulnerability to teratogenic effects from particular drugs. This has made the testing of drugs for teratogenicity (a requirement for the acceptance of any drug for licensing) particularly difficult.

Under these circumstances, even though few drugs have been proven to be teratogenic in humans, no drugs should be given to a woman during the first 3 months of pregnancy unless it is essential to do so. Tetracycline has a limited teratogenic effect on the teeth and skeleton since it is incorporated in calcifying tissues. When the teeth are stained in this way, the effect is permanent and can be disfiguring. Tetracyclines should not be given during the final trimester of pregnancy or until after the 12th year of childhood (Ch. 15), as there are many suitable alternatives.

ADVERSE REACTIONS IN DENTISTRY

These may affect the patient in the following ways:

1. Adverse reactions to drugs given or prescribed for dental purposes
2. Drugs affecting the response to dental operations
3. Interactions between different drugs given for medical and dental purposes
4. Oral reactions to drugs.

Although there is natural concern about adverse reactions to drugs, it is important to appreciate that the disease for which the drug is given may be a more serious source of anxiety. This is particularly important in the case of drugs used to treat heart disease, particularly ischaemic heart disease and hypertension.

Adverse reactions to drugs given for dental purposes

These are rare but usually acute reactions and a cause of emergencies in the dental surgery. Examples are:

1. *Acute anaphylactic shock* following injection of a penicillin
2. *Acute porphyria* (very rarely) after injection of a barbiturate such as methohexitone
3. *Respiratory depression* and sometimes death during anaesthesia, particularly with methohexitone
4. *Acute hypertension* and, occasionally, death from use of high concentrations (1:20 000) of noradrenaline in local anaesthetic solutions.

Adverse reactions to drugs *prescribed* for dental purposes develop after the patient has left the surgery, but are rarely severe. In either case, the dental surgeon will be responsible if he or she has not taken an adequate history. Examples are rashes or other reactions to an oral penicillin, or gastric bleeding due to aspirin.

Drugs which affect the response to dental surgery

Dentistry is, for most people, stressful because of anxiety, pain and, sometimes, loss of blood. Fit patients can usually withstand such stress but drug treatment may affect their resistance in such ways as follows:

1. *Circulatory collapse* (acute hypoadrenal shock) can follow dental surgery, especially under general anaesthesia in a patient receiving systemic corticosteroid therapy
2. *Prolonged bleeding* may occasionally be the result of the patient being on anticoagulant therapy.

Interactions between different drugs given for medical and dental purposes

As discussed earlier (Ch. 3) there is no evidence of clinical interactions between the adrenaline or noradrenaline in dental local anaesthetics and antidepressants, either MAOIs or tricyclics. This is a myth that has arisen as a result of misunderstanding a single series of experiments.

Severe, sometimes fatal interactions can, however, follow the administration of pethidine to a patient concurrently taking MAOI antidepressants. The latter also interact with other opioids with coma as the usual result.

Aspirin can, by its antiplatelet effect, indirectly enhance the effects of anticoagulants. In such patients aspirin, by its action on the gastric mucosa, can also induce dangerous gastric bleeding.

Although a course of amoxycillin can affect the absorption of oestrogens in oral contraceptives, a single dose (as given for prophylaxis of infective endocarditis) probably will not interfere with the action of an oral contraceptive.

Oral reactions to drugs

In relation to the vast range of drugs taken by the population at large, significant oral reactions are uncommon. These reactions are nevertheless important in that patients rarely suspect that the oral symptoms are related to their medical treatment, especially as there is often a long delay between the start of drug therapy and the onset of the reaction. The alert dental surgeon who suspects that an unusual form of stomatitis might be a drug reaction can play an important part in drawing attention to the reaction and, in some cases, be able to prevent the development of more severe or widespread toxic effects.

Oral reactions to drugs are varied in character and, though it is probable that immunological mechanisms often play a part, are frequently of unknown pathogenesis. However, the oral mucosa appears unable to produce any counterpart to the common contact dermatitis or eczematous reactions of the skin. If a patient is sensitive to (say) nickel, a nickel-containing alloy put in the mouth will, if it provokes any reaction at all, produce the characteristic rash on the skin.

When, as is often the case, the patient is taking several drugs it is likely to be difficult or impossible to be certain which of these is the source of trouble.

Oral reactions to drugs include the following:

Local reactions:
1. Chemical irritation
2. Supression of the normal oral flora.

Systemically determined reactions:
1. Depression of any aspect of marrow function (red cells, white cells or platelets)
2. Depression of the immune response
3. Stevens–Johnson syndrome (bullous erythema multiforme)
4. Lichen planus and lichenoid reactions
5. Miscellaneous.

Chemical irritation

The best-known example is an aspirin burn caused by a patient holding a tablet against the gingiva of an aching tooth. Necrosis of superficial epithelial cells produces a white patch.

Elderly and infirm people in hospital can suffer severe mucosal burns from tablets that they are unable to swallow and which stick to the oral mucosa. Such patients should not be expected to swallow tablets without help; they should be given water or milk, and care should be taken to see that the tablets have been swallowed, otherwise the medication may do harm and will certainly do no good.

Suppression of the oral flora

This can be a response to topical use of antibiotics such as tetracycline mouthrinses. After a few days, sufficient numbers of the normal oral bacteria are destroyed to allow the overgrowth of opportunistic organisms, particularly *Candida albicans* which causes acute antibiotic stomatitis, or widespread plaques of thrush.

Topical corticosteroids can also affect local immune responses and promote candidosis. Oropharyngeal thrush is a recognised complication of use of corticosteroid aerosols by asthmatic patients.

Depression of the bone marrow

The red cells. A few drugs can cause anaemia alone (Ch. 7), but this is rarely severe enough to cause glossitis.

Folic acid deficiency leading to macrocytic anaemia can develop in susceptible patients on prolonged treatment with phenytoin. This can occasionally cause aphthous stomatitis which responds rapidly when folic acid is given.

Folic acid deficiency can also follow prolonged treatment with cotrimoxazole, but in fact rarely does so.

The white cells. The leucocytes can be selectively depressed (leucopenia) or with all other bone marrow cells (aplastic anaemia, pancytopenia). Severe neutropenia can progress to agranulocytosis characterised by necrotising bacterial infections especially of the mouth and throat. The mouth is particularly susceptible because of the persistent low-grade infection of the gingival margins and the presence of chronic gingivitis or periodontitis. If resistance is greatly impaired, this infection becomes acute, progressive and destructive.

A wide variety of drugs can have this effect, although it is uncommon. The most notorious are:

1. Antibacterials – chloramphenicol and sulphonamides
2. Analgesics – phenylbutazone and oxyphenbutazone
3. Antidiabetic (hypoglycaemic) agents and antithyroid agents
4. Cytotoxic agents.

Platelets. Purpura due to depression of platelet production may rarely be a selective effect. One of the few drugs causing this effect is apronal (Sedormid), an obsolete hypnotic, but a wide variety of other drugs have been reported to cause purpura on rare occasions.

Drug-induced purpura is more likely to be the result of general marrow aplasia and is frequently the first sign of aplastic anaemia due, for example, to chloramphenicol. In such cases bleeding from the gingival margins or submucosal blood blisters may be conspicuous.

Drugs causing marrow aplasia are essentially those which otherwise cause leucopenia.

Purpura may also result from vascular damage and can result from prolonged corticosteroid therapy, particularly in older patients in whom the vessel walls are already weakly supported.

Depression of immune responses

This may be the result of prolonged corticosteroid therapy for a variety of inflammatory diseases or more intensive immunosuppression for transplant surgery.

Typical effects are infective stomatitis due to viruses (usually herpes simplex) or fungi (*Candida albicans*) or both together as a result of depressed cell-mediated immunity. These infections can be severe in transplant patients, who are given high doses of steroids for long periods.

Stevens–Johnson syndrome (bullous erythema multiforme)

This acute mucocutaneous reaction mainly involves the mouth, eyes and skin. The drugs most often responsible are sulphonamides (particularly the long-acting types) and (rarely) phenobarbitone, but a wide variety of other drugs have been blamed on various occasions as have herpetic and other infections. It is often impossible (as with other types of reaction) to exclude coincidence, and in the majority of cases no precipitating cause can be identified.

The patients are usually young adult males and typical effects are widespread oral ulceration with swollen, cracked, bleeding and crusted lips. There is a rash, often conjunctivitis or more severe ocular inflammation, and other mucous membranes may be involved. The disease is very rarely fatal.

Lichen planus and lichenoid reactions

Lichen planus is a common chronic disease involving the skin and mouth in particular. It is usually without any apparent cause but may occasionally be drug induced.

Oral lichen planus is typically characterised by fine white lines (striae) extending over a variable area of the mucosa, and often ulceration (erosions) which sometimes dominate the picture. Many drugs are capable of causing clinically similar (lichenoid) reactions. They include the following:

1. Allopurinol
2. β blockers (rarely)
3. Captopril (rarely)
4. Chloroquine and other antimalarials
5. Chlorpropamide
6. Gold salts
7. Methyldopa
8. Non-steroidal anti-inflammatory agents, particularly phenylbutazone and indomethacin
9. Penicillamine.

Miscellaneous effects

Gingival hyperplasia. Fibrous overgrowth of the gingivae can complicate the use of a disparate series of drugs, namely:

1. Phenytoin
2. Cyclosporin
3. Nifedipine and other calcium channel blockers.

Phenytoin is the most common cause and like cyclosporin can also cause hypertrichosis. However, any mechanism that these different drugs have in common in order to give this effect is unknown.

Gingival pigmentation. Gingival pigmentation can result from treatment with, or exposure to, heavy metals, particularly mercury, bismuth and lead, but is now rarely seen. Excretion of these metals in gingival pockets leads to the deposition of black (mercury), brown (bismuth) or blue (lead) sulphide deposits. Among currently used drugs, the anticancer agent cisplatin is probably the only one which produces a blue or grey gingival line. Other drugs, notably the phenothiazines, can cause widespread mucosal pigmentation.

Dry mouth. Xerostomia is a side-effect of many drugs, particularly those with an antimuscarinic action. Antimuscarinics such as propantheline have been used to depress gastric acid secretion as an optimistic treatment of peptic ulceration. Tricyclic antidepressants have a strong antimuscarinic action and an unpleasantly dry mouth is often one of the first things a patient notices when starting antidepressant treatment. Antihistamines and antimuscarinic drugs, such as benzhexol used in the treatment of parkinsonism, also have this effect. Ganglion blockers such as mecamylamine (obsolete for the treatment of hypertension), and amphetamines and chemically-related appetite suppressants which are sympathomimetic also (as might be expected) depress salivary secretion. The main groups of drugs likely to cause xerostomia or to have other effects on the salivary glands are summarised in Table 13.1. It should be noted, however, that hypersalivation is not a clinical complaint with any validity, in that any excess of saliva can be swallowed unless some neuromuscular disorder interferes with this process.

Yellow cards

The Committees on Safety of Medicines and Dental and Surgical Materials provide yellow cards on which suspected adverse reactions can – and should – be reported. Dentists should appreciate that they can make a significant contribution to the recognition of the adverse effects of drugs and related substances by completing and sending in these cards.

Doubt as to whether any apparent reaction is no more than coincidental should not deter anyone from sending in a card. The medical assessors are well able to evaluate such problems.

Table 13.1 Drugs affecting the salivary glands

Drug-induced xerostomia

1. Drugs with antimuscarinic effects:
   a. Atropine, ipratropium, oxitropium hyoscine and analogues
   b. Orphenadrine, benzhexol and related antiparkinsonian agents
   c. Tricyclic antidepressants
   d. Antihistamines
   e. Antiemetics (including antihistamines, hyoscine and phenothiazines)
   f. Antipsychotics, particularly phenothiazines
   g. Some antihypertensives, especially ganglion blockers and clonidine (largely obsolete)
2. Drugs with sympathomimetic actions
   a. 'Cold cures' containing ephedrine or phenylpropanolamine
   b. Decongestants
   c. Bronchodilators
   d. Appetite suppressants, particularly amphetamines and diethylpropion

Drugs increasing salivation

Parasympathomimetics such as pilocarpine
Cholinesterase inhibitors (physostigmine, pyridostigmine, etc.)

Drug-associated salivary swelling

Phenylbutazone, iodine compounds, thiouracil, catecholamines, sulphonamides, chlorhexidine and others (uncommon reaction)

Avoidance of adverse reactions

Serious reactions from drugs in common use are rare and a clinician may not, for example, ever see an anaphylactic reaction to penicillin or acute hypotensive shock in a patient on withdrawal from corticosteroid treatment.

At the same time, some of these reactions are so severe that, difficult though it is, the clinician must always be prepared for the unexpected. The chances of a serious drug reaction are much reduced if these precautions are taken:

1. No drug should be given unless absolutely necessary and this is especially important during early pregnancy. Antibiotics and hypnotics in particular are grossly overprescribed.
2. If a drug has to be given, always ask if any other drugs are being taken and try to assess whether there is any danger of interaction.
3. Always ask if the patient has had any ill-effects from any drugs in the past and particularly to the drug that is to be given. This is especially important in relation to the many different penicillins, the names of which differ widely but which all share cross-sensitivity.
4. It is wise to ask if there is any history of allergy, as this may increase the likelihood of sensitisation or reaction to a drug.
5. Try, whenever possible, to use a familiar drug that has stood the test of time.
6. If an adverse reaction is seen, remember to report it on a yellow card when the crisis has been dealt with.

SECTION 2

Clinical drug use in dentistry

14. Prescribing and the Misuse of Drugs Act

Writing prescriptions usually requires no more than common sense and a formulary that gives information such as the forms in which the preparation is available and the usual dose ranges for children and adults.

Pharmacists are not impressed by illegible handwriting and may justifiably regard those who send formless scrawls as either illiterate or trying to disguise their ignorance.

There is no need to use, or try to remember, obscure Latin abbreviations, but it is acceptable and certainly quicker to put 'tds' than to write 'take three times a day' in full.

The essential information to be put on a prescription is obvious enough, namely:

1. The name and address of the prescriber.
2. The name and address of the patient.
3. The date.
4. The preparation, its form (tablets, mixture, or whatever) and the total quantity to be dispensed (in metric units).
5. Instructions as to how and when the drug is to be taken, such as 'take three times a day before meals'. Many dispensing chemists also now have pre-prepared labels based on the coding provided in the *British National Formulary* for any special warnings if, for example, the drug causes drowsiness.
6. The prescriber's signature.

Most drugs are available in some easily taken form that ensures adequate absorption and in amounts that form a convenient dose for taking once, twice or three times a day or more often, as necessary.

Drugs have a full chemical name but this is almost invariably too complicated for everyday use, and no one but a crank would ask for 6-((D)-α-aminophenylacetamido)-penicillanic acid instead of ampicillin, which is the official (approved) name. Manufacturers also have their own proprietary or brand names (Ampilar, Penbritin and others) which are usually patented. Subsequently, other manufacturers often produce the same drug under licence. Chloramphenicol, for example, had no fewer than 45 different proprietary names.

Official (generic) names are incidentally spelt with a small initial letter, e.g. ampicillin. Proprietary names, by contrast, are spelt with an initial capital, e.g. Penbritin (ampicillin).

The prescriber should always use the generic name. If a proprietary name is used the pharmacist has to dispense that particular brand, and clearly he cannot keep perhaps 30 proprietary brands of tetracycline, for example, in stock. Use of the official name allows the pharmacist to dispense whichever brand is cheapest and handiest. Different preparations of the same drug are sometimes absorbed to different degrees. Thus changing brands of the same drug in midtreatment might swing the response to dangerous under- or over-treatment.

Occasionally, it is easier to use a proprietary name, and only the most punctilious refer to Librium by its generic name, chlordiazepoxide.

Aspirin is an odd exception in that it was originally the proprietary name for acetysalicylic acid of the first manufacturer (Bayer of Germany), but has since become the official name.

Sources of reference

The Dental Practitioners' Formulary (DPF). The DPF includes all the drugs that can be prescribed by dentists under the conditions of the British National Health Service at whatever charge the Government of the day has decided. The charge is the same for all drugs and a growing number of drugs such as aspirin are cheaper if bought over the counter.

The DPF contains all the preparations that dental surgeons are likely to prescribe, but not preparations such as local anaesthetics which they themselves administer.

An attempt is made to ensure that there is reasonable evidence that preparations included in the DPF are effective. Although a few oddments hallowed by tradition may remain, they are being progressively discarded.

There is also information regarding the uses, contraindications and adverse reactions of drugs used in dentistry.

Finally, there are full details of the prescribable drugs and their dosage.

Dentists are not, by the way, limited in their prescribing to the contents of the DPF. They can prescribe anything, provided that it does not contravene the Misuse of Drugs Act and that the patient pays the full cost of the prescription of any drugs not included in the DPF.

Currently a combined *Dental Practitioners' Formulary* and *British National Formulary* is issued to practitioners in the Health Service and new editions are published every 2 years.

The British National Formulary (BNF). This handbook (of which the DPF is an offshoot) is for medical prescribing. It contains a much wider formulary, outline information about the drug treatment of a great range of human diseases, and much other information. It is particularly useful to dentists when, for instance, the patient's medical history shows that a complicated regimen of treatment is being followed. These drugs can then be identified and evaluated, both to gain some indication of the patient's physical state and to assess how it may affect the type of dental treatment proposed.

Like the DPF, the BNF tries to include only drugs of proven effectiveness, but also provides basic data on virtually all the different proprietary preparations available.

The BNF is under constant revision and a new edition is published every 6 months. It is thus more up-to-date than any textbook of pharmacology.

Monthly Index of Medical Specialties (MIMS). Basic information about all proprietary preparations available in Britain is also found in MIMS. This gives proprietary and official names for all preparations, formulations and dosage, and also minimal details of side-effects and contraindications. The drugs are grouped according to their main sites and types of action.

Data sheets. Drug companies are required to publish data sheets for their products. These sheets include a bewildering amount of information, including presentation (tablets, capsules or mixtures, as the case may be) and the amounts of the drug in each form, its uses, dosage and administration, possible toxic effects, contra-indications and warnings, effects of overdosage, pharmaceutical precautions, the legal category of the drug, quantities in the manufacturer's packages, further information (which may include information about the pharmacokinetics of the drug), and other facts. Data sheets may sometimes therefore run to two double-sided pages of small print, so that the amount of information provided may unfortunately discourage anyone from reading it.

Misuse of Drugs Regulations 1985

The purpose of these regulations is to control the prescribing of drugs of dependence. Dental surgeons can keep in stock, administer or prescribe Controlled Drugs, but only insofar as they are genuinely needed for dental purposes. In the past a dental surgeon might keep in stock cocaine for example, for use as a topical analgesic for certain special applications, but it would not be justifiable to prescribe the same drug for its systemic effects as there is no dental condition which can be usefully treated in that way.

As discussed earlier (Ch. 4) the important drugs of dependence (addiction) are the opioids, barbiturate hypnotics and stimulants of the CNS, particularly cocaine and the amphetamines. Some morphine derivatives such as codeine are also commonly used drugs which rarely lead to dependence. Similarly, some medicines (for the control of diarrhoea for instance) contain minute amounts of opium and are not controlled.

Under these regulations Controlled Drugs are divided into three classes:

Class A drugs are the most addictive and harmful. Morphine, diamorphine (heroin), cocaine and lysergide (LSD) are examples.

Class B drugs include the oral amphetamines, barbiturates cannabis, codeine and methylphenidate which, although addictive, are less harmful than Class A drugs.

Class C drugs are related to the amphetamines and include benzphetamine and chlorphentamine.

Among the Controlled Drugs, only opioids might be justifiably prescribed in dentistry for control of severe postoperative pain (for example).

Prescribing Controlled Drugs

Controlled Drugs can be dispensed for dental purposes only if certain rules are followed, namely:

1. The address of the prescriber is within the UK.
2. The pharmacist is familiar with the signature of the prescriber.
3. The drug must not be dispensed before, or later than 13 weeks after, the date of the prescription.
4. The entire prescription must be in the prescriber's own handwriting and in ink (or an indelible equivalent) and must show:
   a. The prescriber's name.
   b. The patient's name and address.
   c. The form of preparation (e.g. capsule or tablet) and its strength (unless only one preparation of the drug is available) must be stated.
   d. The total quantity (in both words and figures) of the drug to be supplied must be stated. Alternatively, this may be expressed in terms of the number (in both words and figures) of 'dosage units', such as capsules or tablets.
   e. The prescription must be endorsed with the words *For dental treatment only*.
   f. The prescription must be signed with the usual signature of the prescriber and be dated, and cannot be repeated.

Under the circumstances it is difficult to imagine many occasions in dentistry when Controlled Drus are worth the effort involved in prescribing them. However, it is legitimate to prescribe opioids for patients, including addicts, if they are genuinely in severe pain.

Requisition and possession of Controlled Drugs

To obtain and keep in stock a drug such as pethidine, a dental surgeon must:

1. Order the material on a requisition form which is
   a. Signed by him or her
   b. States his or her name, address and profession
   c. Specifies the purpose for which the drug is required and the total quantity to be supplied.
2. Keep a register of all such Controlled Drugs giving precise details both of what has been obtained and what has been administered, and the dates of both.
3. Store any Controlled Drugs in a fixed, locked container. The dental surgeon must retain the key.

Again, it all seems hardly worth the effort.

Only the main points about prescribing have been discussed, fuller details are provided in the *Dental Practitioners' Formulary* and the *British National Formulary*.

15. Antimicrobial drugs

Different types of antimicrobial drug can be effective against bacteria, viruses, fungi or other types of microorganisms. However, antibacterial drugs are the most numerous and most widely used.

Antimicrobials such as sulphonamides can be entirely synthetic, or like penicillin can be produced by microorganisms (true antibiotics). However, they are equally selective in their actions and the distinction between them has no clinical significance. Some antimicrobials are bacteriostatic (prevent proliferation of microbes) others are bactericidal. Tetracyclines (bacteriostatic) can antagonise the action of penicillins (bactericidal), but many other bacteriostatic and bactericidal drugs can be advantageously used in combination.

Though antimicrobial chemotherapy can sometimes be life-saving, the treatment of many infections, particularly in dentistry, is by traditional surgical means, namely, drainage and elimination of the cause.

PENICILLINS AND OTHER β-LACTAM ANTIBIOTICS

This large group now includes several different types of penicillins and cephalosporins. Their basic structures are shown in Figure 15.1. Some in this group, such as the cephamycins, aztreonam (a monobactam) and imipenem (a carbapenem), are used mainly for uncommon, otherwise resistant Gram-negative infections, particularly *Pseudomonas aeruginosa* infections.

Mode of action

The β-lactam antibiotics are bactericidal. By binding to the D-alanine recognition site on transpeptidase in the bacterial cell wall they inhibit transpeptidisation. This suppresses the cross-linking of mucopeptides which form a major component of bacterial cell walls – a process aptly described as 'causing bacteria to drop stitches in knitting their overcoats' (Fig. 15.2). The defective cell wall is vulnerable to osmotic damage and leakage of electrolytes.

THE PENICILLINS

Penicillin was the first true antibiotic and, with its variants, remains the most widely used. The penicillins are of low toxicity and the only significant hazard is that of allergy. Allergy to one penicillin is shared by all others. About 10% of patients allergic to the penicillins are also allergic to cephalosporins.

Penicillin is inactivated by β-lactamase enzymes (penicillinases) produced by many bacteria, particularly strains of *Staphylococcus aureus*. To counter this, penicillinase-resistant penicillins have been produced. 'Simple' penicillins are also inactive against Gram-negative bacilli which have a phospholipid membrane that impedes their access to the cell wall. Broad-spectrum penicillins such as ampicillin are more hydrophilic, able to penetrate the phospholipid membrane of many Gram-negative bacilli and are active against them.

The penicillins comprise the following main groups:

1. Penicillinase-sensitive penicillins (benzyl and phenoxymethyl penicillin)
2. Penicillinase-resistant penicillins such as flucloxacillin

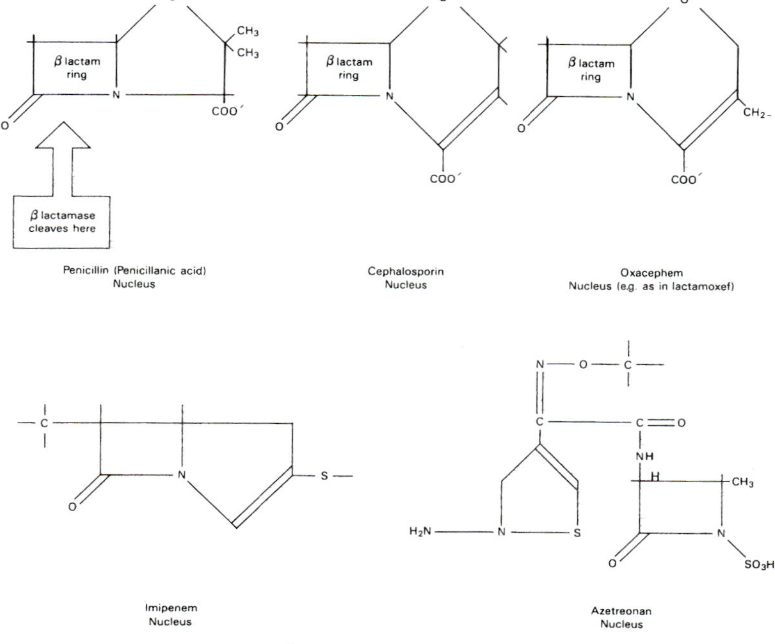

Fig. 15.1 Basic structures of β-lactam antibiotics. (Reproduced with permission from *Aids to Pharmacology*.)

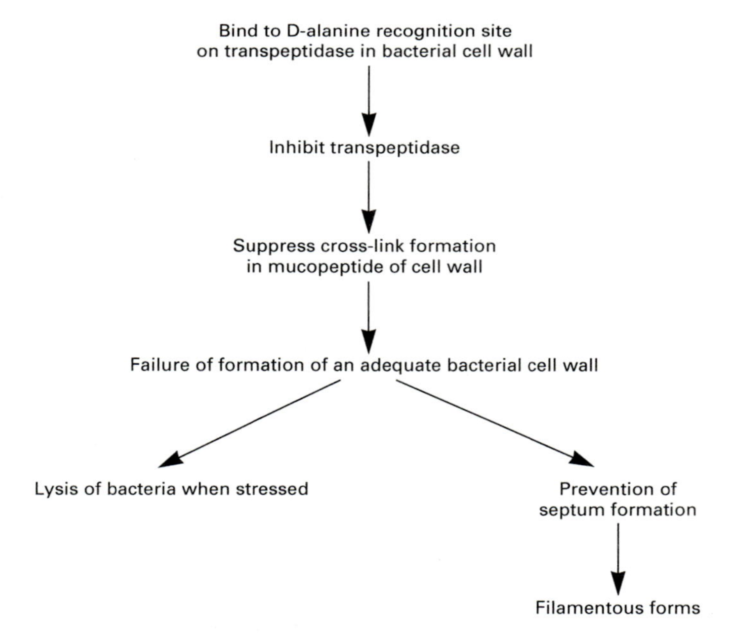

Fig. 15.2 Effect of lactam antibiotics on sensitive bacteria. (Reproduced with permission from *Aids to Pharmacology*.)

3. Broad-spectrum penicillins such as ampicillin and amoxycillin
4. Antipseudomonal penicillins such as ticarcillin and azlocillin.

Penicillins diffuse well into vascular tissues but do not enter the cerebrospinal fluid unless the membranes are inflamed. Penicillins are excreted in the urine.

Benzyl and phenoxymethyl penicillin

Benzyl penicillin is largely destroyed by gastric acid and is given by injection. This produces a high plasma level so that benzyl penicillin is the drug of choice for severe infections such as meningococcal, pneumococcal and severe streptococcal infections. Rapid renal excretion necessitates injections at least four times a day. Probenicid blocks renal excretion and can be used to prolong the action of penicillins and cephalosporins.

Phenoxymethyl penicillin is acid stable. It is given orally but does not achieve such high plasma levels as the benzyl analogue and is used for less severe infections.

Clinical uses

Sensitive organisms include the following:

1. Gram-positive cocci
   a. Some staphylococci (non-penicillinase producers)
   b. *Streptococcus pyogenes*
   c. *Streptococcus pneumoniae*
   d. Viridans streptococci
2. Gram-negative cocci
   a. *Neisseria gonorrhoeae* (some now resistant)
   b. *Neisseria meningitidis*
3. Gram-positive bacilli
   a. *Corynebacterium diphtheriae*
   b. *Bacillus anthracis*
4. Anaerobes
   a. *Clostridia* (e.g. *C. perfringens* and *C. tetani*)
   b. Many bacteroides species
   c. *Fusobacterium nucleatum*
5. Spirochaetes
   a. *Treponema pallidum*
   b. *Borrelia vincentii*
6. Actinomyces.

In dentistry, penicillin may be effective for acute periapical and other dental infections if drainage cannot be carried out immediately. It is also effective for ulcerative gingivitis, but metronidazole is currently the drug of choice.

Toxic effects

The main hazards are:

1. Hypersensitivity
2. Neurotoxicity.

Penicillin is highly allergenic and rashes due to type I reactions are the most common complication. More serious is anaphylaxis characterised by rapid onset of bronchospasm and circulatory failure or laryngeal oedema which can be fatal within minutes. Such reactions are exceedingly rare after oral administration. The immediate treatment is to give 1 ml of 1:1000 adrenaline intramuscularly (Ch. 19). Many more patients think that they are allergic to penicillin than is actually the case, but their word has to be accepted in the absence of any simple confirmatory test.

Type III reactions are less common and usually take the form of serum sickness with fever and joint pains, or severe skin reactions.

Neurotoxicity is seen only after intrathecal injection of anything more than minimal amounts of penicillin, in patients with anuria or if excessive doses are given by injection.

Penicillinase-resistant penicillins

The main example is flucloxacillin which can be given orally or by injection. Its sole use is against penicillinase-producing staphylococci. It is much less effective against other penicillin-sensitive bacteria.

Resistance to penicillinases can also be conferred by the penicillinase inhibitors clavulinic acid and sulbactam. *Co-amoxyclav* consists of amoxycillin with clavulinic acid but sulbactam is no longer available.

A current problem is the emergence of multi- (or methicillin) resistant *Staphylococcus aureus* (MRSA) which may be responsive only to vancomycin, teicoplanin or rifampicin.

Table 15.1 The main features of some important antibiotics

	Special properties	Limitations	Useful activity examples	Side-effects of individual agents	Side-effects of the group	Comments
			THE PENICILLINS			
			Acid-labile penicillins (must be given by injection)			
Natural: Benzyl		Destroyed by penicillinases (especially from staphylococci)	Staphylo-, strepto- pneumo- and gonococci. Actinomyces. *Trep. pallidum.* Clostridia			The most generally useful antibiotic in dentistry
Semisynthetic: Methicillin	Resistant to staphylococcal penicillinase	Much less active than benzyl penicillin against most pathogens other than staphylococci	Staphylococci	Marrow depression (rarely)		Little used; replaced by cloxacillin, etc.
			Acid-resistant penicillins (can be given by mouth)			
Natural: Phenyoxymethyl			Similar to benzyl penicillin			The most generally useful oral penicillin in dentistry and other uses
Semisynthetic: Ampicillin	Broad spectrum	Destroyed by penicillinases	Many Gram-negative (gut) bacilli sensitive	Rash common	Hypersensitisation common to all penicillins which all show cross-allergy to each other	
Amoxycillin	Ditto but better absorption and higher blood levels			Rash common		Replaces ampicillin as a general-purpose broad-spectrum antibiotic
Cloxacillin and flucloxacillin	Penicillinase resistant	Much less active than benzyl and other penicillins against pathogens other than penicillinase-producing staphylococci				Valuable for infections by penicillinase-producing staphylococci for which it should be reserved

Table 15.1 *contd*

	Special properties	Limitations	Useful activity examples	Side-effects of individual agents	Side-effects of the group	Comments
			THE CEPHALOSPORINS			
Cephradine	Broad spectrum. Fairly resistant to penicillinase Acid resistant		Similar to the broad-spectrum penicillins	Risk of renal damage	Hypersensitisation less common than to penicillin but sensitivity to both occasionally	Cross-resistance to both penicillin and cephalosporins, e.g. by viridans streptococci, may develop
Cephalexin						
			OTHER ANTIBIOTICS AND ANTIBACTERIAL AGENTS			
Erythromycin	Acid resistant. Hypersensitivity rare	Fairly rapid development of resistance	Similar to benzyl penicillin but also legionella		GIT disturbances	Often second choice for patients allergic to penicillin
Clindamycin	Good penetration of bone and fibrous tissue, but also better absorbed from the gut than lincomycin		Similar to benzyl penicillin	Diarrhoea common. Occasional cases of colitis	Possible second choice for patients allergic to penicillin	Less used because of risk of colitis
Tetracyclines	Broad spectrum. Absorbed from the gut	Bacteriostatic only. Development of resistance by many pathogens	Widest activity of all	GIT upsets common. Superinfection. Raise the blood urea. Bound to calcium and iron in the diet. Stain developing teeth.		Largely replaced by the broad-spectrum bactericidal antibiotics for general purposes. Still the drug of choice for certain exotic infections
Co-trimoxazole (sulphamethoxazole) and trimethoprim)	Broad spectrum. Absorbed from the gut. Bactericidal		At least as wide a range of bactericidal activity as the broad spectrum penicillins	GIT upsets and rashes. Agranulocytosis (rarely)		Broad-spectrum bactericidal drug, but increasingly widespread resistance
Metronidazole	Absorbed from the gut. Low toxicity. Allergy unknown		Obligate anaerobes including 'Vincent's' organisms	Nausea occasionally. Interaction with alcohol		The drug of choice for ulcerative gingivitis and many other anaerobic infections

GIT, gastrointestinal tract.

Ampicillin and amoxycillin

About 50% of ampicillin is absorbed after oral administration; amoxycillin aborption is unaffected by food in the stomach and gives higher plasma levels.

These penicillins can be used against many Gram-negative urinary infections, exacerbations of chronic bronchitis or cholecystitis. However, about 50% of *Escherichia coli* produce a penillinase as do some *Haemophilus influenzae* strains and pseudomonads are also resistant.

For the prophylaxis of infective endocarditis, amoxycillin is recommended because it gives prolonged bactericidal plasma levels after oral administration, as discussed later. Its broad spectrum of activity is of no relevance in this application.

Toxic effects

In addition to rashes due to penicillin allergy, the broad-spectrum penicillins are prone to cause irritating macular rashes unrelated to allergy. These rashes are particularly frequent in patients with lymphoproliferative diseases such as glandular fever or lymphoma. Nausea and vomiting are more likely to be caused by ampicillin than amoxycillin.

Antipseudomonal penicillins

Infection by *Pseudomonas aeruginosa*, which can cause fatal septicaemia, is a much feared complication of antibiotic treatment. Antipseudomonal penicillins include ticarcillin and carbenicillin. Even more effective are azlocillin and piperacillin which have a broad spectrum of activity. These drugs have little application in dentistry, and though Gram-negative osteomyelitis of the jaw is a recognised condition it is exceedingly rare.

THE CEPHALOSPORINS

The pharmacology of the cephalosporins in terms of absorption, action and excretion is similar to that of the penicillins. Most are acid stable and can be given orally. Their activity resembles that of the broad-spectrum penicillins plus variable resistance to penicillinases. The early cephalosporins, cephradine, cephalexin and cephazolin, have been followed by second- and third-generation analogues with greater activity against penicillinase-producing or particular Gram-negative bacteria.

Clinical applications

Despite their apparent advantages, the cephalosporins have little application in dentistry and are indicated only for severe infections shown by bacteriological testing to be sensitive. Viridans streptococci resistant to penicillin are also resistant to the cephalosporins, which are therefore unsuitable as an alternative in patients who have recently had more than one dose of a penicillin (see Table 15.1).

Toxic effects

Like the penicillins, cephalosporins can cause hypersensitivity reactions, and about 10% of patients allergic to penicillin are also allergic to cephalosporins.

In general, the cephalosporins can cause a considerably wider variety of toxic effects than the penicillins. Several cephalosporins can also interfere with clotting and promote prolonged haemorrhage.

ERYTHROMYCIN AND OTHER MACROLIDES

Erythromycin has a generally similar spectrum of action to penicillin and can be used as an alternative in penicillin-allergic patients.

Mode of action

The macrolides are one of several groups of drugs that include the tetracyclines, aminoglycosides and chloramphenicol, which act on various sites in bacterial ribosomes to inhibit protein synthesis. Erythromycin binds to the 50S subunit (human ribosomes have 40S and 60S ribosomes) to block translocation (Fig. 15.3). It is bacteriosatic.

Clinical applications

Erythromycin is usually given by mouth as the

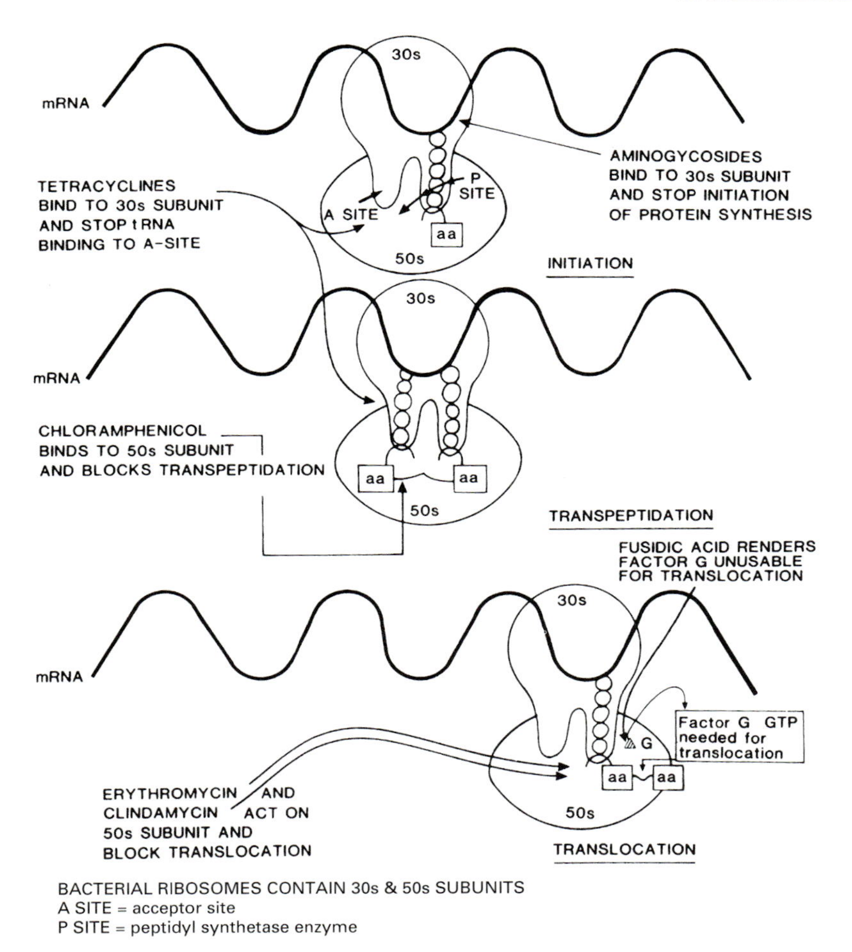

Fig. 15.3 The sites of action of antibacterials on ribosomes. (Reproduced with permission from *Aids to Pharmacology*.)

stearate which is acid stable. The estolate may be better absorbed but can cause a reversible hepatitis-like syndrome.

Erythromycin, as noted above, can be used as an alternative to penicillin-allergic patients, but its absorption is erratic. In large doses especially, it can cause severe nausea and vomiting or diarrhoea, probably in part at least due to its action as a receptor agonist for the gut peptide motilin.

Indications for erythromycin include whooping cough, legionnaires' disease and campylobacter enteritis but erythromycin has few uses in dentistry. It is no longer recommended for the prophylaxis of infective endocarditis in penicillin-allergic patients because of unreliable absorption and the frequency of nausea.

Azithromycin and clarithromycin cause fewer gastrointestinal side-effects, give higher tissue concentrations and have a considerably more prolonged action than erythromycin. Azithromycin has slightly less activity against Gram-positive bacteria but more activity against Gram-negative bacteria than erythromycin.

Toxic effects

The macrolides have low levels of toxicity and little or no allergenic potential. The most frequent complications are gastrointestinal disturbances. As noted earlier, erythromycin estolate can cause a reversible hepatitis-like syndrome.

CLINDAMYCIN

Mode of action

Clindamycin has a similar action to erythromycin on bacterial ribosomes by inhibiting translocation. It therefore competes with erythromycin and shares cross-resistance with it.

Clinical applications

Clindamycin is unusually well absorbed when given by mouth and penetrates well into avascular tissues such as necrotic bone. It has a broadly similar spectrum of antibacterial activity to penicillin but is more effective against many anaerobes such as *Bacteroides fragilis* and some penicillin-resistant staphylococci. It is useful for bone infections, but its main use in dentistry is for prophylaxis of infective endocarditis in penicillin-allergic patients (see Appendix).

Toxic effects

Clindamycin frequently causes diarrhoea, but can occasionally cause pseudomembranous colitis which on rare occasions has been fatal. Virtually any antibiotic, including the penicillins, can cause this complication, but it is more frequent when repeated doses of clindamycin are given to elderly patients. Pseudomembranous colitis is due to overgrowth or superinfection by toxigenic *Clostridium difficile*, but can usually be controlled by giving vancomycin or metronidazole by mouth. Pseudomembranous colitis appears not to be a hazard after the single dose of clindamycin recommended for infective endocarditis prophylaxis.

THE TETRACYCLINES

The tetracyclines have the broadest spectrum of activity of all antimicrobial drugs and even have some activity against mycobacteria and the malaria parasite. Unfortunately, their usefulness has become limited by widespread acquisition of resistance.

Mode of action

The tetracyclines bind to the 30S subunit of bacterial ribosomes and by blocking transfer RNA (tRNA) binding inhibit protein synthesis. They are bacteriostatic.

Clinical applications

The tetracyclines are absorbed from the gut but (with the exception of doxycycline and minocycline) this is hampered by concomitantly administered divalent metals such as calcium and magnesium to which they chelate. Because of the acquisition of resistance to the tetracyclines by so many common bacteria, their main uses are for uncommon or exotic infections. These include chlamydial infections (such as trachoma, psittacosis and lymphogranuloma venereum), rickettsial or mycoplasmal infections, and Lyme disease.

In dentistry, topical tetracycline is sometimes used for oral ulceration due, for instance, to recurrent aphthae. Despite claims, it cannot be said to be reliably effective for this purpose. Tetracycline may also be used to suppress anaerobes and synergistic bacteria for adjuvant treatment of severe chronic periodontal disease. For this purpose various drug-delivery systems have been devised to provide a high concentration of tetracycline in periodontal pockets. Tetracycline may also be appropriate for Lyme disease of the temporomandibular joint, although this is an exceptionally rare cause of temporomandibular arthritis.

Toxic effects

Overall, serious toxic effects from tetracyclines are uncommon but can include the following:

1. Gastrointestinal disturbances
2. Superinfection
3. Renal and metabolic complications
4. Staining of developing teeth.

Minor gastrointestinal disturbances such as nausea, vomiting or diarrhoea are common and are probably due to direct irritation by an unabsorbed drug.

Superinfection is particularly frequently due to *Candida albicans* which is promoted by the wide range of competitors inhibited by tetracyclines. Topical tetracycline for oral ulceration can cause thrush.

Tetracyclines have an antianabolic effect. The resulting increase in nitrogen excretion can raise the blood urea in normal persons. Tetracyclines, apart from doxycycline and minocycline, are therefore contraindicated in patients with poor renal function.

Tetracyclines in high doses can also cause liver damage. They are contraindicated in pregnancy for this reason and for their effects on the fetus' teeth.

By chelating calcium salts, tetracyclines bind to and irreversibly stain teeth and bones during calcification. If given during dental development the teeth appear yellow when they erupt but become a greyish brown. The nature of this pigmentation can be confirmed by microscopy of an undecalcified section under ultraviolet light. Tetracycline fluoresces brilliant yellow where it is deposited along the incremental lines of enamel and dentine. Tetracyclines are therefore contraindicated during the last trimester of pregnancy and during the first 12 years of life.

THE AMINOGLYCOSIDES

Streptomycin, the first member of this group, was the first effective antituberculous drug, but is now only used if resistance is suspected. For other infections it has been superseded by newer analogues such as gentamicin and amikacin.

Mode of action

The aminoglycosides inhibit bacterial protein production by binding to the ribosomal 30S subunit and also by causing misreading of ribosomal messenger RNA (mRNA).

Clinical applications

Aminoglycosides are active against many staphylococci, mycobacteria and Gram-negative bacilli, but have no activity against obligate anaerobes. They are not significantly absorbed from the gut and are given by injection. Their main uses are for the treatment of tuberculosis (in combination with other antimicrobials to prevent emergence of resistance), severe Gram-negative infections and, with penicillin, for the treatment of infective endocarditis by viridans streptococci.

Gentamicin is used in dentistry in combination with intramuscular amoxycillin for prevention of infective endocarditis in patients with a prosthetic valve or who have had a previous episode of endocarditis, who require certain types of dental treatment under a general anaesthetic (see Appendix).

Toxic effects

The aminoglycosides are ototoxic and nephrotoxic to variable degrees. The effect is highly selective: streptomycin can cause deafness, while dihydrostreptomycin (now obsolete) causes loss of balance. These effects are dose related and the elderly are particularly vulnerable. Plasma concentrations should be monitored when a course of an aminoglycoside is given to ensure that the levels are adequate but not excessive. Aminoglycosides also act on the motor end-plate and potentiate muscle relaxants.

Treatment of tuberculosis

The incidence of tuberculosis and non-tuberculous ('atypical') mycobacterioses is no longer declining in the West, and in some countries the mortality is rising. Though the aminoglycosides are effective antituberculous drugs, the emergence of resistance causes difficulties. At least three drugs are therefore given for the initial phase of treatment and two for maintenance, but multiresistant strains are now emerging. Part of this change is due to AIDS in which tuberculosis is common and difficult to treat because of the immunodeficiency. Treatment has to extend over several months because of the slow growth of mycobacteria.

In Britain the standard regimen comprises isoniazid plus rifampicin for 6 months, with pyrazinamide in addition for the first 2 months. If resistance is suspected, ethambutol and streptomycin are added (Fig. 15.4). Treatment is continued for a further 3–6 months for tuberculous meningitis, bone and joint disease and some cases of lymphadenopathy.

Where more obstinate resistance is encountered, second-line drugs such as prothionamide, thiacetazone, cycloserine or capreomycin may

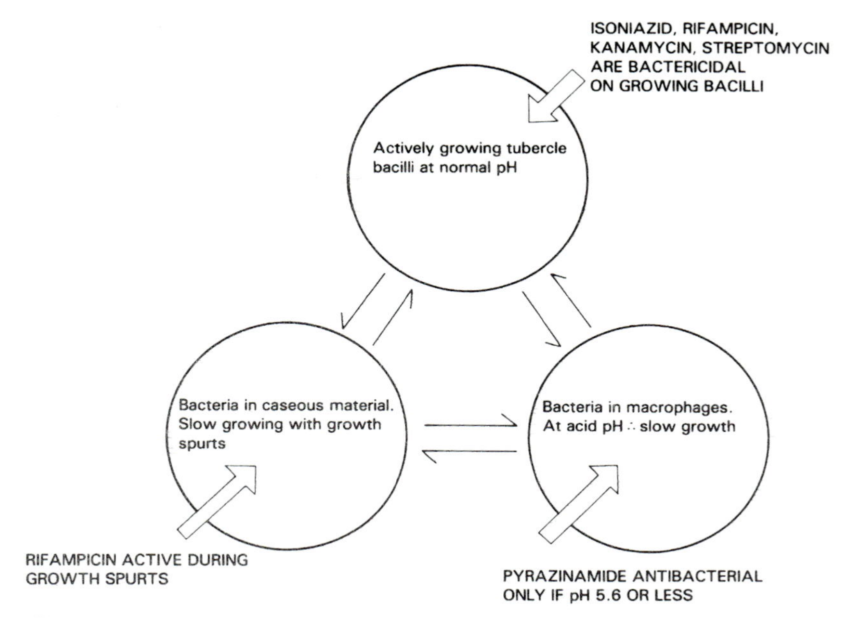

Fig. 15.4 Site of action of antituberculosis drugs. (Reproduced with permission from *Aids to Pharmacology*.)

also have to be given despite their greater toxicity. None of these antituberculous drugs, other than rifampicin, is used for any other purpose.

RIFAMPICIN

Mode of action

Rifampicin inhibits bacterial DNA-dependent RNA polymerase and penetrates virtually all body fluids apart from the CSF.

Clinical applications

Rifampicin is completely absorbed when given orally. Its ability to enter macrophages contributes to its value in antituberculous treatment. In the absence of safer alternatives, rifampicin is also used for other life-threatening infections such as staphylococcal, or legionnaires' disease. It is currently recommended for the prophylaxis of meningococcal meningitis.

Toxic effects

Among numerous other toxic effects, rifampicin can cause a flu-like illness, rashes, liver damage or rarely thrombocytopenia. It turns the saliva, tears, urine and semen pink.

VANCOMYCIN AND TEICOPLANIN

These toxic drugs are mainly used for infections uncontrollable by other means.

Mode of action

Vancomycin and teicoplanin act similarly to the penicillins by blocking bacterial cell-wall synthesis by inhibiting peptidoglycan formation.

Clinical applications

Vancomycin and teicoplanin are bactericidal to many Gram-positive bacteria. They are useful for the treatment of septicaemia or endocarditis due to such bacteria as multiresistant *Staphylococcus aureus*. They are also recommended for prophylaxis of infective endocarditis in certain high risk penicillin-allergic dental patients (see Appendix). Vancomycin given orally is not absorbed from the gut but produces a high local concentration there and, as noted earlier, is the treatment of choice for pseudomembranous colitis due to clindamycin.

Toxic effects

Vancomycin is intensely irritant and has to be given in a dilute infusion extending over at least 100 min. Rapid intravenous injection can induce mast cell degranulation, histamine release and widespread erythema (red man syndrome). It can occasionally cause renal failure or hearing loss. Teicoplanin is very similar but can be given as a simple intravenous or intramuscular injection and has a half-life of 24 h.

CIPROFLOXACIN AND OTHER 4-QUINOLONES

This group which also includes acrosoxacin, nalidixic acid and ofloxacin, has an unusual mode of action. They inhibit bacterial topoisomerase (DNA gyrase) which supercoils bacterial DNA. The uncoiling of bacterial DNA blocks repair and disrupts cellular activity. Theoretically, resistance to this enzyme cannot be acquired, but changes in permeability of the cell membrane can prevent access of the drug to the bacterial cytoplasm.

Clinical applications

The 4-quinolines are well absorbed from the gut but can also be given by intravenous infusion for life-threatening infections. They have little action against Gram-positive or anaerobic bacteria. Ciprofloxacin is used mainly for Gram-negative respiratory and urinary infections and for Gram-negative osteomyelitis. It is also effective for some cases of typhoid fever and penicillin-resistant gonorrhoea. Ofloxacin and acrosaxacin are also effective against the latter, though quinolone-resistant strains are emerging. Oral ciprofloxacin will also eliminate nasal carriage of *Neisseria meningitidis* and will do so when rifampicin has failed.

Toxic effects

Gastrointestinal disturbances are common, and headache, rashes and other hypersensitivity reactions, including anaphylaxis, may also be seen. The 4-quinolones can also lower brain γ-aminobutyric acid (GABA) levels and may precipitate convulsions in those with or without a history of epilepsy. However, the overall frequency of adverse effects does not appear to be more frequent than with the more commonly used antibiotics.

METRONIDAZOLE

Metronidazole is unusual in that it acts only against obligate anaerobes, including some protozoa.

Mode of action

Metonidazole blocks energy production from carbohydrates by inhibiting a reductase in anaerobic bacteria. It also inhibits the anaerobic electron transfer chain (Fig. 15.5). The restriction of its action to anaerobic microbes depends on its reduction to an active derivative which binds to DNA and blocks nucleic acid synthesis.

Clinical applications

Metronidazole is most widely used for vaginal trichomoniasis, but is also useful for many anaerobic bacterial infections. It can be given intravenously for severe infections.

In dentistry, metronidazole is highly effective in ulcerative gingivitis (200 mg, 3 times a day for 3 days is usually sufficient). It is at least as effective as penicillin and has little potential for allergic reactions. Metronidazole is also useful for other dental infections such as acute pericoronitis in which anaerobes play a large part.

Toxic effects

The most common side-effect is a metallic taste due to excretion of metronidazole in the saliva. An interaction with alcohol can cause flushing, sweating, palpitations and nausea. Patients given metronidazole should be warned against taking alcohol during and for a week after completion of treatment.

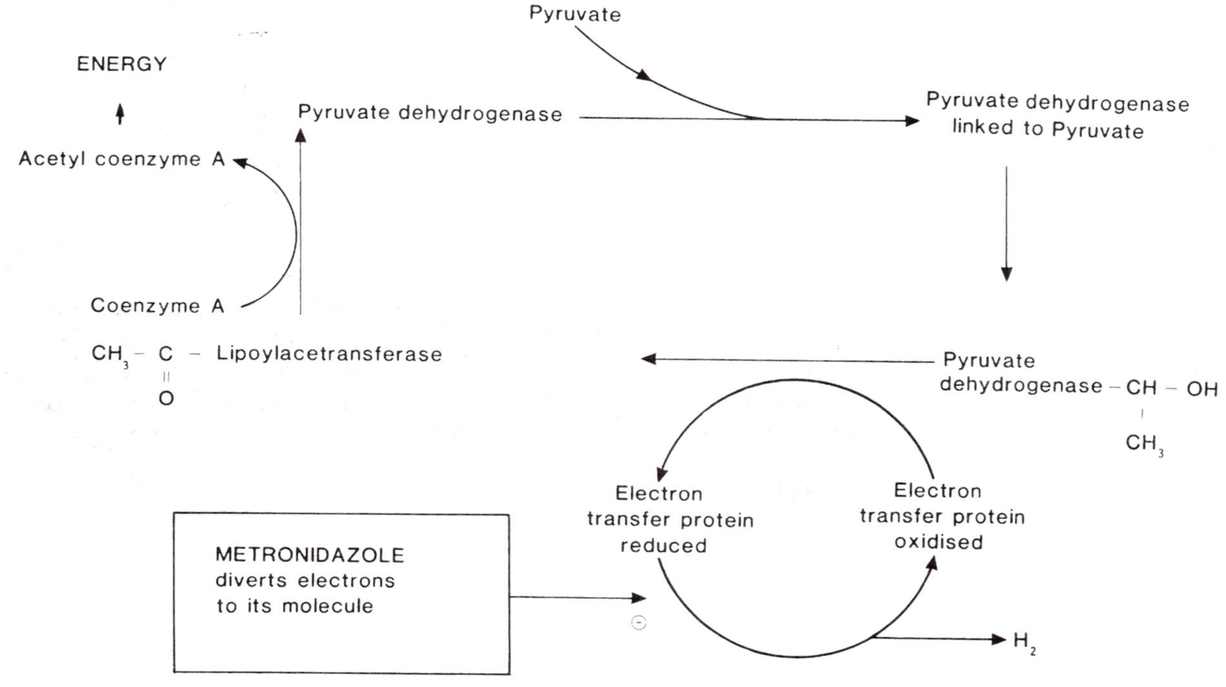

Fig. 15.5 Mode of action of metronidazole. (Reproduced with permission from *Aids to Pharmacology*.)

CHLORAMPHENICOL

This broad-spectrum, bacteriostatic drug is only used for infections where there is no safer alternative.

Mode of action

Chloramphenicol acts on the 50S subunit of bacterial ribosomes to inhibit peptidyl transpeptidase and thus block protein synthesis.

Clinical applications

Chloramphenicol can be given orally or by injection and readily enters body fluids including the CSF. However, because of its toxicity, its use is restricted to typhoid fever and life-threatening haemophilus infections such as meningitis that is unresponsive to other drugs.

Toxic effects

The main complication is marrow aplasia which, though rare is frequently unpredictable, irreversible and fatal. Other side-effects include superinfection (sore mouth due to candidal infection), gastrointestinal disturbances and dose-dependent, reversible marrow depression. In neonates, chloramphenicol can cause circulatory collapse (grey baby syndrome) and depress liver function.

SULPHONAMIDES, TRIMETHOPRIM AND CO-TRIMOXAZOLE

Sulphonamides, the first selective antibacterial drugs, seemed almost miraculously effective when first given for killing diseases such as lobar pneumonia or streptococcal infections. Since then, many bacteria have become resistant and other antimicrobials with fewer toxic effects have become available. The use of sulphonamides was revived by the introduction of co-trimoxazole, a mixture of trimethoprim and sulphamethoxazole in the ratio of 1:5. These drugs both act by blocking bacterial folate production but at different points in the metabolic pathway.

Mode of action

Sulphonamides block folic acid synthesis by binding to pteridine to form an inactive complex. Human folic acid synthesis is unaffected, since this stage in its production is absent.

Trimethoprim also blocks bacterial folic acid production, but as a competitive inhibitor of bacterial dihydrofolate reductase. It has a 50 000-fold greater activity against this bacterial enzyme, than against the human equivalent (Fig. 15.6).

Clinical applications

Sulphonamides and co-trimoxazole have been widely used for urinary tract, respiratory and some gastrointestinal infections, but trimethoprim alone may be as effective, has fewer side-effects and is frequently preferred. However, co-trimoxazole is valuable for the treatment of *Pneumocystis carinii* pneumonia in patients with AIDS.

Sulphonamides appear in high concentration in the CSF. After maxillofacial injuries causing CSF leakage, oral sulphadiazine has traditionally been used for prophylaxis. Unfortunately, most meningococci and staphylococci are now resistant.

Toxic effects

Sulphonamides can cause

1. Rashes and mucocutaneous Stevens–Johnson syndrome (Ch. 13)
2. Renal damage due to crystallisation in the renal tubules if fluid intake is inadequate
3. Bone marrow depression causing agranulocytosis or, rarely, aplastic anaemia

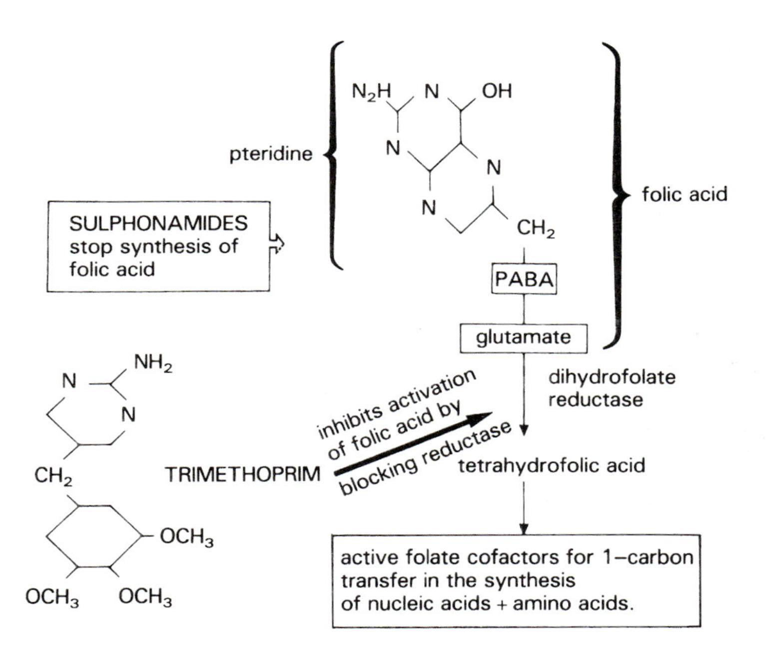

PABA = para amino benzoic acid

SULPHONAMIDES are specifically antibacterial because mammalian cells do not synthesise folic acid but can absorb and utilise the complete molecule. Bacteria have to synthesise the substance intracellularly.

TRIMETHOPRIM acts as a selective antibacterial because it inhibits bacterial dihydrofolate reductase 20 000–60 000 times more powerfully than the mammalian form of the enzyme.

Fig. 15.6 Structural analogy of trimethoprim with the pteridine portion of folic acid and its action as an inhibitor of bacterial dihydrofolate reductase. (Reproduced with permission from *Aids to Pharmacology*.)

4. Hypersensitivity reactions – rashes are the most common effect and topical applications of sulphonamides can cause intractable contact dermatitis.

The adverse effects of co-trimoxazole are mainly due to the sulphonamide component.

Trimethoprim can occasionally cause

1. Nausea vomiting or diarrhoea
2. Rashes
3. Folate deficiency, but only if folate stores are already low; trimethoprim is therefore contraindicated during pregnancy.

ANTIFUNGAL DRUGS

Antifungal drugs are important in dentistry because of the frequency of *Candida albicans* infections under dentures or as oral thrush. Candidosis is common in those with HIV infection and is a sign of a deteriorating prognosis. Deep mycoses are also a recognised but less common complication of AIDS.

The older antifungal drugs fall into two distinct groups. The polyenes (nystatin and amphotericin) are effective against candidosis and the deep mycoses, while griseofulvin is effective only against tinea (ringworm). The newer imidazoles such as fluconazole are effective against both groups. Flucytosine is mainly used for its synergistic effect with amphotericin for otherwise intractable cases of candidosis or for some of the deep mycoses.

Polyene antifungal drugs

These act by binding to ergosterol in the fungal cell membrane to form hydrophilic pores. Sugar and electrolytes leak out and acid leaks in to stop enzymic activity.

Nystatin

Nystatin is not absorbed from the gut and so is used topically for superficial candidosis. Preparations such as the suspension or pastilles should be held in the mouth for as long as possible to allow time for them to act before passage down the bowel and excretion.

Toxic effects

Nystatin is too toxic to be given parentally. Oral preparations and ointments are not absorbed and have no adverse effects.

Amphotericin

Amphotericin is available as lozenges or as a suspension to be used topically like nystatin for candidosis. It is also given intravenously for deep mycoses such as histoplasmosis. Amphotericin encapsulated in liposomes is somewhat less toxic.

Toxic effects

Intravenous amphotericin is nephrotoxic, but renal damage is reversible if treatment is stopped early enough. Other effects are headaches, chills, vomiting, drug fever and hypersensitivity reactions. Nevertheless, amphotericin remains the single most effective drug for treating life-threatening mycoses.

Imidazole and triazole antifungal drugs

Mode of action

These drugs have a somewhat similar mode of action to the polyenes and damage the fungal cell membrane. They inhibit ergosterol synthesis, causing leakage of cytoplasmic fluids, but also block peroxidase to produce lethal accumulation of peroxides in the cell.

Clinical applications

Unlike the polyenes, imidazoles (miconazole, ketoconazole, clotrimazole, etc.) and triazoles (fluconazole, itraconazole) are absorbed when given orally, but intravenous preparations of many of them are also available.

For oral candidosis, miconazole oral gel can be held in the mouth or in the case of denture-induced stomatitis, can be used to coat the fitting surface of the denture. For more resistant oral candidosis as in AIDS, advantage is taken of the systemic action of itraconazole or fluconazole given by mouth.

For deep mycoses, miconazole, fluconazole or

itraconazole, are frequently effective, particularly for aspergillus and cryptococcal infections, and are less toxic than amphotericin. Itraconazole is less well absorbed, but is highly tissue bound. It has a broader spectrum of activity than fluconazole. However, as noted earlier, intravenous amphotericin remains the mainstay for life-threatening infections, with fluconazole or itraconazole mainly used for maintenance therapy.

Toxic effects

Significant oral doses of these drugs can cause nausea, vomiting or abdominal discomfort and rashes. Ketoconazole has rarely caused liver failure and itraconazole, which is metabolised in the liver, should be avoided in those with a history of liver disease.

Flucytosine

Flucytosine is well absorbed when given orally but can also be given intravenously. It is synergistic with amphotericin, but resistance readily develops and it is rarely used alone. It has been used for chronic candidal infections either alone or with amphotericin but has been replaced by the imidazoles and triazoles.

Toxic effects

Nausea, vomiting, diarrhoea, rashes, thrombocytopenia or leucopenia are possible complications.

ANTIVIRAL DRUGS

Viruses colonise host cells and use their enzyme systems for protein synthesis and replication (Fig. 15.7). This intimate relationship has made it difficult to produce drugs that will block viral nucleic acid synthesis without affecting that of the host. The AIDS virus (HIV) possesses reverse transcriptase which is a potential target for drugs and a few other means have been developed to attack viruses.

Acyclovir

Acyclovir is a potent antiherpetic drug.

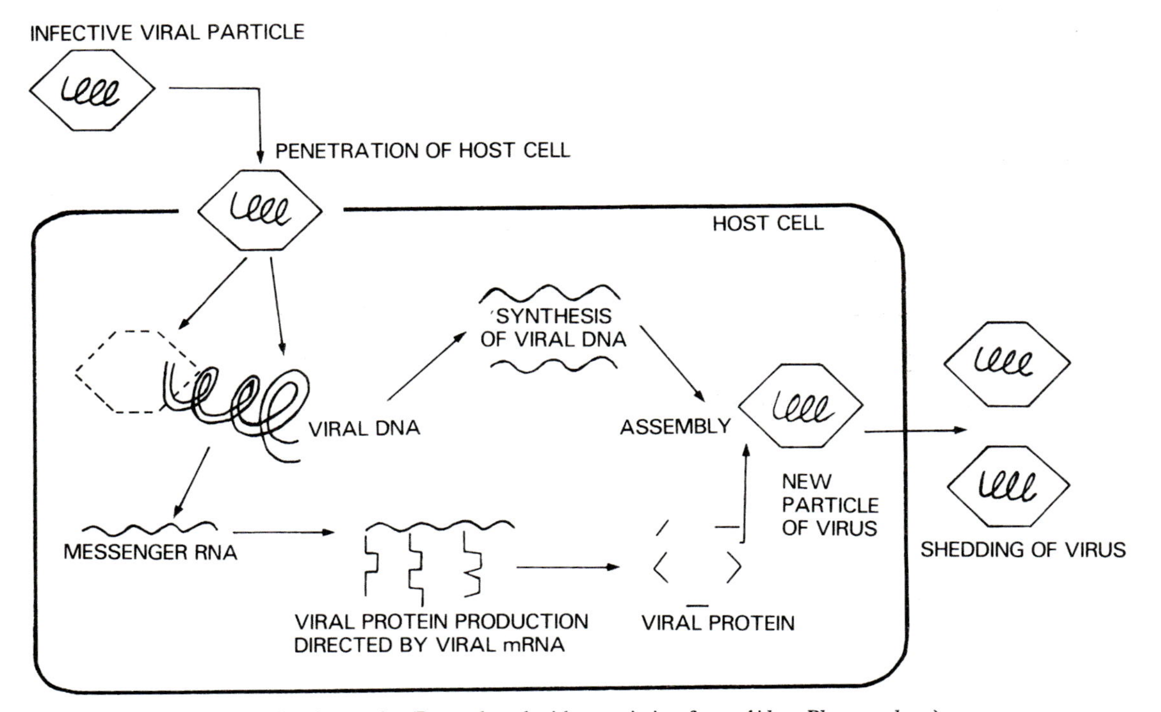

Fig. 15.7 The virus replication cycle. (Reproduced with permission from *Aids to Pharmacology*.)

Mode of action

Acyclovir is a synthetic analogue of deoxyguanosine and readily enters human cells. Herpetic thymidine kinase converts acyclovir to its monophosphate. Acyclovir binds strongly to viral thymidine kinase and is phosphorylated more than a million times faster than by human thymidine kinase, and is unable to escape from the infected cell. Viral DNA polymerase takes up acyclovir triphosphate and incorporates it into viral DNA in place of deoxyguanosine phosphate. This blocks further viral DNA production as no further units can be added to the terminal acyclovir groups (Fig. 15.8).

Since host DNA polymerase will not incorporate acyclovir triphosphate there is no interference with host DNA production. This gives acyclovir a high degree of specificity and an unusually low toxicity.

Clinical applications

Acyclovir is highly effective against *herpes simplex* and *herpes zoster viruses*, but less effective against other viruses of the herpes group such as Epstein–Barr or cytomegalovirus. It can be given orally or intravenously for severe infections.

The effectiveness of acyclovir is demonstrated

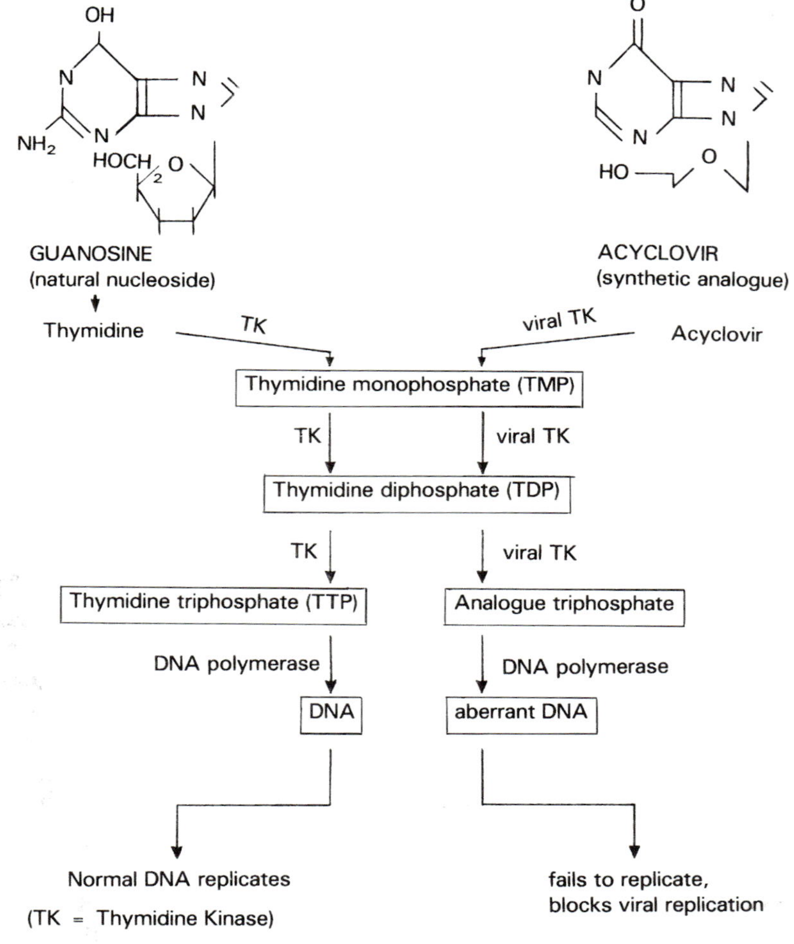

Fig. 15.8 Action of acyclovir on nucleic acid synthesis by virally infected cells. (Reproduced with permission from *Aids to Pharmacology*.)

by the fact that it is effective when given prophylactically or therapeutically for life-threatening herpetic infections, particularly herpes zoster in immunodeficient patients. The incidence, morbidity and mortality from such infections has been reduced significantly as a consequence. Herpetic encephalitis, the most common cause of encephalitis in temperate climates, can be diagnosed reliably only by brain biopsy. Acyclovir, given on suspicion, has largely eliminated the need for this procedure and has significantly lowered the mortality.

In the case of primary herpetic stomatitis or recurrent herpes labialis, the value of acyclovir is limited by the rapidity of viral damage to the tissues, the epithelium being destroyed before the diagnosis is made. However, patients prone to recurrent attacks of herpes labialis should be able to recognise the prodromal stages and apply acyclovir cream with benefit.

Herpes zoster infection of the trigeminal area can cause intense pain and, in elderly patients especially, a debilitating illness. High-dose oral or even intravenous acyclovir should therefore be given. Early administration of high-dose acyclovir may possibly also lessen the risk of postherpetic neuralgia, but this has not been widely confirmed. Intravenous acyclovir should be given for herpes zoster in AIDS patients in whom the infection is life-threatening.

In long-term treatment, such as in patients with AIDS, resistance to acyclovir may be acquired.

Toxic effects

With high doses, and particularly with prolonged intravenous administration, blood urea and creatinine are raised. This effect is reversible and in patients in renal failure, acyclovir can be given in lower dosage. Liver enzyme levels may also rise, but hepatotoxicity is not a major risk. Rashes, gastrointestinal disturbances, depression of haematological indices and neurological dysfunction are other possible effects of high-dose systemic treatment. Extravasation of acyclovir during injection can cause severe local inflammation.

Ganciclovir

Ganciclovir is chemically related to acylovir, but has greater activity against cytomegalovirus (CMV).

Cytomegalovirus can cause serious infections such as retinitis in AIDS or other immunodeficiencies. Despite its toxicity, ganciclovir is recommended for life- or sight-threatening cytomegalovirus infections.

Toxic effects

Ganciclovir is also considerably more toxic than acyclovir, can cause bone marrow depression, is a potential carcinogen and should only be given when the possible benefits outweigh the risks.

Idoxuridine

Idoxuridine is an antimetabolite that was used as a superficial application for mucocutaneous herpetic infections. Acyclovir has largely replaced it, but idoxuridine in dimethyl sulphoxide for cutaneous application to herpes labialis and idoxuridine ointment for herpetic ocular ulceration are available.

Zidovudine (azidothymidine, AZT)

Zidovudine is used only for HIV infection.

Mode of action

Zidovudine triphosphate produced in the cell, competes with thymidine triphosphate for binding sites on viral reverse transcriptase (Fig. 15.9). It is also incorporated into the proviral DNA chain and terminates it.

Clinical applications

Zidovudine is given orally or intravenously. It was thought to be the only drug that had any effect on the progress of AIDS, but at best does no more than slow the progress of the disease. Currently, there is doubt as to whether it has

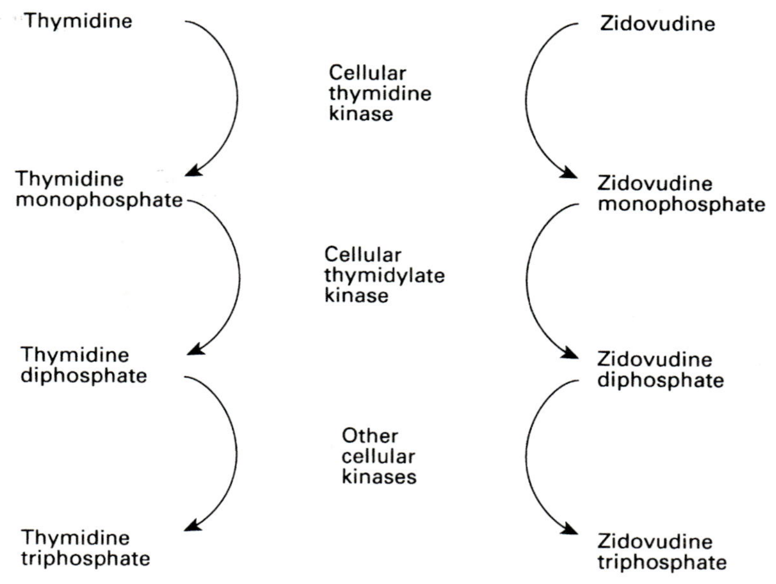

Fig. 15.9 Phosphorylation of zidovudine and thymidine to their triphosphates. Zidovudine triphosphate interferes with proviral synthesis by (1) competition with thymidine triphosphate for binding sites on the enzyme reverese transcriptase, and (2) incorporation into and termination of the proviral DNA chain. (Reproduced with permission from *Aids to Pharmacology*.)

has any value for treatment or prophylaxis. However, in the absence of any more effective drug, zidovudine will probably continue to be given to patients with AIDS and to health workers who have received needle-stick injuries while treating HIV-infected patients.

These considerations aside, treatment of the many bacterial and fungal infections, that are the major feature of AIDS, by specific antimicrobial drugs is essential and can prolong life to a variable degree.

Toxic effects

Bone marrow depression is the main adverse effect, particularly with high doses and advanced HIV infection. Anaemia may be severe enough to require transfusion. Marrow depression is enhanced by concomittant ganciclovir administration, and the two drugs should not be given together. Gastrointestinal disturbance, headache, rashes and myalgia may also be induced by zidovudine.

Foscarnet

Foscarnet is recommended only for CMV retinitis in patients with AIDS in whom ganciclovir is inappropriate. Foscarnet can cause renal toxicity in up to 50% of patients.

INTERFERONS

α-, β- and γ-interferons are a family of proteins produced by many body cells in response to viral infections. They are not virus-specific but are species specific and rabbit interferon, for example, is effective only for infection in rabbits. However, human α-interferon has been produced by recombinant DNA techniques and has some anti-tumour as well as antiviral actions.

Mode of action

The antiviral action of interferon depends on its binding to surface receptors to induce the synthesis of inhibitory proteins which interfere with translation of viral mRNA to viral protein.

Clinical applications

α-interferon is licensed for the treatment of chronic active hepatitis B, for hairy cell leukaemia (associated with HTLV, an oncorna virus unrelated to HIV), AIDS-related Kaposi's sarcoma, and for maintenance treatment of multiple myeloma.

Toxic effects

The toxic effects can be formidable, although less now that purer preparations are available. They include a flu-like illness with joint pains, lethargy but insomnia, and depression. Marrow depression, cardiovascular disorders, hepatotoxicity, rashes, coma and convulsions have also been reported.

Amantadine

Amantadine has an antiviral action by blocking uncoating of virus in preparation to cell entry. It is highly specific and useful only for prophylaxis or lessening the severity of influenza A_2 in high-risk patients. Its claimed value for herpes zoster is unconfirmed.

Amantadine also has mild antiparksonian effects and is sometimes used for that disease (Ch. 3).

Toxic effects

In high doses amantadine has amphetamine-like effects of restlessness, anxiety, insomnia and anorexia.

PRACTICAL ASPECTS OF MANAGEMENT OF INFECTIONS

Antimicrobial chemotherapy has revolutionised the control of many, but by no means all, otherwise lethal infections. A recent illustration of the limitations of chemotherapy has been the outbreak of the AIDS epidemic. The latter illustrates the limited variety of antiviral drugs available. That most AIDS patients die from overwhelming infections also underlines the fact that antimicrobial chemotherapy may be ineffective when the immune system fails.

In the case of surgery, postoperative infection has largely been abolished by strict aseptic technique. In the case of established infections, drainage of pus or exudate, which acts as a reservoir of infection, is essential. It may be sterilised by an antibiotic but not removed. If the infection is very acute, as in the case of cervicofacial cellulitis, an arbitrary choice of antibiotic, such as a penicillin, has to be made and given as soon as a specimen has been obtained for bacteriological examination. The antibiotic may then have to be changed according to the bacteriological findings.

USE OF ANTIBIOTICS IN DENTISTRY

Pericoronitis

Pericoronitis is an infection of the blind pocket round a third molar which has started to erupt into the mouth. Pericoronitis usually responds quickly to local measures, namely irrigation under the flap and frequent hot mouthwashes. Severe infection can, however, spread quickly and there may already be lymphadenitis when the patient is first seen. In this case metronidazole or penicillin (if there are no contraindications) should be given. When the infection has subsided the tooth can, if necessary, be extracted.

Prophylactic use of antibiotics for oral surgery

Prophylactic antibiotics are given with the aim of preventing infection in the following circumstances:

1. Major jaw surgery
2. Difficult disimpactions of third molars
3. Severe maxillofacial injuries.

In the case of orthognathic surgery, such as resections of the jaw followed by grafting or 'push back' operations for prognathism, it is vital to get vascularisation of the graft and union either of the graft to adjacent bone or between newly exposed bone surfaces. All this must happen in the presence of considerable amounts of blood clot. The consequences of bone infection can be disastrous and treatment is more difficult than prevention. Nevertheless, the value of prophylactic antibiotics for this purpose is unproven when good aseptic technique is practised.

In the case of third molar disimpactions, the prophylactic use of antibiotics is also controversial. Many believe that without them the incidence of painful infected sockets is much higher. Once a socket has become infected localised osteitis does not respond to antibiotics; their prophylactic use here is therefore possibly justifiable. On the other hand, good aseptic technique probably renders antibiotics unnecessary for this type of operation.

Postoperative oedema

After extensive oral surgery there is, not surprisingly, often considerable facial swelling. The main consideration is to make sure that there is no postoperative infection. A short course of a systemic corticosteroid such as dexamethasone taken with non-steroidal anti-inflammatory agents preoperatively can often abolish postoperative pain and swelling.

Maxillofacial injuries. Penicillin (600 mg) is usually given routinely to patients who have had severe maxillofacial injuries. In these patients there is a greater chance of infection of blood clot from the exterior by way of a periodontal pocket when this is in the fracture line.

If the cranial cavity has been opened by a fracture passing through the cribriform plate of the ethmoid, then rifampicin is probably the antibiotic of choice.

ANTIBIOTIC RESISTANCE – ACQUISITION AND MECHANISMS

Bacteria can become resistant to antimicrobial drugs by several mechanisms. Acquired resistance depends, in essence, on genetic material which encodes the information necessary to direct the process. Acquisition of resistance to antibiotics, in turn, is by two main mechanisms, namely:

1. Mutation and therapeutic selection
2. Transmission of new genetic material from other bacteria.

Mutation

In bacterial populations, mutants naturally resistant to an antibiotic, appear at a rate of less than one per million bacteria for each division. This type of resistance is referred to as *chromosomal resistance* since it depends on changes in the bacterial chromosome.

Once such mutants appear, they can proliferate freely without competition after removal of the dominant antibiotic-sensitive strains by antibiotic. This phenomenon is well recognised in the case of oral viridans streptococci where a single dose of penicillin produces a resistant population within 24 h.

Transmission of new genetic material

Antibiotic resistance can be transmitted by bacteriophages (bacterial viruses) or by plasmids. The latter consist of extrachromosomal DNA which is transmitted between bacteria during conjugation. Such DNA, known as an r-determinant, directs the production of enzymes which can inactivate one or several antibiotics and is perpetuated by division of the bacterium.

Mechanisms of enhanced bacterial resistance to antibacterials

The main mechanisms by which bacteria can become resistant are as follows:

1. *Altered permeability of the bacterial cell for the drug.* An antimicrobial has to penetrate the cell membrane to reach target sites in the bacterial cell to exert its action, but the ways in which permeability of the cell can be altered are poorly understood.

2. *Changes in the target sites for the drug in the bacterial cell.* Typical mechanisms of action of several antibiotics are by binding to and inactivating bacterial enzymes or nucleic acids. Mutation or episome transfer can, however, change an amino acid or base component of these target substances with the result that the drug can no longer bind to them. Resistance of staphylococci and streptococci to erythromycin and clindamycin, for example, depends on transfer of plasmid-

mediated methylase which interferes with the binding of these antibiotics to ribosomal RNA.

3. *Bypassing metabolic reactions blocked by the drug.* Essential metabolic reactions of bacteria depend on chromosome-coded enzymes which can be blocked by antimicrobials. However, another enzyme, resistant to the drug, may be acquired by plasmid transfer and confer resistance to the antibiotic.

A major example is the blocking of bacterial folic acid production by sulphonamides which inhibit chromosomal-coded dihydrofolate reductase. However, episome-mediated dihydrofolate reductase can be acquired and is not blocked by sulphonamides; such bacteria become sulphonamide resistant as a result.

4. *Drug inactivation.* This important mechanism is usually mediated by the transmission of r-determinant episomes, as described earlier. Inactivation of many of the penicillins by β-lactamases and of chloramphenicol by acetyl transferase are well-known examples.

Broadly speaking, therefore, the mechanisms of bacterial antibiotic resistance are as follows:

1. *Antibiotic tolerance* – reduced permeability to the drug, changes in target substances within bacteria and bypassing blocked metabolic pathways all render bacteria tolerant to an antibiotic
2. *Antibiotic destruction* – the best-known example of induced enzymic antibiotic destruction is the production of penicillinases (β-lactamases), but other enzymes can inactivate cephalosporins, aminoglycosides and chloramphenicol.

Cross-resistance. In most cases bacteria resistant to an antibiotic are resistant to variants of the antibiotic which are chemically closely related. Staphylococci resistant to benzyl penicillin, for example, are resistant to most other related penicillins, but are sensitive to the penicillinase-resistant penicillins (cloxacillin and its relatives). Bacteria resistant to penicillins may also show resistance to the cephalosporins which chemically resemble the penicillins. For all practical purposes, bacteria resistant to one tetracycline are resistant to all. The same principle applies to the sulphonamides and other agents, where different members of the group have been formed by relatively minor chemical modifications to the basic substance.

Antibiotic resistance – preventive measures

1. Avoid the use of antibiotics unless they are essential. The overuse of antibiotics has contributed to the increasing number of antibiotic-resistant infections in hospitals. Even worse, chloramphenicol-resistant *Salmonella typhi* have infected some 100 000 patients in Mexico in recent years and caused more than 14 000 deaths. Resistant strains of *S. typhi* are also widespread in other countries where there is unrestricted public sale of antibiotics, particularly in India, Thailand and Vietnam.

2. When an antibiotic has to be given, give it in adequate doses and for long enough to be reasonably certain that the infection has been eliminated. Inadequate treatment can allow resistant survivors to proliferate.

3. In the case of life-threatening infections, emergence of resistant strains may be prevented by combination therapy, as discussed in relation to tuberculosis. Combination chemotherapy is also used in the treatment of infective endocarditis.

16. Antiseptics, anticaries agents and related drugs used in routine dentistry

In the lay mind, Victorian concepts about spread of infection die hard and it still seems to be believed that bacteria leap out of drains and lavatory pans to attack anyone nearby. This strange belief enables the manufacturers of antiseptics to achieve what must be the purest and most complete apotheosis of capitalism. Advertisements therefore exhort housewives to protect their families by pouring antiseptics (literally) down the drain and, as a corollary, to hasten out to buy more in order to repeat the process ad infinitum. The benefits from this cycle of events come, of course, solely to the manufacturers and their advertising agents.

Historically, antiseptics played a crucial role in the early victories against infection. The name of Lister is inseparably associated with his introduction of antiseptics into the operating room and his success in reducing infection introduced by surgeons.

Antiseptics must be clearly distinguished from antibiotics and their synthetic analogues. Antiseptics have a relatively crude toxic effect on living cells, but in high concentration, and *given enough time*, can kill a variety of accessible bacteria when circumstances are favourable.

Antibiotics, by contrast, act in exceedingly low concentrations and have selective actions which interfere with the metabolism of microorganisms in such a way as to have bacteriostatic or bactericidal effects. Unlike antiseptics, antibiotics are effective and generally innocuous when given systemically.

Disinfectants and antiseptics

There is no real difference between antiseptics and disinfectants. Disinfection refers to the *cleansing* of any item and implies the removal of bacterial contamination, particularly by antiseptics. However, the latter will only kill some of these contaminants and are generally ineffective against bacterial spores. Antiseptics are often little more effective than thorough mechanical cleansing with soap and water, and should in general only be used in conjunction with the latter.

Antiseptics poison living tissues, whether human or bacterial, and their limitations are as follows:

1. They are non-selective in their action on cells and need to be used in relatively high concentrations
2. They require considerable time (usually many hours) to destroy significant numbers of bacteria
3. They are usually inhibited by organic matter such as blood or pus
4. They are usually ineffective against bacterial spores and will not necessarily destroy viruses.

As a consequence of these limitations, antiseptics are only of value in disinfecting contaminated surfaces. They are ineffective or poisonous if given internally and their differences from antibiotics and related antimicrobials have been described in the previous chapter. Antiseptics will also not sterilise instruments; this can only be achieved by autoclaving. However, it may sometimes be acceptable to store *sterilised* instruments in an antiseptic solution temporarily.

Mode of action of antiseptics

Antiseptics can act in a variety of ways including:

1. *Coagulation and precipitation of cell proteins.* Phenols are an example.

2. *Damage to cell membranes.* This allows leakage of cell contents, particularly electrolytes, and cell death. Detergents in particular affect cell membranes.

3. *Oxidation of thiol (SH) groups.* Many cell enzymes are dependent on free SH groups. When these are oxidised by agents such as the halogens, cell damge is severe and the cell usually dies.

Antiseptics are therefore toxic to cells in general. These effects are not specific to microorganisms, but severe damage to host cells can be limited by restricting the use of antiseptics in man to superficial application where the intact epithelium is protective, or to hard dental tissues which are resistant to chemical damage. Some antiseptics can be used to irrigate wounds but must be used in dilute solution and only if they have no toxic effect if absorbed.

The effectiveness of an antiseptic depends upon:

1. The properties of the agent itself
2. The degree of dilution
3. The time for which it is allowed to act
4. The degree of interference by other materials, either organic contaminants such as blood or pus or chemicals such as soap.

Some antiseptics are relatively unstable and after a time break down; antibacterial power is then lost or the solution will actually support bacterial growth.

Uses of antiseptics

Antiseptics should only supplement and are not a substitute for adequate mechanical cleansing. They can be used for two main purposes, namely:

1. Disinfection of non-living surfaces – often termed 'environmental disinfectants'
2. For use on living surfaces, namely skin, mucous membranes and teeth.

Typical applications of antiseptics in hospital are therefore:

1. Disinfection of surfaces in high-risk areas such as operating areas
2. Disinfection of faecally or other heavily contaminated articles
3. Disinfection of food preparation areas
4. Preoperative cleansing of surgeons' and patients' skin.

INDIVIDUAL ANTISEPTICS

Phenolics

Phenol derivatives such as Sudol or Hycolin are cresols in soap solution used for environmental disinfection of such things as floors or bedpans. They are cheap and effective, have a wide range of antibacterial activity and are not easily inactivated, but tend to be irritant or caustic.

Cresols of various sorts, beechwood creosote (which contains cresols) and other phenolics such as paramonochlorphenol have been used as dressings to disinfect root canals. They are strongly antiseptic, but agents such as paramonochlorphenol nevertheless seem to do little harm and (surprisingly) do not appear to irritate periapical tissues.

Alcohols

Ethyl and isopropyl alcohol are effective and rapidly active. At the optimal concentration of 70%, alcohol is useful for preparing clean skin for injections. It is, however, ineffective on the oral mucosa.

Surgical spirit (a mixture of methyl and ethyl alcohol) is used for wiping down surfaces such as trolley tops or bracket tables.

Halogens

Hypochlorites have a wide range of antibacterial activity by releasing chlorine. Their action is rapid but they are inactivated by organic matter. Strong solutions (e.g. Chloros) have a characteristic smell and bleaching power. Milder compounds such as Milton (1% sodium hypochlorite) can be used for irrigation of root canals to wash out infected debris after reaming and for disinfecting acrylic dentures in patients with denture stomatitis (candidosis).

Sodium hypochlorite (2%) is also recommended for cleaning work surfaces where there is a risk of contamination by hepatitis viruses. Hypochlorites are effectively virucidal (if allowed sufficient time), but are corrosive and may blunt some stainless-steel instruments.

Iodine. Iodine (2.5%) in 70% alcohol is a strong and rapidly acting bactericidal agent, and will kill some spores and viruses in addition to most bacteria and fungi. It is not greatly inhibited by organic matter and is effective for surgical preparation of clean skin. It stains the skin and can, rarely, cause sensitisation or severe rashes in an already sensitised person.

Organic halogen compounds

Iodophors. Iodophors are combinations of iodine and surface-active detergents which act together to have a cleansing and enhanced germicidal effect. Iodine is slowly released and the action is prolonged. These preparations are non-irritant, are said not to cause sensitisation and are non-staining. Povidone iodine (Betadine) is widely used for preparation of patients' skin and operators' hands before surgery.

Chloroxylenols. Chloroxylenols have a pleasant smell but are greatly inactivated by organic matter. Their antibacterial activity is relatively weak and unreliable. Dettol is the best-known example. This is so ineffective against one opportunistic pathogen (*Pseudomonas aeruginosa*) that it is used in culture media as a selective agent to encourage the growth of this organism.

Hexachlorophane. Hexachlorophane is effective mainly against Gram-positive cocci, particularly *Staphylococcus aureus*. It is non-irritant and rarely causes sensitisation, but in babies absorption through the skin can be toxic. Hexachlorophane leaves a germicidal residue to the skin and is an effective preparation widely used for disinfection of patients' skin and surgeons' hands before operation. For this purpose hexachlorophane is incorporated into soap or used as a detergent cream (e.g. Phisohex). Disinfection is slower than with chlorhexidine so that hexachlorophane must be applied repeatedly to achieve a useful effect by cumulative action. Despite its antiseptic properties hexachlorophane can become contaminated and permit the growth of bacteria.

Chlorhexidine (Hibitane). Chlorhexidine, a biguanide, is a highly effective antiseptic with a wide and rapid antibacterial action, especially when in alcoholic solution. It is as effective as iodine in alcohol, both of which when rubbed firmly on to the skin on gauze for 2 min remove about 80% of skin organisms. Chlorhexidine is non-irritant and non-toxic. It is inactivated by soap but cationic detergent preparations such as Hibiscrub are available.

Chlorhexidine (0.5%) in 70% alcohol and Hibiscrub are both widely used for preoperative skin preparation of both patient and surgeon. It is non-corrosive so that it can be used for storing sterile instruments or burs and is an effective and useful general purpose antiseptic for dental purposes.

The effectiveness of chlorhexidine in aqueous solution is enhanced by the cationic detergent cetrimide. This preparation known as Savlon can be used for a wide variety of purposes from irrigation of wounds to the cleansing of instrument trolleys.

Chlorhexidine in alcohol also has a rapid antiseptic action on the oral mucosa and in aqueous solution inhibits dental plaque formation. However, it does not of course remove existing plaque.

Aldehydes

Aldehydes are potent bactericidal agents, but *formaldehyde* is little used now.

Glutaraldehyde is more potent, more rapidly acting, less irritant and lacks the unpleasant smell of formaldehyde. 2% glutaraldehyde in 70% isopropyl alcohol may be used for so-called 'cold sterilisation' of delicate instruments such as glass-fibre optic endoscopes. Many bacteria are killed after a 30 min exposure and many spores are destroyed after 7–10 h. Nevertheless, full sterilisation is not achieved, and the action of glutaraldehyde against *M. tuberculosis*, for example, is weak.

Glutaraldehyde (2%) may be used for treatment of articles, such as impressions contaminated by HIV or hepatitis B virus, but which cannot be autoclaved. Exposure to 2% glutaraldehyde for this purpose should be for at least 1 h, but preferably for 12 h.

Glutaraldehyde should not be used on body surfaces as it is irritant and allergenic and a pollutant.

Dyes

Aniline dyes such as crystal (gentian) violet and brilliant green are active against some Gram-positive organisms, but are easily inactivated by organic matter. Application of gentian violet was a traditional treatment for infantile thrush, but it is potentially irritant and its use on mucous membranes or unbroken skin is no longer advised. In any case it is also so messy as to be obsolete.

Acridine dyes, particularly acriflavine and proflavine, have a wider range of antibacterial activity than the aniline dyes, are bactericidal and are not appreciably inactivated by organic matter. They can be used for application to superficial wounds or burns.

Quaternary ammonium compounds

Benzalkonium chloride (Roccal) and *cetrimide* (Cetavlon) are examples. They are good detergents, but poor antiseptics. Their action is mainly bacteriostatic and is against only a narrow range of microorganisms. They also support the growth of *Pseudomonas aeruginosa*. They are inhibited by organic matter and completely inactivated by soap.

DISINFECTION POLICIES

Policies determining the choice and uses of antiseptics vary from one hospital to another but a typical example is as follows:

1. *Environmental disinfectants*:
   a. Hycolin (2%) for routine use apart from food preparation surfaces;
   b. Sodium hypochlorite (1%) (must be freshly prepared); especially indicated for clearing up blood or other discharges from hepatitis or AIDS patients.
2. *Staff handwashing*:
   a. The hands should be washed thoroughly in liquid soap and water;
   b. Povidone iodine (7.5%) (Betadine) surgical scrub or, especially by those sensitive to iodine, chlorhexidine (4%) surgical scrub (Hibiscrub) should be used.

   The hands cannot be sterilised, but scrubbing up in this way will significantly reduce the bacterial count on the skin surface for a limited period. Surgical gloves give added protection, but microbes readily leak out through minute perforations. For extra protection, in high-risk situations, two pairs of gloves may need to be worn.
3. *Preoperative preparation of patients' skin:*
   a. Thorough washing with soap and water;
   b. Paint with povidone iodine (10%) in alcohol *or* chlorhexidine (0.5%) in alcohol.
4. *Skin cleaning before injections:* wipe with 70% isopropyl alcohol.

USES OF ANTISEPTICS IN DENTISTRY

The main occasions when antiseptics are used in dentistry can be summarised as follows:

1. For storing sterilised surgical instruments and operating equipment
2. For preparation of the skin before surgery
3. For preparation of the surgeon's hands
4. For preparation of the skin before injections or venepuncture
5. For preparation of the oral mucosa before injections
6. For dressing infected sockets
7. For superficial infections of the mouth in lozenges or mouthwashes
8. In dentifrices
9. For inhibition of bacterial plaque (chlorhexidine)
10. In endodontic treatment
11. For irrigation of infected areas, such as pericoronitis
12. In cross-infection control.

These uses will not all be discussed in detail, but antiseptics will be considered in relation to other measures used in the management of some of the more important infections of the mouth and teeth.

Instruments and operating equipment

Antiseptics should not be used in an attempt to

sterilise instruments. Sterilisation should preferably be by autoclaving (134°C for 3 min). Antiseptics can, at most, be used for short-term storage of heat-sterilised instruments.

Antiseptics are used for cleaning the surface of bracket tables or operating trolleys. But even then an operating trolley should be covered by a sterile towel on which the instruments lie.

Preparation of surgeons' hands

Surgeons' hands often carry pathogens. Wearing surgical gloves gives partial protection to the patient but microbes can escape through minute perforations. 'Scrubbing up' for surgery involves thorough washing followed by the use of antiseptics, and similar methods are used as for preparation of the skin of the operating site.

As mentioned earlier, a typical regimen would be to wash the hands thoroughly with running water and a detergent antiseptic containing hexachlorophane, chlorhexidine or povidone–iodine followed by application of 10 ml of 0.5% chlorhexidine in alcohol rubbed on the hands until dry. In spite of extreme care and the use of potent antiseptics, patients' skin and surgeons' hands cannot be sterilised. The best that can be achieved in practical terms is a significant reduction in the resident bacteria for a limited period.

Preparation of the skin for surgery

Before a skin incision is made, the patient's own dermal bacteria must be eliminated as far as possible from the field of operation. The usual skin flora often include staphylococci and other pathogens, but these tend to be deeply entrenched, particularly in hair follicles.

Adequate skin preparation requires thorough washing, for which purpose an antiseptic soap, such as *Hibiscrub* (*chlorhexidine* in detergent) can be used. This is followed by applications of potent, but not irritant, antiseptics. This can be done by firm swabbing with alcoholic chlorhexidine for several minutes. When the skin is deeply contaminated or the risks of infection are high (as in poorly vascular tissue) repeated compresses of an *iodophor* (*povidone–iodine*) for 30 min at a time will give better clearance of skin bacteria. Where applicable, the skin must be shaved just before antiseptic preparation.

Preparation of skin surfaces for injection or venepuncture

It is traditional to cleanse the skin with 70% isopropyl alcohol.

Preparation of the oral mucous membrane

The oral mucosa represents a much less severe problem than the skin. Virulent pathogens are virtually only found in periodontal pockets, and are inaccessible to antiseptics. However, local immunity is high and, as a consequence, teeth are extracted with minimal aseptic or antiseptic precautions. The residual bony wound, with rare exceptions, heals remarkably rapidly. Infected sockets are usually due to other causes.

It may be considered desirable to prepare the oral mucosa before injecting a local anaesthetic but, if this is to be anything more than a gesture, the antiseptic must (1) act very quickly (within 30 s) and (2) have a drying effect on the mucosa to prevent recontamination with saliva. The only preparations which are at all effective are therefore those in alcoholic solution such as iodine or (better) 2% chlorhexidine. Seventy per cent alcohol which is effective as a skin antiseptic is ineffective on the oral mucosa.

Preparation of the oral mucosa for surgery is not a practical proposition as contamination with saliva is inevitable.

Infected sockets

These are generally spoken of as 'dry' sockets because of the absence of clot. The main predisposing factors may be (1) poor local blood supply, (2) operative trauma, and (3) local fibrinolytic activity. The lower molar region is usually affected and infection was a common complication of disimpaction of third molars in the era before the introduction of antibiotics.

An infected socket is an area of localised osteitis where part of the bone of the lamina dura dies and eventually sequestrates. These sequestra are usually small, however, and are eventually shed unnoticed.

The clot having been destroyed, the socket fills with debris from the mouth and there is persistent low-grade infection. Once this has happened, antibiotics have no useful effect.

The usual measures are to:

1. Irrigate the socket thoroughly with warm dilute antiseptic or normal saline to remove debris
2. Lightly pack the socket with Whitehead's varnish on ribbon gauze or an appropriate proprietary preparation
3. Repeat daily if pain remains severe and persistent
4. Prescribe a hot salt mouthwash to keep the rest of the mouth clean
5. Prescribe an analgesic such as aspirin.

Healing takes its own time and the socket eventually fills with granulation tissue. This may take 10 or more days, in its initial stages at least, is very painful, and there is so far no effective way of hastening resolution. Hence, where there is a strong chance of this complication – as after difficult disimpaction of third molars – prophylactic use of an antibiotic may be justified, although its value is unproven. Infected sockets are, by contrast, so uncommon a complication of ordinary dental extractions that the routine use of antibiotics is pointless and undesirable.

Superficial injections of the mouth and throat

Antiseptic lozenges. These contain antiseptics such as cetyl pyridinium or benzalkonium chloride and are popular over-the-counter preparations used for conditions ranging from aphthous stomatitis to sore throats. There is no evidence that these lozenges are of any benefit and they can cause harm by chemical irritation or by inducing superinfection if used persistently. Worse still, diagnosis of serious diseases, especially cancer, can be delayed if the patient chooses to treat himself rather than get expert help.

Mouthwashes. Mouthwashes have a mechanical cleansing effect. Any antiseptic that they contain has little effect since it is in the mouth for so short a time. The warmth of a mouthwash may also be comforting and is traditionally thought to improve the local circulation. Again any such effect is transient.

CROSS-INFECTION CONTROL

The two most serious infections from which the dental surgeon is currently at risk are hepatitis B and AIDS. Vaccination against hepatitis B is particularly important, and gives adequate protection to most (but not all) of those that receive it. There is also a small risk of transmission of hepatitis C. HIV infection can be acquired via needle-stick injuries. At least one general surgeon has died from this disease acquired occupationally and it has been transmitted by a dentist in the USA to several of his patients. The possibility of HIV transmission to or from a dental patient cannot therefore be dismissed, though the risk is of a very low order. The following are basic precautions to lessen these hazards, but it must be borne in mind that carriers of these viruses will frequently be treated unknowingly.

1. The patient should be treated at the end of the working day.

2. Dental staff should wear gloves (preferably two pairs), mask, gown and paper apron. Any skin wounds should be adequately protected.

3. Disposable instruments should be used wherever possible and all non-disposable instruments should be autoclaved (121°C for 20 min, or 134°C for 3 min) after decontamination in fresh 1% sodium hypochlorite.

4. Air turbines can be used, but goggles should be worn to protect against aerosol spread of microbes and where there is any risk of splatter. As with all other procedures, high volume aspiration should be used.

5. Needles should not be resheathed (except into a special receiver), broken or bent, or removed from disposable syringes.

6. All disposable instruments should be put in puncture-proof boxes, double wrapped in plastic bags which are clearly labelled as a biohazard, for transmission to the incinerator.

7. All working surfaces should be covered with plastic sheeting.

8. Any spilt blood or other discharge should be quickly wiped up using fresh 1% sodium hypochlorite.

9. Instruments and impressions which cannot be autoclaved should be soaked in 2% glutaraldehyde or a proprietary alternative for at least an hour, but preferably overnight.

Hepatitis B vaccines

Hepatitis B is more readily transmitted than is HIV and, once acquired, can lead to chronic liver disease or be fatal. Dental surgeons are at high risk of infection by the hepatitis B virus and the even more dangerous delta agent. Active immunisation is highly advisable as it protects against both agents.

The vaccines consist of a suspension of hepatitis B surface antigen. The latter is made biosynthetically by recombinant DNA techniques. Three doses are given over 6 months and a booster dose may be given later. Adverse effects are uncommon and mild, but include soreness at the injection site, headache, malaise or joint pains.

If there has been exposure or suspected exposure to the virus, specific hepatitis B immune globulin (HBIG) should be given for immediate passive protection and followed by active immunisation.

PREVENTION OF DENTAL CARIES

Dental decay is an infective process. It is the result of a localised attack on the enamel and dentine by bacteria concentrated within an adhesive plaque. It is mediated by bacterial acids produced by the metabolism of sugar from the diet.

The main components of dental plaque are bacteria and polysaccharides (polyglucans) synthesised particularly by the *Streptococcus mutans* group. Essential properties of cariogenic bacteria appear to be an ability both to produce acid and to synthesise polysaccharides. The latter give the plaque its adhesive properties, prevent dilution or neutralisation of bacterial acid by saliva, and form a reserve nutrient supply for the bacteria.

Plaque forms on all surfaces of the teeth, but caries develops only in stagnation areas where plaque can form thickly and remain undisturbed. The main factors necessary for caries to develop are as follows:

1. Cariogenic bacteria
2. Bacterial plaque
3. Substrate (dietary sugar) for acid production
4. Stagnation areas on the teeth
5. Susceptible dental tissues.

Prevention of dental caries may, as a consequence, be based in theory or in practice on use of one or more of the following measures:

1. Antibacterial (antiseptics, antibiotics or vaccines)
2. Restriction of substrate (limitation of frequency of sugar intake)
3. Obliteration of stagnation areas (fissure sealants)
4. Raising the resistance of the dental tissues (fluorides).

Of these, the main practicable measures are limitation of frequency of sugar intake and use of fluorides. Fissure sealants are effective but relatively labour intensive. Chlorhexidine has a possible role.

Antiseptics

Chlorhexidine mouth rinses can inhibit plaque formation if used regularly, but do not penetrate stagnation areas. However, it has been suggested that chlorhexidine may have a preventive effect once caries activity has been controlled by restorations and other means.

Fissure sealants

Fissure sealants are plastics which are either bonded to dental hard tissue by the so-called 'acid-etch technique' (to form a submicroscopic mechanical key) or by direct (chemical) adhesion to the tissues. Examples include methacrylate and polyurethane compounds, some of which also incorporate fluoride salts.

These agents seal the pits and fissures with a protective layer resistant to acid attack. They cannot be used on interproximal surfaces, but the occlusal pits and fissures are the most vulnerable zones and the first to be attacked in children. These areas are also the least well protected by fluorides.

FLUORIDES AND THEIR ACTIONS ON THE DENTAL TISSUES

Fluoride was detected in human dental enamel in 1805 and waterborne fluoride was detected by Berzelius in 1822. By 1897 it had not merely been hypothesised that fluoride would make teeth more caries resistant but it was also postulated that this effect might be mediated by an anti-enzymic or antibacterial effect. Fluoride-containing dentifrices became available at least as early as 1902. The whole matter was more or less forgotten until the 1930s when it was confirmed that fluorides had a caries-prevention action. They are as yet the only effective drug for this purpose.

Absorption and distribution

Fluorides are rapidly absorbed from the gut. They have a strong affinity for calcium salts, particularly calcium phosphate, and become incorporated into bones and teeth. Any remaining fluoride is excreted in the urine. Fluorides continue to enter bone after development is complete but, after the teeth have been fully formed, negligible amounts of fluoride are incorporated by continued apposition of cementum. In these tissues fluorides replace hydroxyl groups to form calcium fluorapatite.

Effects of fluorides on the teeth

The optimal effect is achieved when drinking-water containing about 1 part per million (ppm) of fluoride, is ingested throughout the period of dental development. These persons have about 50% less dental caries than those from non-fluoride areas. This finding has been confirmed on so vast a scale in many parts of the world that all other variables that might affect these results can reasonably be excluded.

Inhibition of dental caries by fluorides

Mechanism of action. The means by which fluoride reduces dental caries appear to be as follows:

1. By a direct effect on the development of dental enamel as follows:

a. Fluorapatite is more resistant to solution by acid than hydroxyapatite. The initial rate of dissolution of these two compounds may be similar but there is secondary precipitation of insoluble calcium fluoride from fluorapatite on the surface of the enamel crystallites. This reduces the rate of movement of hydrogen ions into the crystals and slows further dissolution.

b. Larger crystallites are formed. These have fewer imperfections, the crystalline lattice is more stable and a smaller surface area per unit volume is accessible for attack by hydrogen ions.

c. The enamel has a lower carbonate content. This also lowers solubility.

d. Calcium phosphates are reprecipitated when enamel is attacked and fluoride enhances the possibility of their crystallising as apatite. Remineralisation of enamel after attack is therefore favoured.

2. Effects on the enamel surface. Fluorides may reduce the tendency of the enamel surface to adsorb proteins. In this way plaque may not build up so quickly.

3. Effects of fluoride on bacterial plaque. Fluoride is incorporated into bacterial plaque in relatively high concentrations but mostly bound to organic material. Were the fluoride in plaque mainly unbound (in ionised form), the concentration might be high enough to affect bacterial metabolism, and possibly inhibit acid production, or synthesis of polysaccharides. However, it is questionable whether the small proportion of free fluoride in plaque is sufficient to have any of these effects.

Methods of fluoride use

Fluorides can act systemically or locally on the teeth. Both effects can be achieved when fluoride salts are ingested after the teeth have erupted. Methods of using fluorides are:

1. *Ingestion*
   a. In drinking-water, other fluids or foods
   b. Fluoride tablets
2. *Local applications*
   a. Toothpastes
   b. Mouth rinses
   c. Topical application.

Fluoride in drinking-water

Fluorides are most effective when ingested throughout the period of dental development. This is most conveniently, effectively, reliably, economically and safely achieved by the addition of sodium fluoride to the water supply to maintain a concentration of one part per million (1 mg/l). In addition to its effects on the development and maturation of enamel, fluorides ingested in the drinking-water can also have a topical effect on the teeth.

No effort is needed by recipients and since daily fluid intake is relatively constant, the daily dose level is equally constant. Overdose is practically impossible, since about 2500 l of water would have to be swallowed in a short period to cause acute poisoning. Chronic overdose is almost equally difficult to achieve.

Fluorides in food

An expressed objection to fluoridation of water is that adults who are at a lower risk from dental caries continue to take in fluorides unnecessarily. Although there is no evidence of any harmful effect, long-term exposure might conceivably have as yet unrecognised actions.

Fluoride salts can be added to school milk or to table salt. Both are effective, but both are less reliable than fluoride added to the water, as intake can vary widely.

Fluoride tablets

Where water is not fluoridated infants and children can be given fluoride tablets. These contain 0.55–1.1 mg of sodium fluoride (250–500 µg F^-), usually in a lactose base. When taken by the mother during pregnancy, the fetus benefits little as the placenta acts as an effective barrier to the fluoride ion. Even more important, the fluoride is taken up in maternal bone.

Mottling of enamel can be a complication even of conventional dosage of fluoride tablets, especially as a fluoridised dentifrice is likely also to be used. Because of wide individual susceptibility to mottling, a balance has to be struck between adequate protection and the risk of discoloration of the teeth. The currently *suggested* regimen is as follows:

1. To be used only where fluoride in the drinking-water is less than 0.7 ppm.
2. To be taken as soon as teeth start to erupt.
3. Tablets should be chewed to get a local effect also, and taken before retiring.
4. Dosage:

a. Water content less than 0.3 ppm

Up to 6 months	none
6 months to 2 years	0.5 mg NaF (250 µg F^-)/day
2–4 years	1.1 mg NaF (500 µg F^-)/day
Over 4 years	2.2 mg NaF (1 mg F^-)/day.

b. Water content 0.3–0.7 ppm

Up to 2 years	none
2–4 years	0.5 mg NaF (250 µg F^-)/day
Over 4 years	1.1. mg NaF (500 µg F^-)/day.

If the child allows a tablet of fluoride to dissolve slowly in the mouth at night just before going to sleep, it can produce a concentration of fluoride of 500–1000 ppm locally. It also allows the fluoride a long period to act. Pleasantly flavoured fluoride tablets are available, and by this means reductions in caries of up to 90% or greater have been reported.

Fluoridised toothpastes

If the teeth are brushed regularly and efficiently then the fluoride salt is brought by a mildly abrasive vehicle into intimate contact with the enamel once or twice daily. Fluoride toothpastes can reduce caries by 20–30%.

In the past, fluoride salts tended to become rapidly bound to calcium carbonate (the commonly used abrasive) and a satisfactory alternative abrasive was not easy to find. Some fluoride salts, notably stannous fluoride, stain the teeth and some fluoride toothpastes have an unpleasant flavour.

Current fluoride toothpastes contain sodium fluoride and sodium monofluorophosphate with a relatively inert abrasive. Nevertheless, the amount of available fluoride declines gradually during storage as it reacts with other components.

Infants using fluoride toothpastes swallow a significant amount of fluoride. The worst that can be expected from this small quantity of ingested fluoride is mild mottling of the enamel. On the other hand, greater resistance to caries may result from incorporation of the ingested fluoride into the forming enamel.

However, virtually only fluoride-containing dentifrices are currently available, and following their introduction there has been a remarkable decline in the prevalence of dental caries in children, with little or no evidence of adverse effects. Admittedly there are other possible explanations for this phenomenon, but it seems likely that the widespread use of fluoride dentifrices, encouraged by persuasive advertising, has had a major effect.

Fluoride mouth rinses

This method can also be effective. The best results have been obtained from daily use of a 0.05% sodium fluoride solution rinsed round the mouth for 1 or 2 min.

Supervision is needed to ensure that the rinse is used for an adequate period and to see that the rinse is not swallowed. The effort needed is therefore considerable and the procedure is too labour intensive to be used except domestically, where a parent can supervise the child.

Fluoride salts for topical application

Sodium fluoride. This is usually applied as a 2% solution. The advantages of sodium fluoride are: (1) it is stable chemically but has to be stored in plastic containers as glass may be attacked; (2) the taste is not too unpleasant; (3) it is not irritating to the gingivae; and (4) it does not stain the teeth.

Stannous fluoride. Stannous fluoride is used in a 2–8% solution. It is widely believed to be more effective than 2% sodium fluoride. In vitro stannous fluoride apparently also slows the rate of solution of enamel by acid. Disadvantages of stannous fluoride are: (1) it is unstable in aqueous solution (its effectiveness is rapidly reduced and a fresh solution must be made up on each occasion); (2) it has an unpleasant and astringent flavour; (3) it sometimes causes gingival irritation and blanching; and (4) it often stains the teeth. To overcome some of these disadvantages, a stable 0.4% stannous fluoride gel (Omnigel) is available.

Acidulated phosphate fluoride (APF). APF is a solution of sodium fluoride in weak phosphoric acid. Laboratory studies suggest that APF enhances uptake by enamel of fluoride as compared with a stannous or neutral sodium fluoride.

Clinical trials have shown that APF gives a greater reduction in caries than other topically applied fluorides. As seems to be usual, the striking improvements noted in the initial trials have not been entirely repeated in later trials, but APF may have a significantly better effect than sodium or stannous fluoride.

Fluoride gels. APF has been incorporated into a gel which is applied to the teeth in specially designed trays. Fluoride gels applied in commercially made trays have also been proposed for home use by parents of caries-prone children. However, unsupervised application of fluorides in this way can lead to undesirable amounts of fluoride being ingested; this may cause nausea. Home use of fluoride gels in this way should therefore be discouraged.*

In several areas of the country the prevalence of caries in children has declined so greatly that there now is little need for topical application of fluorides. The chief indications for these preparations are:

1. Highly caries-susceptible children, not responsive to other preventive measures
2. Patients with xerostomia, particularly those who have been irradiated for cancer.

Patients whose salivary glands have been destroyed by irradiation are not merely highly susceptible to dental caries, but also to osteoradionecrosis of the jaws and osteomyelitis secondary to infection from the teeth or to extractions. Prevention of caries and periodontal disease is therefore essential.

In such circumstances as these, where topical application of fluorides is indicated, APF gel is probably most widely favoured.

Toxic effects of fluorides

Ingestion of an overdose of sodium fluoride can cause acute poisoning, but is rare. More com-

*As one group of investigators quaintly expressed it, 'Home gelling should not be undertaken'.

monly there is continued intake of relatively large amounts of fluoride, either as an occupational hazard or as a result of high natural fluoride content of water which can give rise to chronic endemic fluorosis.

Acute fluoride poisoning

Sodium fluoride has been used as a rat poison and an insecticide. It is white powder which can be mistaken for such foods as flour or powdered milk. Acute poisoning has resulted from addition of sodium fluoride powder into food. The lethal dose of fluoride for man is probably about 2.5 g. Sodium fluoride in high concentrations is strongly irritant and some of the effects of ingestion of large amounts of this compound are nausea, vomiting, diarrhoea and bleeding from the gut.

In fatal cases death has usually been ascribed to poisoning of enzyme and transport systems. With massive overdose the blood has been noticed to be uncoagulated at autopsy. This presumably is due to calcium binding by fluoride which would also lead to tetany and cardiorespiratory failure.

Chronic endemic fluorosis

Chronic endemic fluorosis affects the teeth, the skeleton and, to a lesser extent, other organs.

Dental fluorosis – mottled enamel. Mottling of enamel is the most sensitive indicator of excess fluoride intake. It is seen when the fluoride content of the drinking-water exceeds 2–4 ppm. At such levels, changes in the skeleton may be difficult to detect.

The mildest form of dental fluorosis appears as chalky white patches in the enamel, though the surface is intact and of normal texture. These white patches become stained a brownish colour. With more severe fluorosis the enamel becomes rough or pitted and brittle. In spite of these defects the teeth retain an enhanced resistance to dental caries.

At a fluoride level of 1 ppm there is a significant, but invisible, effect on the teeth in terms of caries resistance and the skeleton shows no detectable change.

Skeletal fluorosis. Skeletal fluorosis develops when the fluoride content of the drinking-water exceeds 4 ppm, and this is seen particularly in north India and North and South Africa. The main features are excessive calcification. Osteophytes form at the margins of joints, tendons, ligaments, and fascia become calcified and joints become fused. The vertebral column in particular can become completely rigid. Radiologically the bone is dense; the structure is indistinct but, in spite of its greater density, fractures are common.

Clinical effects include stiffness of the back and legs and limitation or slowing of movement. Progressive osteosclerosis of the spine leads to narrowing of the neural canal and compression of the spinal cord. This can cause neurological complications of which the most severe is paraplegia.

Fluorides and osteoporosis

Osteoporosis is common in non-fluoride areas, but uncommon in areas where the water fluoride content is at least 4 ppm; the skeleton is of greater density than in non-fluoride areas. Osteoporosis is probably part of the ageing process and consists of progressive loss of osseous tissue from the skeleton. There is progressive thinning of trabeculae, increased radiolucency of the skeleton and weakening of bones. Common complications are collapse of vertebrae or fractures of the neck of the femur in the elderly, with delayed healing.

Fluorides stimulate osteoblasts and increase trabecular bone mass if given with additional calcium. However, the doses required to correct osteoporosis cause gastrointestinal side-effects and thus fluorides are obsolete for this purpose in Britain.

Fluorides in other drugs

Although the value of the fluorine ion is well-known in dentistry, its importance in pharmacology is less obvious. It is an essential element in all modern inhalational anaesthetic agents where it confers the valuable property of non-inflammability without the toxicity of other halogens. Fluoride is also an important component of many other drugs such as benzodiazepines, the benzodiazepine antagonist flumazenil and more than 20 other drugs with the prefix 'flu-'.

DENTIFRICES

The functions of dentifrices may be summarised as follows:

1. To assist removal of bacterial plaque
2. To reduce dental caries
3. To prevent gingivitis
4. To achieve other effects (e.g. desensitisation of exposed dentine).

Brushing teeth with a dentifrice will remove plaque, but only from accessible surfaces of the teeth (not from pits, fissures, or interstitial surfaces) and only if carried out carefully and conscientiously. Toothbrushing alone will remove plaque but a dentifrice aids the process and makes the whole dull business considerably more pleasant. Long-term comparative trials of toothbrushing with and without dentifrices have proved not to be feasible, because volunteers will not willingly forego the use of a dentifrice for more than a few days. Flavouring agents are therefore important components.

Thorough and regular toothbrushing will control or prevent marginal gingivitis, but has little or no effect on dental caries unless a fluoride is present in the dentifrice.

Composition

The basic components of toothpastes are:

1. Abrasive
2. Soap or detergent
3. Binding agents
4. Flavouring agents
5. Humectant
6. Preservative
7. Colouring.

In addition there may be ingredients with some pharmacological activity such as:

8. Fluoride salts
9. Antiseptics and antacids
10. Agents to desensitise exposed dentine.

Abrasives. These, with a detergent, materially aid removal of plaque. An abrasive is also essential for removal of stains from the teeth. It must be hard enough to remove deposits, but not so hard as to cause excessive wear of the enamel surface. Calcium carbonate (precipitated chalk) has been the most widely used, but this binds fluorides. Dicalcium phosphate, calcium pyrophosphate and other materials, including chemically inert plastic particles, have been used to overcome this difficulty.

The mechanical effect of the abrasive on the teeth depends on several variables. The amount of abrasive trapped among the toothbrush filaments depends both on the amount used and the effectiveness of the binding agent. The effect is enhanced by the stiffness of the filaments and the muscular effort put into the operation. Finally, once dentine is exposed, it is worn away more quickly than enamel.

Soaps and detergents. In the past, simple soaps were used, but synthetic detergents such as sodium lauryl sarcosinate are now more general.

Binding agents. A common example is carboxymethyl cellulose. This compound, used in commodities as diverse as wallpaper adhesive, purgatives and ice cream, forms a mildly adhesive gel. Imbibition of water from the saliva is slow so that the gel does not quickly wash away. This gel helps to keep the toothpaste in the toothbrush.

Flavouring agents. The importance of these agents, which make a tedious process more pleasant, have been emphasised. Flavouring agents are chosen to give, in advertisers' terms, sensations of 'freshness' or even 'tingling freshness'. Essential oils, particularly peppermint or spearmint, are common examples.

Non-fermentable sweeteners such as saccharine or sorbitol are also included. For obvious reasons, sucrose should not be used.

Humectants. These hygroscopic, or moisture-retaining, agents such as glycerine or sorbitol keep the paste soft and prevent it from solidifying.

Preservative. This is a non-toxic antiseptic, such as sodium benzoate, to inhibit bacterial proliferation in the preparation. It has no useful antibacterial action in the mouth.

Colouring. The dentifrice should look attractive, especially if children are to use it. Appropriately chosen colours also have a strong subjective effect in convincing the user how beneficial the preparation is – and what could be better than a multicoloured, striped toothpaste.

Fluoride salts. The use of fluorides in the inhibition of caries has been discussed. They are probably the only pharmacologically effective agent used in toothpastes.

Antiseptics and antacids. Antiseptics in toothpastes and mouthwashes have too weak an action and are too transiently in the mouth to have any significant effect. Chlorhexidine, by inhibiting plaque formation, may possibly have a useful effect, but there is as yet no positive evidence of effect when it is incorporated in a dentifrice.

Antacids such as magnesium hydroxide are incorporated in some dentifrices. However, plaque is very resistant to external changes in pH and is unaffected by transient changes in its immediate environment.

Desensitising agents. These are more or less irritant compounds which are designed to promote secondary dentine formation. If used in a dentifrice, however, they must not be so irritant as to damage the adjacent tissues. One commercial preparation contains 10% strontium chloride, and another 1.4% formalin, for this purpose.

Other desensitising agents have been applied directly to the area after it has been isolated with cotton wool rolls. These included silver nitrate, formalin, zinc chloride, fluoride salts and corticosteroids. The variety of agents recommended suggests that perhaps there is some uncertainty as to their effectiveness.

ANTIBACTERIAL EFFECTS OF TOOTHPASTES

Antiseptics present in toothpastes do not have any significant effect on dental disease. More important is the role of toothpastes in assisting mechanical removal of plaque and as a vehicle for fluorides.

Chlorhexidine and its derivative hexetidine are available in dentifrices and have a more persistent effect. Chlorhexidine 1% gel has the greatest effect and depression of salivary bacteria persists for up to 5 h. A hexetidine-containing, commercially available toothpaste has a lesser effect than chlorhexidine gel, but a still significantly greater effect than that of conventional antiseptics. Whether this effect is of any clinical value has not been shown.

Chlorhexidine

Chlorhexidine has proven to be a useful, effective and safe antiseptic with many applications. As mentioned earlier, it is one of the few agents which have been shown to clear the oral mucosa of bacteria as a preparation for injections.

Aqueous chlorhexidine has also been shown to inhibit dental bacterial plaque formation. It is active against oral streptococci, is absorbed on enamel, and may also bind to the polysaccharides of the plaque.

Chlorhexidine will not remove plaque but, if the teeth have been carefully scaled and polished, a mouthrinse of 0.1% or 0.2% chlorhexidine, preferably used at least twice daily, will diminish the amount of plaque formed. As long as chlorhexidine is used this effect is maintained and trials have shown this measure to be effective for 2 years or more. On the other hand, plaque formation quickly reverts to normal as soon as chlorhexidine is stopped.

Staining of the teeth may discourage some from using chlorhexidine, but the stain can usually be removed by toothbrushing with a conventional dentifrice. In many cases, however, it is the patient's failure to use a toothbrush and dentifrice effectively which has created the need to use chlorhexidine.

Although chlorhexidine can be shown to have a plaque-inhibiting effect, it is not as effective as toothbrushing. If the patient is an efficient and regular toothbrusher, chlorhexidine brings no additional benefits. Some trials have not confirmed the effectiveness of chlorhexidine in reducing plaque or gingivitis. The quantitation of plaque and gingivitis is notoriously subjective, and therefore it is not too surprising that findings have not been consistent.

Chlorhexidine is available commercially as a gel (1%) and as a 0.2% mouthwash. The gel has the advantage of having a more pleasant flavour but its effectiveness in the control of plaque seems not to have been convincingly established. The mouthwash appears to be more effective, but is probably best regarded as an aid to toothbrushing when the latter is substandard.

Before a course of chlorhexidine is started, all dental plaque and calculus should be removed to allow the drug a fair start.

An important limitation of chlorhexidine is that it does not penetrate into subgingival pockets or into stagnation areas in general. Hence it seems to have little effect on periodontal pockets, even though it may mitigate supragingival plaque formation.

The effect of chlorhexidine on dental caries seems to be no more than marginal, as mentioned earlier.

PERIODONTAL DISEASE

Drugs have little place in the routine prevention management of chronic periodontal disease.

Acute ulcerative gingivitis. This predominantly affects neglected mouths. Restoration of oral hygiene, with removal of deposits which harbour a vast number of bacteria, is the first essential. Such measures are important because anaerobes typically depend on other bacteria to maintain a low local oxygen tension. Oral hygiene can therefore be effective alone, but antimicrobials greatly hasten resolution. Metronidazole (three 200 mg tablets a day for 3 days) is usually given for its antianaerobic activity and is highly effective.

Chronic gingivitis and periodontitis. The most important aspect of the management of periodontal disease is control of bacterial plaque. This depends on regular conscientious toothbrushing. In periodontal pockets removal of sepsis depends primarily on mechanical cleansing measures such as root planing. Regular use of chlorhexidine as a mouth rinse (or possibly in a dentifrice) depresses dental plaque formation, but does not improve on effective toothbrushing.

Antibiotics, particularly tetracycline, have been used, usually as topical applications, for control of pocket bacteria in periodontal disease. Tetracycline may be effective for such diseases as accelerated periodontitis or suppurating pockets unresponsive to conventional treatment. Its exceptionally broad spectrum of activity may discourage proliferation of pathogenic Gram-negative and anaerobic bacteria which may not readily re-establish themselves. However, long-term use of tetracycline is likely to create a resistant bacterial population.

17. Local analgesia

The term 'analgesia' is used since *anaesthesia* implies unconsciousness. This may or may not be pedantic, but the term 'local anaesthetic' persists and both 'local anaesthesia' and 'local analgesia' are currently used and equivalent terms.

Mechanism of conduction of the nerve impulse

A nerve impulse (irrespective of whether it is afferent from a sense organ or efferent to a neuromuscular junction) is in effect a wave of electrical activity passing along the fibre. This electrical activity results from exchange of Na^+ and K^+ across the nerve cell membrane.

In the resting state the nerve cell membrane is permeable to potassium ions but relatively impermeable to sodium ions, so that there is a minute potential difference between the inside and the outside of the cell. In this resting state, sodium ions are forced outwards (by the so-called sodium pump) and the intracellular concentration of sodium kept at a low level. As a result, the concentration of sodium ions outside the cell is approximately 10 times higher than inside.

When a nerve impulse is initiated the permeability of a short length of an axon is momentarily but greatly increased. Sodium ions diffuse rapidly into the cell, overwhelming the sodium pump and suddenly reversing the polarity of the interior of the fibre relative to the exterior. The inrush of sodium ions is then balanced by escape of potassium ions. This membrane change, with resulting reversal in polarity of the interior relative to the exterior of the cell, is referred to as a *wave of depolarisation*. Its rapid movement along the fibre constitutes the nerve impulse (Fig. 17.1).

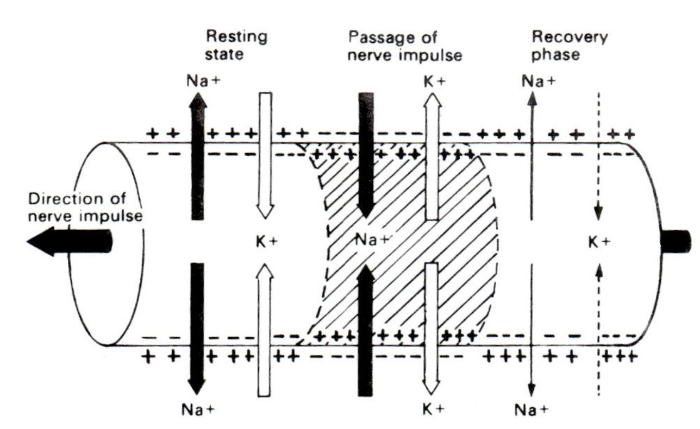

1. Resting state. The intracellular concentration of potassium ions greatly exceeds the extracellular concentration. The opposite is true for sodium which is actively 'pumped' out

2. Passage of impulse. There is a transient inrush of sodium ions and outflow of potassium ions and the polarity of the interior of the cell relative to the exterior is reversed (depolarisation).

3. Recovery phase. Sodium ions are ejected and replaced by potassium ions until the relative concentration of these two ions inside and outside the cell is restored to that of the resting state.

Fig. 17.1 Conduction of a nerve impulse.

In the immediate wake of the wave of depolarisation, the membrane starts to recover. Sodium ions are ejected by the sodium pump and potassium ions flow in. The relative concentration of these two ions inside and outside the cell is quickly restored to the levels characteristic of the resting state.

Mode of action of local analgesics

The mode of action of local analgesics is complex, but in essence they can be regarded as reversibly blocking sodium channels and thus the rapid inflow of sodium ions on which neural transmission depends.

The fact that local analgesics appear to act

selectively on sensory fibres is due to the stronger diffusion barriers around A fibres (motor and other functions) than around C fibres. Motor fibres are thickly myelinated.. An unusual local analgesic, etidocaine, is highly lipid soluble. Therefore it rapidly causes both motor and sensory blockade and, since an intraoral injection can, for example, paralyse the soft palate, etidocaine is no longer used. Most local analgesics are poorly soluble in lipids and rapidly enter C fibres, but penetration of the diffusion barriers around motor fibres is so slow that, normally, no significant block develops.

As a result of this process, clinical loss of function follows a consistent order. Autonomic functions and pain are lost first, followed by loss of sensations of cold, heat and light touch. Sensation of deep nerve pressure, and finally proprioception, and skeletal muscle tone and activity are lost.

Toxic effects of local analgesics

Though dental local analgesics such as lignocaine used in normal doses are remarkably harmless, most local analgesics if absorbed in sufficient quantity into the circulation have toxic effects on the CNS and heart.

Effects on the heart

With the exception of cocaine and bupivacaine, most local analgesics have a depressant action on the heart. This may sometimes be sufficient to cause a significant fall in cardiac output by reducing the rate and force of contraction. Nevertheless, advantage is taken of this action therapeutically, in that intravenous lignocaine is currently used to reduce the risk of ventricular fibrillation after a myocardial infarction. After ischaemic damage, hyperexcitability of the myocardium can result in such ineffective contractions that cardiac output falls to zero (Ch. 5). The stabilising action of lignocaine maximises the effectiveness of contractions and so raises cardiac output.

In contrast to such effects, cocaine is strongly sympathomimetic (Ch. 2) and increases heart rate and excitability to such an extent that a major cause of death among addicts is ventricular fibrillation. Bupivacaine can also cause cardiac arrhythmias which have caused over 50 deaths in the USA, mostly as a consequence of extradural blocks for obstetrics.

However, the toxic effects of dental local analgesics cannot be predicted in any simple way, because they are usually given with a vasoconstrictor (such as adrenaline) to prevent rapid absorption and to give a prolonged effect. Any cardiotoxic effect of a local analgesic is therefore the combined action of both substances. If some or all of the local analgesic preparation enters a blood vessel, the adrenaline – small though the amount is – may have a significant cardiovascular effect, namely palpitations and *possibly* cardiac irregularities, outweighing any toxic action of the local analgesic itself. Catecholamine vasoconstrictors have a slight but detectable systemic effect, even when they are localised to the site of injection by their own vasoconstrictor effect.

CNS effects

The typical toxic effects of local analgesics on the CNS are stimulation followed by depression. Again, cocaine is an exception in that it is so potent a central stimulant that overdose can result in convulsions and death. The action of lignocaine on the nervous system seems somewhat paradoxical in that intravenous injection of it for myocardial infarction can cause fits, but smaller doses of intravenous lignocaine have been used as an anticonvulsant for status epilepticus.

Despite these comments, modern local analgesics are remarkably safe and effective. Significant toxic effects are exceedingly rare if overdose is avoided.

Effectiveness of local analgesics

The effectiveness of a local analgesic under clinical conditions is affected by several variables, including:

1. The analgesic potency of the agent itself
2. The proximity of the point of injection to the appropriate nerves, i.e. the skill of the operator

3. The persistence of the agent at the site of injection (this mainly depends on the concentration and effectiveness of the added vasoconstrictor)
4. The rate at which the agent is metabolised at the site of injection
5. The extent of spread of anaesthesia.

In addition to the operator's skill, anatomical variations may result in the local analgesic being injected further from the nerve trunk than expected when a regional block is being carried out. Some spread of the analgesic effect is therefore desirable to cover such contingencies and also to provide an adequate field of analgesia, without having to give too many injections. Lignocaine in particular gives an excellent spread of anaesthesia. None of the more recently introduced agents seems to be so effective in this respect as 2% lignocaine with 1:80 000 adrenaline which, as a consequence, has retained a well-deserved popularity.

To try to obtain an effective inferior dental nerve block using procaine was (for those who can remember it) an experience which makes the advances in local analgesics only too apparent.

LOCAL ANALGESIC AGENTS

The main types are as follows:

1. *Esters*
   a. Cocaine
   b. Procaine
   c. Amethocaine
   d. Benzocaine
2. *Amides*
   a. Lignocaine
   b. Mepivacaine
   c. Prilocaine
   d. Bupivacaine.

Of these, the esters (with the exception of procaine) are used solely as surface anaesthetics. By contrast, only members of the amide group are used as injectable local analgesics for dental and medical purposes. Both ester and amide local analgesics are synthetic, apart from cocaine which is a natural product present in the leaves of the shrub *Erythroxylon coca*.

Therapeutic formulation of local analgesics

To enable local analgesics to be injected, they need to be soluble in both fats, to facilitate binding to neuronal lipids, and in water for formulation in stable solutions. Molecules of local analgesics are therefore usually composed of both hydrophilic and hydrophobic components joined by an ester or amide link. The hydrophilic component permits the preparation of hydrochloride salts that are both suitable for injection and able to dissociate at physiological pH to bind to nerves. Benzocaine which does not possess a hydrophilic component to its molecule is insoluble and, therefore, not injectable.

For clinical purposes, the composition of a typical local analgesic solution is as follows:

1. Lignocaine hydrochloride (usually 2%) or other local analgesic agent
2. Adrenaline (usually 1:80 000 = 12.5 μg/ml) or other vasoconstrictor
3. Modified Ringer's solution.

Termination of local analgesic action

The action of local analgesics is terminated by their removal by the circulation from their site of action and by enzymatic degradation. Esters are broken down by plasma cholinesterase. Amides, by contrast, are metabolised by hepatic amidases and the products excreted by the kidneys.

ESTERS

Cocaine

Cocaine was the first effective local analgesic. Its properties were the subject of early research by Sigmund Freud.* However, after a relatively short time Freud handed these investigations over to an ophthalmologist colleague, Koller, and went on to what he regarded as more interesting and important matters. After Koller's introduction of

*Freud himself was not apparently averse to taking cocaine from time to time (and who can blame him), but the suggestion by a recent biographer, that the whole of Freudian sexual and psychoanalytic theory is no more than the vapourings of a cocaine addict, seems a somewhat extreme view.

cocaine as a local analgesic for ophthalmology, Freud (with tedious facetiousness) used to refer to his friend as 'Coca Koller'.

Cocaine is probably the most effective surface analgesic, but is too toxic for use by injection.

Since cocaine has both direct and indirect sympathomimetic actions, it is unique as a local analgesic in being a strong vasoconstrictor. Hence cocaine produces not merely a localised and persistent effect but also protects the patient againsts its own systemic actions to some degree.

Applications. Cocaine should only be used as a surface analgesic but is so effective for this purpose that an ointment containing 20% of cocaine on cotton wool placed against the antral wall allows the underlying bone to be painlessly opened with a trocar. Topical cocaine has therefore remained in use for this purpose in ENT departments and is still sometimes used in ophthalmology.

In dentistry cocaine was occasionally, in the past, used topically in the depths of an apicectomy cavity when an orthodox local analgesic failed.

Toxic effects. The toxic effects of cocaine are mainly those of sympathetic overactivity and central stimulation. In addition to the effects on the CNS mentioned above, heart and respiration rates accelerate. Heightened myocardial excitability leads to progressively more severe disturbance of rhythm. Ventricular fibrillation or convulsions may be fatal.

The cerebral stimulant effect of cocaine makes it liable to addiction and it has become one of the most widely abused drugs (Ch. 4). It resembles the amphetamines in this respect, but dependence has considerably more serious effects. Cocaine is, therefore, a Controlled Drug and a Class A poison. Overdose causes restlessness, excitement and convulsions or ventricular fibrillation.

Incidentally, patients are not very likely to become addicted to cocaine used clinically. If that were so, all our parents or grandparents in the cocaine era would have become addicts. It would have been the dentist, who had access to the drug, who was more likely to become dependent.

Procaine

Procaine consists of a *p*-amino benzoic acid residue linked to an ester group (Fig. 17.2). The linking group is readily hydrolysed by cholinesterase and this contributes to the short duration of action of procaine when given by local infiltration. Procaine is also a weak vasodilator and is rapidly absorbed. Thus the much lower toxicity of procaine compared with cocaine is counterbalanced by its rapid absorption into the circulation. As a consequence, procaine must be given

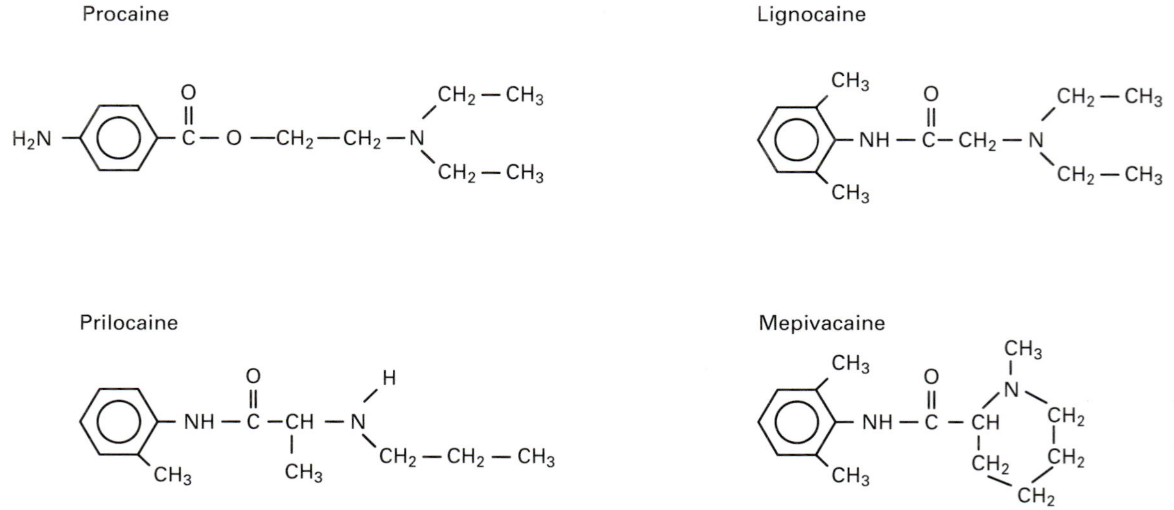

Fig. 17.2 The chemical differences between the ester local analgesic procaine and the amide, lignocaine. Also shown are two other amide analgesics: prilocaine and mepivacaine.

with a vasoconstrictor to ensure adequate duration of action and to minimise systemic toxic effects.

Procaine has no surface analgesic action.

Applications. Until the 1940s, procaine was the principal agent used for local analgesia, but since the introduction of the superior amide analgesics procaine has become obsolete for dental and other clinical purposes.

Toxic effects. The main effect is cerebral stimulation or excitement and restlessness going on to depression and ultimately, coma.

The cardiovascular effects are depression of myocardial excitability and of cardiac output. In addition there may be peripheral vasodilatation with the overall result that the blood pressure falls severely.

Hypersensitivity to procaine, like all other ester agents, can develop, particularly among those who handle it frequently.

AMIDES

Lignocaine

Lignocaine differs from procaine in that an amide group links the two parts of the molecule (Fig. 17.2). As a result it is not affected by plasma cholinesterase and is less rapidly metabolised than procaine. Lignocaine has no vasoconstrictor effect. As a consequence, a vasoconstrictor (usually adrenaline at a concentration of 1:100 000 or 1:80 000) is needed to give lignocaine adequate duration and reliability of action.

Applications. The combination of 2% lignocaine with 1:100 000 or 1:80 000 adrenaline in 2-ml cartridges provides an outstandingly effective, reliable and safe local analgesic for dental purposes.

Lignocaine without adrenaline can be given when thought necessary, but its action is unreliable and brief. If analgesia is inadequate, pain will cause endogenous catecholamine secretion. If, therefore, the patient is thought to be at risk from cardiovascular disease, omission of adrenaline has no practical advantages. Theoretically, prilocaine, with or without felypressin, may be safer, but its advantages in such situations are unproven and it provides no more than a false sense of security.*

Lignocaine has some surface analgesic activity (although this is weak in comparison with cocaine and amethocaine) and is widely used for this purpose, as discussed later.

Toxic effects.

1. *Cerebral.* Lignocaine in overdose usually causes cerebral depression without preliminary excitement. Moderate doses of lignocaine, as mentioned earlier, may be anticonvulsant.

2. *Cardiovascular.* In gross overdose lignocaine causes cardiac depression, but depresses cardiac excitability before it significantly weakens the force of contraction. Lignocaine, as a consequence, is the first choice for the control of dangerous tachyarrhythmias after myocardial infarction. For this purpose 100 mg is given intravenously.

3. *'Lignocaine allergy'.* Although isolated cases of 'lignocaine allergy' have very occasionally been reported, it is doubtful whether there have ever been any fully authenticated and immunologically confirmed cases. This is particularly surprising in that local analgesics are often given repeatedly to the same individuals (some of whom inevitably are susceptible to such reactions) for successive sessions of treatment. These conditions are ideal for the induction of hypersensitivity.

In most cases of so-called allergy to lignocaine it has usually been unclear which component of the solution has caused the trouble. In particular, most local analgesic solutions used to contain, as a preservative, a benzoic acid derivative (a parabens) which is a well-recognised sensitising agent. As a consequence, parabens-free local analgesics are now generally used.

Despite the persistence of the belief in lignocaine allergy in some circles, the use of literally billions of cartridges for well over a quarter of a century in the UK, USA and other countries with such a rarity of reports of adverse reactions indicates that hypersensitivity to this drug is more likely to be a theoretical rather than a real possibility.

*In the 10 years 1980–89 there were only three deaths in any way associated with dental local anaesthetics. In *all* these cases, prilocaine was given. This does not of course mean that prilocaine was the cause of death, but at the same time it hardly fails to confirm that it is safer than lignocaine which was probably used in many more cases.

Although lignocaine and adrenaline have been shown to be remarkably safe in practice, they should not and do not need to be given in unlimited quantities. If a couple of cartridges in any given area fail to produce the desired effect, then there is something wrong with the solution, the patient, or (most often) the operator, and the attempt should be abandoned until the problem has been investigated.

The maximum dose of lignocaine with adrenaline that should be given to a healthy adult is 10 2-ml cartridges (500 mg of lignocaine) over the space of an hour. When lignocaine is used without adrenaline the maximum dose should not exceed 200 mg (five cartridges).

Prilocaine

Prilocaine is chemically similar to lignocaine (Fig. 17.2) and has very similar properties, apart from the fact that it has weak vasoconstrictor activity. Prilocaine is rapidly redistributed around the body and metabolised after absorption; as a result it has a lower nominal toxicity than lignocaine. Prilocaine is therefore used in a higher concentration (3%) than lignocaine; this also makes use of the weak vasoconstrictor action and only a very low concentration of adrenaline (1:300 000) is added.

Applications. Three per cent prilocaine with 1:300 000 adrenaline is almost as effective as 2% lignocaine with 1:80 000 adrenaline. Its action is briefer, but this is sometimes an advantage. An alternative (as described later) is 3% prilocaine with felypressin, a synthetic, non-catecholamine vasoconstrictor. Only prilocaine is available with felypressin, since they are both produced by the same manufacturer. Another is prilocaine (4%) without any vasoconstrictor. Under such circumstances it provides more reliable analgesia than lignocaine alone, but is only suitable for brief procedures.

Toxicity. Prilocaine can cause methaemoglobinaemia and cyanosis, but in general is as safe as lignocaine. Though allergy to prilocaine has also been reported, as with lignocaine this is probably not a significant hazard.

The claim that prilocaine, with or without felypressin, is safer than lignocaine with adrenaline is unsupported by the morbidity and mortality data on local analgesics, as discussed earlier.

Mepivacaine

Mepivacaine is also similar to lignocaine in chemical constitution and properties.

Applications. Mepivacaine can be used as a 3% solution without a vasoconstrictor to provide local analgesia of short duration. It is not clear whether this preparation has any advantages over 4% prilocaine used in the same way.

Two per cent mepivacaine with 1:200 000 adrenaline is available and has the theoretical advantage of a lower vasoconstrictor content.

Toxicity. Allergy to mepivacaine has also been reported as it has to virtually every other substance known to humankind.

Bupivacaine

Bupivacaine is an ultralong-acting local analgesic.

Applications. The main use of bupivacaine is for spinal or epidural analgesia for surgery or childbirth. In dentistry bupivacaine is only useful for some forms of otherwise intractable pain. Complete analgesia of the related area after an inferior block may last for 8–12 h.

Toxicity. As mentioned earlier, bupivacaine is considerably more cardiotoxic than other currently used local analgesics, but probably only in the larger doses required for extradural regional analgesia.

VASOCONSTRICTORS FOR USE WITH LOCAL ANALGESICS

The purpose of adding a vasoconstrictor to local analgesics is to reduce the local circulation at the site of injection sufficiently to prevent the agent from diffusing away too rapidly.

The delayed absorption is often said to minimise any toxic effects of the local analgesic entering the general circulation. Such statements seem, however, to betray a certain confusion of thought, in that the most feared component of analgesic solutions is the vasoconstrictor itself. Nevertheless, the vasoconstrictor effect of catecholamines (such as adrenaline or noradrenaline) is protective, since vasoconstriction slows their own absorption. If, however, the injection accidentally enters a blood vessel, a catecholamine vasoconstrictor might possibly have more serious effects than the local analgesic.

Another effect of the vasoconstrictor with a local analgesic is that, when given as a local infiltration, it provides a relatively bloodless field of operation.

The main agents that have been used are adrenaline, felypressin and, in the past, noradrenaline.

Adrenaline

Adrenaline is an effective and generally safe vasoconstrictor.

Applications. In the usual concentration of 1:80 000 adrenaline reliably prolongs the effect of a local analgesic, and by slowing absorption makes it possible to increase the amount of local analgesic that can be safely given.

Toxicity. The chief adverse effects of adrenaline result from its adrenergic activity and, in particular, heightened myocardial excitability. In overdose this can lead to disturbance of cardiac rhythm and even ventricular fibrillation. Adrenaline also increases the rate and force of contraction of the heart. It raises the systolic pressure transiently, but tends to lower the diastolic pressure.

In spite of these drawbacks, clinical evidence of serious adverse reactions to adrenaline-containing local analgesics is very hard to find.

The main systemic effect of adrenaline in dental local analgesics is to cause, in some patients, transient tachycardia (palpitations).

Drug interactions. When given in large doses, adrenaline can interact with drugs such as propranolol to raise the blood pressure. This results from the fact that adrenaline causes constriction of skin and visceral vessels (the α effect), but dilatation of muscle arterioles (the β effect). Since the muscles contain the larger vascular bed, the net effect is that peripheral resistance is slightly lowered and, typically, the diastolic pressure falls.

When, however, adrenaline is administered to a person receiving propranolol (for example) its β effect of dilating muscle vessels is blocked but the α effect on skin and visceral vessels is unopposed. The consequent constriction of both muscle and skin vessels raises the peripheral resistance and blood pressure.

Clinically, occasional cases of hypertensive interactions between adrenaline and propranolol have been, as yet, reported only in patients receiving relatively large amounts of adrenaline in local analgesics for plastic surgery.

Unsubstantiated interactions.

1. *Monoamine oxidase inhibitors (MAOIs).* As discussed in Chapter 3, there is no evidence that either adrenaline or noradrenaline is potentiated by monoamine oxidase inhibitors since they are broken down by another enzyme, catechol-*O*-methyl transferase (COMT).

2. *Tricyclic antidepressants.* As discussed earlier, interactions between adrenaline and tricyclic antidepressants have been demonstrated only by giving volunteers tricyclic antidepressants and then infusing them with *intravenous* adrenaline at the rate of 18 µg/min for 25 min. One can only wonder both at the heroism of the participating volunteers and also that the consequences were so slight.

3. There is *no* clinical evidence that adrenaline in the amounts used in dental local analgesics has any significant interaction with antidepressant drugs.

Noradrenaline

Noradrenaline has only slight effects on cardiac activity, but since it is α adrenergic it causes widespread vasoconstriction.

Applications. Noradrenaline has no advantages as a vasoconstrictor and, unlike adrenaline (in spite of the latter's *theoretical* disadvantages), has been shown to cause serious clinical complications, as discussed below.

There are no indications for the use of noradrenaline as a vasoconstrictor in local analgesic preparations for dentistry.

Toxic effects. Several cases of acute hypertension, including some deaths, have resulted from the use of *high* concentrations (1:20 000) of noradrenaline or from the use of four or more cartridges containing 1:80 000 noradrenaline.

Noradrenaline can therefore cause severe complications, particularly when used in excessive amounts.

Felypressin

Felypressin is a synthetic analogue of the pituitary hormone vasopressin. It is an effective vasoconstrictor, although less powerful than adrenaline.

Applications. Felypressin is available commercially only with prilocaine (3%), but has only *theoretical* advantages over adrenaline. When a bloodless field is needed for oral surgery under anaesthesia, felypressin is so much less effective that adrenaline is still preferred.

Toxicity. Felypressin appears to have no adverse systemic effects in normally used concentrations. It does not appear to have any untoward effects on the heart and does not seem to increase myocardial excitability. It has been suggested that, because of its close structural resemblance to oxytocin, felypressin could cause premature contraction of the pregnant uterus, but this has not been substantiated. As far as is known, felypressin does not seem to have any adverse interactions with other drugs.

The periodontal ligament injection

An alternative to local infiltration or regional blocks is intraligamentary injection. The latter depends on special syringes to facilitate the injection of a local analgesic into the periodontal ligament. Only a minute amount of solution is injected, but great pressure and a fine-bore (30 gauge) short needle have to be used.

The mechanism of production of analgesia by intraligamentary injection is unknown, but experiments have shown that with this technique sterile normal saline or adrenaline alone is effective as 2% lignocaine with 1:80 000 adrenaline. The pressure used seems to be the determining factor, and is so high with an intraligamentary injection that the solution may either interrupt the blood supply to the pulp or simply compress the sensory nerve fibres.

Intraligamentary injection for local analgesia has the following advantages:

1. It can produce effective pulpal anaesthesia or analgesia for extractions when conventional injections have failed.
2. Single-tooth anaesthesia is possible and enables individual teeth in different quadrants to be treated without the widespread numbness that results from conventional injections.
3. The onset of analgesia can be very rapid – sometimes immediate or within 30 s. The duration is typically up to an hour.
4. The injection can be painless.
5. Using the special syringes the amount of local analgesic solution injected is small, usually about 0.2 ml, although this is usually no more than of theoretical benefit.

Intraligamentary injection has both its enthusiasts and its opponents. Its main applications are those where its advantages are important considerations and, in particular, when a conventional injection has failed to produce adequate pulpal anaesthesia.

On the debit side, intraligamentary injections can cause significant bacteraemias. Before giving an intraligamentary injection, it may be desirable to irrigate the gingival sulcus with an antiseptic such as chlorhexidine in alcohol in order to avoid propelling bacteria into the bloodstream. There is, however, no evidence as yet that intraligamentary injections are a cause of infective endocarditis.

Surface analgesics

The usefulness of surface analgesics is limited. Painful conditions of the mouth should not be treated symptomatically and untreatable disease such as hopelessly advanced cancer needs to be managed by generous use of opioids.

A 'sensitive palate' (a tendency to retch during dental treatment) is mainly caused by anxiety, so that an anxiolytic such as diazepam by mouth is usually more effective than a surface analgesic. Benzocaine lozenges are available for this problem or for painful oral lesions unresponsive to other treatment.

Surface analgesics are also used as ointments or sprays to lessen the pain of injection of local analgesics.

Cocaine is a potent surface analgesic but, as

discussed earlier, has no current applications in dentistry. *Amethocaine* is an effective surface analgesic, but is too toxic for injection and a potent sensitiser. If used as an ointment, the operator can develop contact dermatitis of the fingers. Amethocaine is included in some surface analgesic sprays but is not used in dentistry.

Lignocaine has some surface analgesic action on the mucosa and is available as gels and sprays. Unlike cocaine its action is relatively superficial, and enough time (preferably 1 or 2 min) must be allowed for a lignocaine-based surface analgesic to act. During this time it should be protected from being washed away by saliva. However, most of the discomfort from a local analgesic comes during the injection itself when the tissues are being pulled apart by the injected fluid. A surface analgesic such as lignocaine has little effect at this level and the main precaution is to make the injection very slowly. This is particularly important when injections are made into the palate where the tissues are tightly bound down to bone.

Lignocaine gel is useful for painful oral lesions such as major aphthae, for which no satisfactory or specific treatment is available, and allows eating and swallowing in relative comfort.

Local analgesics are ineffective on healthy skin because of their inability to penetrate the stratum corneum. This limitation has been overcome by use of *EMLA* (eutectic mixture of local analgesics) cream which contains high concentrations of lignocaine and prilocaine in an oil/water emulsion. Five per cent EMLA cream can penetrate intact skin and lessen injection pain, provided that it is applied about an hour before the procedure. Its principal use is in paediatrics and for needle-phobic adults.

EMLA should not be used on wounds or damaged skin or on mucous membranes which allow excessive absorption. Similarly, toxic levels may be reached when used on infants, and methaemoglobinaemia can result.

18. General anaesthesia and sedation

The introduction of general anaesthesia has been one of the greatest advances in medicine. It is easy to forget that it has made possible the enormous range of complex surgical operations that are now taken for granted.

Humphrey Davy noticed the analgesic effects of nitrous oxide in 1799 and suggested its value for lessening the pain of surgery. However, it was not put to any practical use until an American dentist Horace Wells demonstrated the effectiveness of nitrous oxide in 1844; another, William Morton did the same for ether in 1846. The first general anaesthetic administered in Britain was also given by a dentist, James Robinson, who used ether in December 1846.

Dentists have undoubtedly, therefore, made one major contribution to reducing suffering and to the physical welfare of the world.

The use of drugs to produce a state of depression of the CNS short of unconsciousness (conscious sedation) has become increasingly important in the second half of the present century. Unlike general anaesthesia, the use of which is now restricted to medically qualified specialists, the provision of conscious sedation is accepted as part of the dentist's role.

GENERAL ANAESTHESIA

General anaesthesia provides a controlled and reversible state of unconsciousness from which the patient cannot be aroused by external stimuli. All nervous system depressants, in overdose, produce unconsciousness, but it is not readily reversible and natural recovery is usually very slow.

Anaesthetic agents, by contrast, induce unconsciousness rapidly and, ideally, without depression of respiratory or cardiovascular function.

An ideal general anaesthetic agent should therefore:

1. Produce a controllable and rapidly reversible level of unconsciousness, together with analgesia and muscle relaxation.
2. Have a wide margin of dosage between that inducing unconsciousness and that causing medullary paralysis.
3. Give a rapid, smooth and pleasant induction.
4. Have no adverse effects on the cardiovascular system causing either significant disturbances of cardiac rhythm or depression of blood pressure.
5. Have no toxic effects on other organs such as the liver.
6. Have no irritant effect on the respiratory tract (if an inhalational agent).
7. Cause no local irritant effect at the site of injection (if an intravenous agent).
8. Be non-inflammable. Inflammable agents with oxygen produce a powerful explosive mixture that can be ignited even by an invisible spark of static electricity.
9. Have no undesirable interactions with other drugs likely to be given before or during anaesthesia.
10. Be quickly metabolised and/or excreted.
11. Allow pleasant and (preferably) rapid recovery.

In practical terms, the main requirements of a general anaesthetic for major surgery comprise

1. Unconsciousness
2. Freedom from pain

3. Abolition of reflex movements and muscular relaxation.

These can all be achieved by heavy dosage of a single potent anaesthetic agent sufficient to cause deep anaesthesia. However, this is at the price of greater risks, a prolonged recovery period and, usually, unpleasant after-effects.

In modern anaesthesia, therefore, a combination of drugs, each having a specific effect, is used to achieve these aims with greater control and fewer risks. This technique is termed *balanced anaesthesia.*

DRUGS PRODUCING UNCONSCIOUSNESS

Most drugs which produce unconsciousness are highly lipid soluble or are converted into lipid-soluble metabolites in the body. Since the site of action of general anaesthetic agents is the brain, it has been suggested that the anaesthetic effect is due to a direct effect on cell membranes within the brain and is related to their ability to bind to these lipid structures.

Certainly, the potency of individual drugs appears to be related to their degree of lipid solubility. However, it may be that the binding sites for some anaesthetics are specific proteins or synapses rather than lipids. Anaesthetic drugs produce the following physiological changes in brain neurones:

1. No change in resting potential
2. A rise in action potential threshold and inhibition of rapid increases in sodium permeability, resulting in inhibition of action potentials
3. Inhibition of excitatory synaptic transmission.

Although both the efficacy of the drugs used to produce general anaesthesia and their effects on brain physiology are well documented, the exact physical or chemical mechanisms by which different drugs achieve these effects are unclear.

Stages of anaesthesia

General anaesthetic agents, like other depressants, subdue the CNS in stages from the higher centres downwards until the brainstem is reached (Ch. 3). This process can be seen as the four stages of anaesthesia which, during the slow induction with open ether, could easily be identified. Nowadays, particularly when powerful intravenous agents are used, the stages often merge so smoothly and quickly as to be barely identifiable.

Stage 1: Analgesia. Analgesia is initially incomplete but varies with the drug used. Nitrous oxide, for example, is strongly analgesic, while barbiturates have no analgesic action.

Stage 2: Excitement. The patient is unconscious, reflexes are intact and there may be automatic movements or sometimes violent struggling.

Stage 3: Surgical anaesthesia. Reflex activity and muscle tone are progressively lost until in the fourth stage there is complete muscular relaxation.

Stage 4: Medullary paralysis. This is the result of overdose or may be a complication of hypoxia or both. Immediate resuscitative measures must be started.

INHALATIONAL ANAESTHETIC AGENTS

These include gases and volatile liquids which can be vaporised for inhalation. They are carried in blood to the brain. Their relative potencies are measured as their minimum alveolar concentration (MAC) value. This refers to the concentration of the drug in lung alveoli which is needed for 50% of an experimental population to be sufficiently anaesthetised to tolerate a standard surgical stimulus. As a rough guide, drug concentrations approximately 1.5 times the MAC will anaesthetise most patients. The MAC value for a drug depends on whether it is measured in air or oxygen, or mixed with other agents such as nitrous oxide, which frequently constitutes up to 60% of anaesthetic mixtures.

The time to the onset of anaesthesia with any particular agent depends upon how quickly the concentration in the alveoli equilibrates with that of the blood and, particularly, the brain. Agents with low tissue solubility equilibrate faster than very soluble drugs. Similarly, drugs which are excreted simply via the lungs result in a much quicker recovery than those which have to undergo complex redistribution, metabolism and excretion processes.

Gases

Gases are used for two purposes in anaesthesia. First, they replace the normally respired volume of air (a mixture of gases) with an artificial mixture of gases that will permit normal respiration. Oxygen must always be present as at least 30% of the gas mixture to maintain adequate tissue oxygenation.

Second, gases are used to provide desirable pharmacological effects.

Nitrous oxide

Nitrous oxide was the first anaesthetic agent, but has remained in use for 150 years. It is one of the safest agents available, but this is partly because it is so weak an anaesthetic that in the highest acceptable concentration (80% with 20% oxygen) it is unable to depress the medulla.

Nitrous oxide has the following properties:

1. Colourless, non-irritant gas with a faint odour
2. Neither inflammable nor explosive but will support combustion
3. Induction is rapid and pleasant
4. No adverse effects on the heart, respiratory tract, liver or kidneys
5. Potent analgesic and anxiolytic, even in subanaesthetic doses
6. Recovery is rapid as the gas in excreted unchanged from the lungs.

The rapid equilibration of nitrous oxide in blood and brain and equally rapid elimination are due to its very poor solubility in body tissues. It has the great advantage that it causes no respiratory depression and its effects can be reversed instantly.

At concentrations between 50% and 80% the analgesic potency of nitrous oxide is probably comparable to that of morphine, and it has at least as great an anxiolytic effect.

Adverse effects. Nitrous oxide occasionally causes *nausea* or *vomiting* if given too rapidly in high concentration. The mechanisms are unknown, but it may be a central effect like that of opioids, with which nitrous oxide has properties in common.

Nitrous oxide *inactivates vitamin* B_{12} in the form of methyl cobalamin and can, on prolonged exposure, cause depletion of methionine and cause megaloblastic anaemia, leukopenia and neurological damage. This effect is not normally significant in fit patients, as megaloblastic marrow changes are not detectable until after a 5–6 h exposure to 50% nitrous oxide. However, in the past, patients requiring prolonged sedation have been exposed to nitrous oxide continuously for many days, or, in some cases, intermittently, for months – itself a remarkable tribute to the safety of this drug in other respects. The dyshaemopoietic effect of nitrous oxide can be prevented or reversed by giving folinic acid.

This toxic effect of nitrous oxide is a cause for concern for clinical staff (especially women who are or are likely to be pregnant) exposed to traces of nitrous oxide in the atmosphere. Although there is little firm evidence of significant adverse effects, effective scavenging is desirable. Paradoxically, in long-term abusers of nitrous oxide, neurological complications are the main effect, but megaloblastic anaemia is rare. Therefore some compensatory mechanism seems to be able to develop and overcome the effect of nitrous oxide on the bone marrow.

Entonox

Entonox is premixed, 50:50 nitrous oxide and oxygen. It is used as an analgesic and sedative for such purposes as the immediate management of myocardial infarction or obstetric analgesia. Cylinders of Entonox are standard equipment in many ambulances and it is given by ambulance personnel for patients in transit to intensive care units. Entonox has also been used for dental sedation, mixed with air, to provide a fixed output of 25% nitrous oxide.

Volatile agents

These vaporised liquids have very little volume. They are taken up by the mixture of anaesthetic gases flowing to the patient which provides their vehicle for transport to the lungs. Volatile agents do not contribute significantly to the volume of 'air' respired by the patient, but have potent pharmacological effects.

Ether and chloroform

Chloroform is now obsolete but ether is still used in developing countries. Ether is highly soluble but irritant, so that induction of anaesthesia is slow and uncomfortable for patients. It is very inflammable and has been responsible for operating theatre explosions. However, ether has a good safety record and, in particular, is not cardiotoxic.

Chloroform, a hydrocarbon, is not explosive and much less irritant, but can induce fatal cardiac dysrhythmias. The modern halogenated hydrocarbons and ethers described below are safer modifications of these two prototype drugs.

Halothane

Halothane, a halogenated hydrocarbon, has been the standard inhalational anaesthetic agent for nearly half a century and has been widely used in dentistry. It has the following properties:

1. Non-inflammable and non-explosive
2. More smooth and pleasant than newer agents
3. Minimal excitement and surgical anaesthesia can be induced in 2–3 min
4. Provides some muscle relaxation, but muscle relaxants can be given if necessary
5. Overdose depresses the respiratory centre, but depression of the vasomotor centre is more delayed
6. Recovery is usually rapid, but depends on the total dose given.

In practice, halothane is given with nitrous oxide and oxygen, at a concentration of 2–3% for induction, then continued at 0.5–2%. For this purpose a calibrated vaporiser has to be used to ensure accurate regulation of the concentration.

Adverse effects. Halothane sensitises the heart to catecholamines such as adrenaline, which may be given in oral and plastic surgery to produce a bloodless field. Hypoxia or excessive accumulation of CO_2 increase the tendency to *dysrhythmias*. β blockers are effective against these dysrhythmias but are rarely used, as a brief period of controlled ventilation is usually sufficient to stop them.

Like most anaesthetics, halothane also causes dose-related depression of blood pressure.

Liver damage can very occasionally follow administration of halothane. Reactions range from abnormalities of liver function, detectable only by laboratory tests, to fatal massive hepatic necrosis. The latter is so uncommon, however, that surveys on an immense scale have had to be carried out to confirm whether there was any cause-and-effect relationship. Remarkably, the incidence of hepatic reactions to halothane is considerably lower than the incidence of unexpected abnormalities of liver function found preoperatively.

It is clear that a minority of patients can have hepatotoxic reactions to halothane, particularly after repeated exposure, but after years of intensive study, the mechanism of the hepatotoxic effects remains unclear and controversial. An immunological mechanism of unknown nature appears to be responsible because repeated exposure presents the greatest risk and because only a minority of individuals appear to be susceptible.

In summary:

1. Halothane can rarely cause fulminant and occasionally fatal hepatitis
2. Only certain individuals appear to be at risk from halothane hepatitis, but cannot be identified beforehand
3. It appears to be particularly important to avoid hypoxia or circulatory depression when halothane is given
4. Halothane should never be given again to anyone who has had a reaction to it
5. Even when there has been no reaction, halothane should not be given again for 6 months after any exposure.

Although there is no doubt about its potential hepatotoxicity, halothane has been used and investigated on so vast a scale over so many years that no other anaesthetic agent is known with certainty to be safer and halothane has not been made obsolete by newer agents.

With regard to other adverse effects, nausea and vomiting are rare, but there may be shivering during recovery.

Enflurane and isoflurane

Enflurane and *isoflurane* are halogenated ethers.

Enflurane has the following properties:

1. Relatively pleasant induction, but less pleasant than with halothane
2. Very rapid onset of action
3. Only about 2.5% of enflurane is metabolised and systemic effects seem to be minimal
4. Cardiac rhythm is more stable than with halothane and less sensitive to injected adrenaline
5. No firm evidence that enflurane can cause hepatitis
6. Depresses respiration more than halothane
7. Is potentially epileptogenic.

Enflurane has been used satisfactorily for brief dental operations. Its advantages for this purpose are the low risk of dysrhythmias, the rapid induction, which is complete in about a minute and a half, and the more rapid recovery than with halothane.

Isoflurane is an isomer of enflurane and has the following properties:

1. Very rapid induction but it is pungent and cause undesirable salivation, coughing and laryngospasm; induction is therefore considerably less pleasant than with halothane
2. Less respiratory depression than enflurane, but nevertheless more than halothane
3. Minimal adverse cardiac effects and it is a coronary vasodilator
4. Not epileptogenic
5. Not hepatotoxic
6. Recovery is slower than with halothane.

Isoflurane is a valuable anaesthetic agent for anyone with heart disease or who has had a hepatic reaction to halothane. However, both enflurane and isoflurane are considerably more expensive than halothane. Newer volatile agents being developed in the search for the ideal anaesthetic, include *sevoflurane* and *desflurane*. Their advantages include quicker recovery due to minimal metabolism, but their much greater cost than established drugs is likely to limit widespread adoption.

INTRAVENOUS ANAESTHETIC AGENTS

These drugs can provide very rapid and pleasant induction. Intravenous anaesthesia also causes no pollution of the operating theatre atmosphere. A consideration is that even mild respiratory obstruction can interfere with the giving of inhalational agents but intravenous agents can be injected, irrespective of the state of the airway. They include:

1. Barbiturates – thiopentone and methohexitone
2. Non-barbiturates – propofol and ketamine.

Barbiturates

The ultrashort-acting barbiturates were the first intravenous induction agents and remain the most widely used. Short operations, where neither analgesia nor muscle relaxation is essential, can be carried out with these agents alone.

Disadvantages of intravenous barbiturates include the following:

1. They are very powerful anaesthetics. Overdose is easy to give and once injected their action is not reversed until they have been metabolised.

2. They are potent respiratory depressants and severe hypoxia can result if there is any respiratory obstruction. The latter is a major hazard in operations, such as dental surgery, at the upper end of the airway.

3. They depress cardiac output and this can aggravate the effects of hypoxia.

4. Intravenous barbiturates can occasionally cause severe hypersensitivity reactions which may not be recognised as such.

Thiopentone

Thiopentone has remained the standard induction agent in general surgical practice since its introduction in the 1930s. It is almost universally used in general surgical practice for induction of anaesthesia which can then be continued with the more readily controllable inhalational agents. It is usually given as a 2.5% solution and has the following properties:

1. Induces unconsciousness smoothly and pleasantly in little more than the arm to brain circulation time.

2. No analgesia in moderate dosage so that surgical stimulation causes reflex movements.

3. Higher doses readily cause respiratory depression and the airway must be maintained with absolute certainty.

4. Causes circulatory depression which makes it particularly dangerous for patients with poor cardiac function or in shock.*

5. Immediate recovery after a moderate dose of thiopentone is rapid, but largely due to redistribution. Metabolism is slower, so that variable degrees of sedation persist for up to 24 h and is further delayed if liver function is poor.

Adverse effects.

1. *Laryngeal spasm.* This is a hazard of induction and probably due to overactive laryngeal reflexes. Spasm is usually brief but administration should stop until it relaxes. If it persists a muscle relaxant and artificial ventilation may need to be given.

2. *Extravascular injection.* Thiopentone is irritant, so that extravascular injection can cause pain, swelling and local tissue necrosis. Local infiltration of the area with procaine and hyaluronidase may help to relieve symptoms and disperse the drug.

3. *Intra-arterial injection.* The irritant effect of thiopentone on arterial walls is such that accidental intra-arterial injection can cause intense arterial spasm. The risk was mainly with strong (5%) solutions, which are now obsolete. Typical symptoms are sudden pain in the arm and, if the spasm leads to thrombosis, blanching of the fingers. In extreme cases this has terminated in gangrene necessitating amputation. An α blocking agent and anticoagulants may help to relieve the spasm.

4. *Overdose.* Respiratory depression is the first and most important effect. Immediate positive pressure mechanical ventilation must be given as there is no specific antagonist. Respiratory stimulants are of little value.

5. *Hypersensitivity reactions.* Thiopentone can cause histamine release or, rarely, hypersensitivity reactions of various types which have occasionally been fatal. In a typical severe reaction, there is bronchospasm, flushing, oedema, vasodilatation, and a sharp fall in blood pressure. The treatment is essentially the same as that for similar reactions to penicillin.

In spite of these hazards, thiopentone has over many years proved, in expert hands, to be a safe and useful drug which has not been displaced by newer agents. However, its safety record, despite its low therapeutic index, is largely a reflection of anaesthetists' skill.

*Thiopentone is reputed to have caused more deaths among American troops injured during the bombing of Pearl Harbour than did the enemy.

Methohexitone

Methohexitone is in most respects similar to thiopentone. The chief differences are as follows:

1. It is 2.5 times as potent as thiopentone
2. Recovery is more rapid, but mainly because of more rapid redistribution
3. It causes excitatory activity (involuntary movements and hiccup)
4. It has epileptogenic potential
5. It is less prone than thiopentone to cause laryngeal spasm
6. It is much less irritant when an accidental intravascular injection is given.

Methohexitone has not displaced thiopentone as an induction agent in general surgical practice, probably because of the involuntary movements it causes and lack of any significant advantages. In dental practice, methohexitone has had widespread use in the past because of the apparently rapid recovery and the lesser dangers from extravenous injection than with thiopentone. However, methohexitone was implicated in a significant number of deaths during dental anaesthesia.

Non-barbiturates

Etomidate

This induction agent causes less hypotension than comparable agents. Recovery is rapid, but injection is painful and involuntary movements are common. Repeated doses or continuous infusions of etomidate may also cause adrenocortical suppression.

Ketamine

Ketamine differs from other anaesthetic agents in that it produces a state of *dissociative anaesthesia* in which, apart from loss of consciousness and analgesia, bodily responses are quite different from those to conventional anaesthetics. Reflexes typically remain intact so that there is increased muscle tone instead of relaxation. There is also cardiovascular stimulation, rather than depression.

Analgesia is intense but the main limitation of ketamine is that, without premedication, it is prone to cause vivid and terrifying nightmares or hallucinations during recovery, particularly in adults. Ketamine is sometimes useful for dental anaesthesia of children or handicapped patients, particularly if repeated anaesthetics are needed. It also has the advantage that it can be given by intramuscular injection, which is valuable for otherwise uncontrollable patients. Recovery is slower after ketamine than other non-barbiturates.

Propofol

This agent is used for induction or maintenance of anaesthesia, with very rapid recovery with few after-effects and little involuntary movement. It has the advantage that it seems to be antiemetic. Propofol is the only non-barbiturate induction agent in regular current use for dental anaesthesia.

Injection can be painful and the drug is sometimes mixed with lignocaine to overcome this problem. Propofol is also used by controlled infusion or patient-controlled systems to provide sedation rather than anaesthesia for dentistry.

DRUGS PROVIDING ANALGESIA

Analgesia may be produced to a greater or lesser extent by the same drugs which produce unconsciousness but also by other drugs given expressly for this purpose. Since the patient is deeply unconscious during anaesthesia, there is little obvious benefit from the agents having an analgesic action. However, the latter property is valuable in that it allows surgery to be carried out under light anaesthesia by preventing reflex autonomic responses to pain. If muscular relaxation is required, a relaxant can be given.

INHALATIONAL ANALGESIC AGENTS

Nitrous oxide (see above).

INTRAVENOUS ANALGESIC AGENTS

Ketamine (see above).

Opioid and non-opioid analgesics (Ch. 4)

Opioids and other analgesics are mainly used for control of pre- and post-operative pain, as discussed below.

DRUGS PRODUCING MUSCULAR RELAXATION

Drugs which produce unconsciousness may cause or potentiate muscular relaxation to a greater or lesser degree. However tailor-made drugs are usually given to provide controlled muscular relaxation. They comprise:

1. Depolarising muscle relaxants
2. Non-depolarising muscle relaxants.

The mechanisms of action of muscle relaxants have been described earlier (Ch. 2).

DEPOLARISING (NON-COMPETITIVE) BLOCKERS

Suxamethonium is the only depolarising blocker used in current clinical practice. It acts quickly and its action is short-lived (2–3 min). Its principal use is to paralyse the vocal cords to enable an endotracheal tube to be passed easily and without causing laryngospasm. After recovery from suxamethonium, anaesthesia can proceed with the patient breathing spontaneously.

If mechanical ventilation is required a longer-acting relaxant must be given.

Reversal. Reversal of suxamethonium blockade is by enzymatic degradation of the drug by circulating plasma pseudocholinesterase. The suxamethonium molecule consists of two fused acetylcholine molecules, but it is not degraded by normal cholinesterases. As there is no pharmacological means of reversing suxamethonium paralysis, individuals with inherited pseudocholinesterase deficiency may remain paralysed for many hours. This phenomenon is termed *suxamethonium apnoea* and necessitates prolonged artificial ventilation until recovery is complete.

NON-DEPOLARISING (COMPETITIVE) BLOCKERS

Tubocurarine was the first of these agents to be used, but newer drugs offering more flexibility in use are constantly being developed. This variety of drugs with different properties enables the anaesthetist to tailor his or her choice to provide adequate paralysis for specific indications. Currently used relaxants include *pancuronium*, *atracurium* and *vecuronium*. Details of these drugs have been given in Chapter 4.

Reversal. Most of these require reversal with an anticholinesterase such as neostigmine. This allows flooding of the neuromuscular junction with acetylcholine which displaces the relaxant and re-establishes normal neuromuscular activity. The drugs are then metabolised in the liver and excreted via the kidneys.

Since anticholinesterases cause a generalised rise in acetylcholine levels throughout the body, the patient must be protected against unwanted and excessive cholinergic activity at muscarinic sites within the autonomic nervous system. This leads to vagal stimulation with bradycardia, increased secretions and gut motility. All these effects are dangerous during emergence from anaesthesia. For this reason reversal agents are administered with a specific antimuscarinic such as atropine or glycopyrronium.

Atracurium does not depend upon pharmacological reversal to terminate its action as the molecule undergoes spontaneous degradation after about 20 min of action. This makes it useful for patients with hepatic or renal disease.

OTHER DRUGS USED IN CONJUNCTION WITH GENERAL ANAESTHESIA

The drugs described above are given immediately preoperatively and during the operation. Other drugs, given pre- or post-operatively can be considered as being part of the anaesthetic. These include premedication, drugs used to reverse the effects of drugs given intraoperatively such as muscle relaxants and drugs to control post-operative pain or nausea and vomiting.

PREMEDICATION

In addition to the anaesthetic agents themselves it is usual in hospital practice to give drugs before the operation (premedication) and sometimes also afterwards, to assist recovery or to make it more pleasant.

Premedication is not usually given for dental outpatient anaesthesia, partly because it is rarely necessary and partly because it tends to delay recovery.

The purposes of premedication are:

1. To allay anxiety
2. To make induction more pleasant
3. To minimise oral and bronchial secretions
4. To reduce the amount of anaesthetic agent needed
5. To protect against some of the possible adverse effects of the anaesthetic agents
6. To control preoperative pain.

Anxiolysis

Since anxiety about the anaesthetic or operation may increase production of adrenaline or noradrenaline, anxiolytic premedication may also protect the patient against their cardiovascular effects. This is particularly important with agents such as halothane which sensitise the heart to catecholamines.

For general surgery, opioids are often used. They are sedative and analgesic, and valuable if the patient is already in pain. Analgesics also diminish reflex movements during light anaesthesia and reduce postoperative restlessness due to pain. The disadvantages of opioids are that they are respiratory and, to a lesser extent, cardiac depressants. They also increase the likelihood of postoperative nausea and vomiting.

For anxiety alone, a benzodiazepine is useful. Diazepam (5 or 10 mg) or temazepam (10–20 mg) can be given orally on the night before the operation and repeated an hour before operation.

An antihistamine such as promethazine, which is also a phenothiazine, is another alternative popular for children since it has a strong and prolonged sedative effect but it tends to cause postoperative restlessness.

Inhibition of secretions

Atropine may be given to reduce salivary, pharyngeal, bronchial and gastric secretions. This reduces aspiration of saliva, mucus and gastric contents and lessens the chance of postoperative pulmonary collapse and aspiration pneumonia. Modern anaesthetic agents are, however, very much less likely to induce excessive secretions compared with ether. Hyoscine has the same peripheral actions as atropine, but is also sedative and depresses the vomiting centre.

Anticholinergic drugs, such as atropine and hyoscine, may possibly also reduce the chance of sudden death due to excessive vagal slowing of the heart during induction of anaesthesia. This was particularly important in the past, when chloroform was used.

An opioid analgesic and anticholinergic drug have traditionally been given together. Common combinations were papaveretum or pethidine with hyoscine or atropine. However, a benzodiazepine is, probably, overall the most satisfactory choice today and many anaesthetists use no other premedication, unless the patient is already in pain.

GENERAL REQUIREMENTS FOR THE PROVISION OF GENERAL ANAESTHESIA

Fewer general anaesthetics are being performed for dentistry and, since the publication of an expert working party report on General Anaesthesia, Sedation & Resuscitation in Dentistry (the Poswillo Report), dental anaesthetics are increasingly being provided in hospitals or clinics, or practices which are specially equipped and staffed. Nonetheless, dentists need to recommend general anaesthesia to some of their patients and should be able to pass on appropriate and relevant information when referring them to specialist centres. For these reasons the following concepts should be understood.

The management of a general anaesthetic is, to large degree, acute applied pharmacology. The pharmacological effects are exceptionally rapid and the patients' reactions almost immediate, as are the many complications that can arise. Generally speaking too, the level of dosage needed to produce deep unconsciousness is close to that which depresses the respiratory or cardiovascular centres. General anaesthetic agents vary widely in their toxicity, but anaesthesia is a craft where the skill of the anaesthetist is generally more important than the nature of the drugs used. Naturally, however, expert anaesthetists choose agents the potentialities of which they know and are also prepared for and skilled in the management of emergencies.

Precautions

General anaesthesia should only be provided where the premises, equipment and staff are of the highest standard.

1. *Before administration of the anaesthetic* – a general anaesthetic should only be given when:

a. The patient is fit enough to withstand it and has no history of adverse reactions to anaesthesia

b. There are no serious problems relating to any drugs the patient is taking

c. The patient has had nothing to eat or drink for 4 h previously

d. The patient or a parent or guardian is able to give informed consent, which should be obtained in writing

e. Another person is available to accompany the patient home afterwards.

In the case of outpatient anaesthesia, it is also a good idea to make sure that the patient's bladder has been emptied.

2. *After the operation the patient must be*:

a. Placed in a position where blood or saliva do not drain back into the pharynx

b. Kept under supervision until conscious

c. Allowed home when conscious provided that it is reasonably certain that the accompanying adult can be responsible for the patient

d. Forbidden to drive a car or operate unguarded machinery until the following day at the earliest.

CONSCIOUS SEDATION

The term 'conscious sedation' or 'dental sedation' refers to the abolition or obtunding of anxiety by drugs for the duration of a dental procedure. Only a few agents have suitable properties, as most of the commonly used sedatives taken by mouth are slow in onset and too long-acting to be useful for this purpose.

The practice of sedation by a dentist treating his or her own patients, the operator-sedationist, is well established and dentistry has led the way in improving safety standards and regulating practice in this area.

The currently accepted definition of sedation is:

> A technique in which the use of a drug, or drugs, produces a state of depression of the central nervous system enabling treatment to be carried out, but during which communication is maintained such that the patient will respond to command throughout the period of sedation. The drugs and techniques used should carry a margin of safety wide enough to render loss of consciousness unlikely.

Dental sedation is usually provided by a single drug administered by the oral, inhalational or intravenous route. The main drugs used are benzodiazepines and nitrous oxide.

Benzodiazepines

Benzodiazepines (Ch. 3) are currently used for oral or intravenous sedation. They act at specific receptors throughout the central nervous system, modifying synaptic transmission to reduce the impact of stressful sensory information. The effects of benzodiazepines relevant to dental sedation are:

1. Sedation
2. Anxiolysis
3. Amnesia.

The considerable amnesia produced by intravenous benzodiazepines is advantageous to the patient facing a single unpleasant procedure, but may be counterproductive if sedation is being used to rehabilitate chronically anxious patients to accept normal dental treatment.

Nitrous oxide

For inhalational sedation the only agent in routine use is nitrous oxide, the properties of which have been described earlier in relation to general anaesthesia. However, its anxiolytic effects, rather than its analgesic or anaesthetic properties, are particularly useful in the technique of inhalational sedation.

Patient assessment

A thorough assessment including an up-to-date medical history must be made of each patient's dental needs, their fears of treatment or unpleasant past experiences, their willingness and ability to comply with treatment, and their social circumstances. It is most important to assess the likelihood of sedation being the best way to make effective treatment acceptable. Sedation should not be used outside specialist clinics or practices if there is any doubt about a patient's fitness for the type of sedation proposed. As sedation is given solely to make treatment acceptable, no patient should be put at added risk from any adverse effects due to any pre-existing medical condition or its treatment.

A useful rule of thumb grading of medical suitability for sedation is the American Society of Anesthesiologists' Classification of Risk (Table 18.1). Outside specialist areas sedation should only be used for those falling into Classes I or II.

Oral sedation

The use of oral diazepam as an anxiolytic for therapy or premedication before general anaesthesia has been discussed. The clinical effects of diazepam are maximal about an hour after an oral dose and are more reliable in cumulative or repeated doses. Its disadvantage is its very long half-life (20–50 h) and resulting prolonged recovery time.

Table 18.1 American Society of Anesthesiologists' Classification

Class I	A normal healthy patient
Class II	A patient with mild systemic disease
Class III	A patient with severe systemic disease which limits activity but is not incapacitating
Class IV	A patient with incapacitating systemic disease that is a constant threat to life
Class V	A moribund patient not expected to live 24 h with or without an operation

Oral diazepam can be effective for moderately anxious individuals who are facing particularly stressful treatment or for those whose principal difficulty is plucking up the courage to attend for an appointment.

Diazepam (5–10 mg) is given on the night before an appointment followed by 5 mg on waking and, if treatment is not scheduled until later in the day, a further 5 mg 1 h before treatment.

Alternatively, temazepam, which has a shorter half-life, can be used in a similar way to diazepam in a dose of 10 mg the night before an appointment and a further 10 mg an hour before treatment.

If either drug is used in this way, careful instructions must be given to patients and their escorts, who must of course accompany a sedated patient to the surgery.

Temazepam can also be used to provide more controlled and profound sedation in a dose of 30 mg (for a fit adult), given in a readily absorbable form such as a gelatine capsule or elixir. Given about 45 min before treatment, this provides more acute sedation than do smaller divided doses. The drug must be administered by the dentist and the patient should be supervised and monitored while it takes effect.

The advantage of oral sedation is its ease of administration, but this may be outweighed by the unpredictability of its effect. Absorption of oral drugs is dependent upon such factors as the formulation of the drug, the time when it is taken, whether or not the stomach is full, and any interference with normal gut activity or absorption. Autonomic stimulation by anxiety may delay absorption or cause vomiting. Once absorbed, oral drugs can be further reduced in efficacy by first-pass liver metabolism.

If sedation is to be taken at home, the dentist must rely on the patient's compliance and that of his or her escort with instructions.

Both diazepam and temazepam are long-acting drugs and patients must adhere to the same postoperative instructions as those receiving intravenous sedation.

Intravenous sedation

Among the many benzodiazepines, only diazepam and midazolam (Fig. 18.1) have proved suitable for intravenous sedation.

Diazepam

The advantages of diazepam as a safe sedative are so great that, despite the disadvantage of an irritant solvent, it quickly became the most widely used drug for intravenous dental sedation after its first use in 1966. Provided that a careful slow injection technique is used, accidental loss of consciousness is very unlikely and respiratory or cardiac depression are minimal.

The replacement of the early irritant propylene glycol solvent by a soya bean oil emulsion overcame the problems of pain on injection and occasional thrombophlebitis.

A disadvantage of diazepam is its prolonged action. Even after a single intravenous dose, the drug and its active metabolites (and thus its

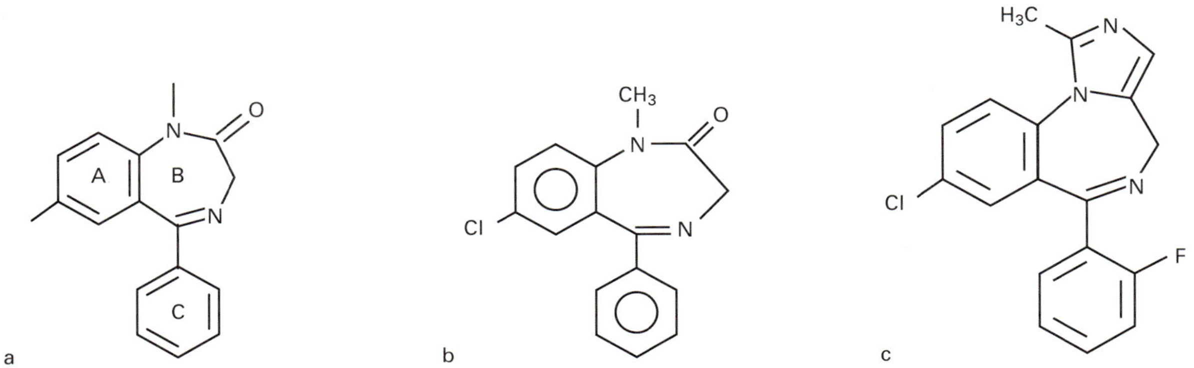

Fig. 18.1 **a** The basic benzodiazepine molecule consists of the benzodiazepine grouping (A–B) to which is attached a benzene ring (C). The latter is common to all the sedating benzodiazepines. **b** Diazepam has modifications to the diazepine ring, while midazolam (**c**) differs in the diazepine side-chain and the benzene ring is fluorinated.

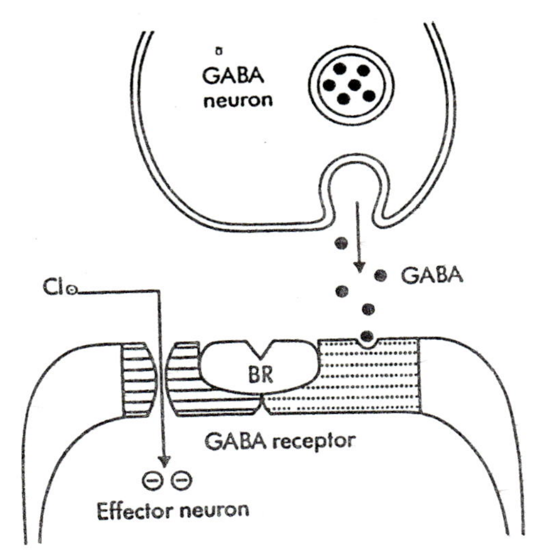

Fig. 18.2 Schematic diagram of a GABAergic synapse. The GABA receptor is part of the postsynaptic membrane and consists of three functional components: the GABA receptor; a chloride channel (effector system); and a modulating component, the benzodiazepine receptor (BR). (Reproduced with permission from Roche Products Ltd.)

potential to impair an individual's judgement or motor function) may not be cleared for 2 or more days. Moreover, the second peak effect due to hepatic recirculation can cause sudden drowsiness hours after wakening.

Midazolam

The introduction of this imidazobenzodiazepine has overcome some of the limitations of diazepam. Midazolam has an elimination half-life of only 1.5–2 h (compared with 20–50 h for diazepam) and none of its breakdown products contribute any clinical effects after those of the drug itself.

In addition, midazolam is water soluble and, unlike diazepam, provides reliable sedation when given by intramuscular injection.

Midazolam is 2–3 times as potent as diazepam and must be given slowly, as described below, in order to avoid the possibility of overdose.

It must be emphasised that the quality and duration of clinical sedation are similar for the two drugs. Sedation is usually effective for at least 20–30 min and treatment can often be continued for up to an hour on a relaxed and cooperative patient. The similar duration of clinical sedation of diazepam and midazolam is because it is related to the time that drugs are bound to receptors rather than to how long it takes for their complete elimination. The distribution half-life (the time taken for the drugs to be shifted from receptors) is 15–30 min for diazepam compared with 6–15 min for midazolam. Because of its overall quicker recovery time and other advantages, midazolam is now the drug of choice for intravenous sedation for dentistry.

Flumazenil

Flumazenil is a specific benzodiazepine antagonist. The drug is itself also an imidazobenzodiazepine, sharing a common core molecular structure with all other (Fig 18.3) benzodiazepines. Since flumazenil has stronger affinity for receptors than sedative benzodiazepines it is able to displace them (Figs 18.2 and 18.4). Once bound to receptors, flumazenil exerts no clinical depressant

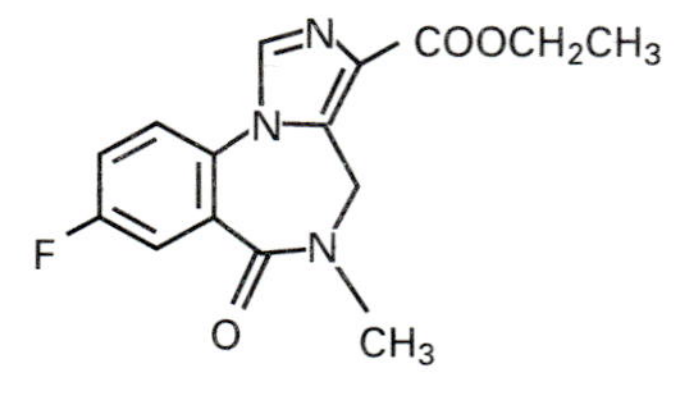

Fig. 18.3 Flumazenil shows the benzodiazepine group which enables it to bind to the benzodiazepine receptor, but it lacks the benzene side-chain of the sedating benzodiazepines.

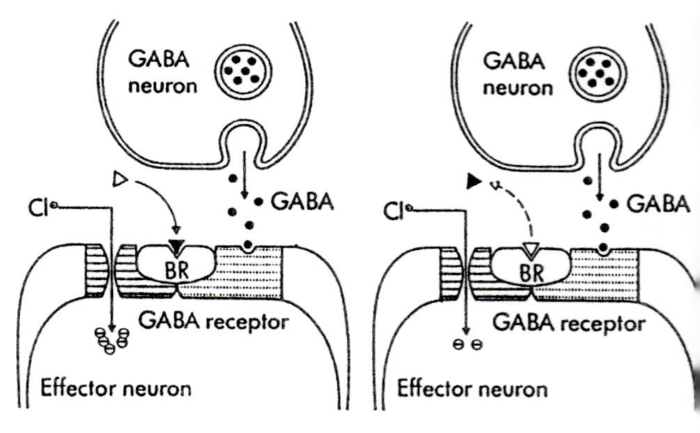

Fig. 18.4 Competitive displacement of a benzodiazepine agonist by flumazenil at the specific receptor, with abolition of benzodiazepine effect in the chloride channel. (Reproduced with permission from Roche Products Ltd.)

or stimulant effects on the CNS but restores a previously sedated patient to a non-sedated state. Flumazenil can therefore be used to reverse undesirable effects of benzodiazepines such as respiratory or cardiovascular depression due to overdose.

The elimination half-life of flumazenil (about 50–60 min) is shorter than that of the sedating benzodiazepines. Once displaced from their receptors, midazolam and diazepam continue to be redistributed and metabolised whilst flumazenil is active. Sudden resedation when the antagonist wears off is therefore not seen after the single dose sedation used in dentistry, although this can be a problem if repeated and cumulative doses of benzodiazepine are used, for example, in intensive care.

The technique of intravenous sedation

Patients should be supine and well supported in the dental chair. The dentist and a trained assistant must be present throughout the sedation and treatment.

Blood pressure and pulse are recorded preoperatively and a pulse oximeter should be used to monitor oxygen saturation throughout the induction and duration of the sedation.

Midazolam must be administered via an indwelling intravenous line. A teflon cannula provides the surest means of maintaining venous access. Small increments of drug are given slowly as individual responses vary widely. For beginners the manufacturer's data sheet recommendations are an excellent guide and are summarised as follows:

1. An initial 2 mg midazolam is given over 30 s.
2. The sedationist watches for signs of drowsiness, physical and mental relaxation and, by reassuring conversation, monitors the level of consciousness. Midazolam must always be titrated to such responses. Drooping of the eyelids — Verrill's sign — is a useful and consistent sign of adequate sedation with diazepam, but is very unreliable with midazolam. *Patients must respond to verbal commands at all times.*
3. After 2 min, if sedation is inadequate, increments of 1 mg are given every 30 s until a satisfactory result is achieved. Average size, fit adults usually require between 4 and 8 mg, but this is very variable.

Local analgesia must be given for dental treatment, because benzodiazepines are not analgesic.

Every patient must be discharged into the care of a responsible adult who should be given written and verbal instructions for postsedation care. No patient who has been sedated should drive a vehicle, use unguarded machinery, sign important documents, drink alcohol, care for children, or undertake other responsible duties until the following day.

Inhalational sedation

Nitrous oxide is the only drug in regular use for inhalational sedation. It is most commonly used in a technique termed *relative analgesia.* In fact, nitrous oxide is used in dentistry principally for its anxiolytic effects rather than for analgesia. Effective pain control is more reliably achieved by local analgesia.

Nitrous oxide is given from specially designed machines in combination with oxygen. These machines must be able to provide it in precise concentrations to suit different patients, must provide a minimum of 30% oxygen at all times and have appropriate tubing, nose-pieces and scavenging systems to minimise surgery pollution.

Nitrous oxide provides very flexible and safe sedation for patients of all ages. It is suitable for children, in whom benzodiazepines are unpredictable, and elderly patients who may be very susceptible to the depressant effects of benzodiazepines.

Nitrous oxide is also safer for patients with respiratory or cardiac disease and, as the drug is excreted unchanged through the lungs, may be used for those with liver or kidney disease.

The technique of inhalational sedation

Nitrous oxide is administered in an incremental fashion similar to intravenous midazolam as follows:

1. The patient becomes familiar with the apparatus by breathing oxygen, the flow of

which is adjusted to match the minute volume requirement
2. 10% nitrous oxide is allowed to flow for 1 min
3. A further 10% is introduced, as above
4. Further increments of 5% are added at 1-min intervals until sedation is satisfactory.

The technique of nitrous oxide sedation also requires a continuous flow of quiet reassuring conversation by the sedationist. Most adults are adequately sedated at concentrations of 20–40% nitrous oxide in oxygen, but children may require higher concentrations.

Nitrous oxide produces physical changes as well as mood-altering effects. Patients may experience any of the following symptoms:

1. Warmth due to vasodilatation
2. Paraesthesia of limbs
3. Visual or auditory changes.

Objective signs of sedation include:

1. Hesitancy in replying to questions
2. Slowing or slurring of speech
3. Facial muscle relaxation
4. Infrequent blinking.

Nitrous oxide must be inhaled continuously to have an effect and, once discontinued, recovery is fast. Most patients feel normal within 5 min, and the gas is almost completely eliminated within 20 min. Residual effects are minimal compared with oral or intravenous benzodiazepines. Nonetheless, for safety, patients must be accompanied home from the surgery.

Alternative methods of dental sedation

Both midazolam and propofol provide reliable sedation when administered by continuous infusion or patient-controlled systems.

These and others, including sublingual or intranasal administration, may eventually prove as, or more, effective than current methods. Both enflurane and isoflurane have been used successfully for inhalational sedation, but care is necessary to prevent patients becoming anaesthetised.

THE DENTIST'S ROLE IN ASSESSMENT AND SELECTION OF PATIENTS FOR GENERAL ANAESTHESIA OR SEDATION

The following questions must be addressed before a patient is advised to have treatment under anaesthesia or sedation:

1. *The dental treatment*
   a. Is anaesthesia/sedation the most appropriate way to provide the necessary treatment?
   b. Can the proposed treatment be successfully completed under anaesthesia/sedation?
2. *The patient*
   a. Is the patient fit for anaesthesia/sedation?
   b. Has the patient understood the possible risks of the planned procedure and given written consent?
3. *The facilities*
   a. Are the premises, staff and equipment suitable for the proposed anaesthesia/sedation and dental treatment?

19. Emergencies in dental practice

Dentists must know how to recognise and manage medical emergencies, rare though they may be. Their professional skill and equipment should enable them to make a useful contribution and sometimes even save patients' lives. Dentists are also required to ensure that all members of their staff are able to provide practical assistance in these circumstances.

Medical emergencies do not obey strict rules and do not always manifest themselves in the expected way. However, the main hazards that may have to be faced, usually take the following forms:

1. *Sudden loss of consciousness (collapse)*
   a. Fainting
   b. Acute hypoglycaemia
   c. Circulatory collapse of a patient on corticosteroid therapy
   d. Anaphylactic shock
   e. Myocardial infarction
   f. Cardiac arrest
   g. Stroke
2. *Acute chest pain or difficulty in breathing*
   a. Angina
   b. Myocardial infarction
   c. Asthma
   d. Anaphylactic shock
3. *Convulsions*
   a. Epilepsy
   b. Any other cause of loss of consciousness, including fainting
4. *Other emergencies*
   a. Haemorrhage
   b. Drug reactions and interactions.

SUDDEN LOSS OF CONCIOUSNESS (COLLAPSE)

Fainting

Fainting is the most common cause of sudden loss of consciousness in the dental surgery. It is caused by transient hypotension and cerebral ischaemia. Most patients who faint are otherwise healthy adults and the attack is precipitated by anxiety. Some patients are, however, particularly prone to fainting and frequently do so. Predisposing factors include:

1. Anxiety
2. Pain
3. Fatigue
4. Hunger.

Probably the most common precipitating factor is an injection and young fit adult males in particular are particularly susceptible to react in this way.

Signs and symptoms

1. Premonitory dizziness, weakness or nausea
2. Pale, cold moist skin
3. Initially slow and weak pulse becoming full and bounding
4. Loss of consciousness.

The premonitory symptoms usually make the nature of a fainting attack obvious, but sometimes consciousness is lost almost instantaneously.

Management

1. Lower the head, preferably by laying the patient flat. It is harmful to keep a fainting patient upright (this worsens cerebral anoxia)
2. Loosen any tight clothing round the neck
3. Give a sweetened drink when consciousness has been recovered.

Recovery usually comes within a few minutes, but if not other causes of loss of consciousness must be considered, particularly if the patient is elderly. These are discussed below but a persistently rapid, thready or irregular pulse suggests cardiac disease. Alternatively, the pulse may be abnormally slow (bradycardia) if the patient is suffering from heart block as a result of such causes as an earlier myocardial infarct.

Prevention

Regular fainters are frequently helped by being given an anxiolytic, such as temazepam 10 mg orally, on the night before and again an hour before treatment.

Acute hypoglycaemia

Hypoglycaemia affects diabetic patients who have had an overdose of insulin or who have been prevented from eating at the expected time. This in turn may be because of dental treatment.

Signs and symptoms

1. Premonitory signs are similar to those of a faint, but there is little response to laying the patient flat
2. Unconsciousness steadily deepens.

Management

1. The patient is often aware of what is happening and able to warn the dentist. The treatment is then to give glucose tablets or powder, or sugar (at least four lumps) as a sweetened drink, repeated if symptoms are not completely relieved.

2. If consciousness has been lost, give sterile intravenous glucose (up to 50 ml of a 50% solution).

3. Subcutaneous *glucagon* (1 mg) is a satisfactory alternative if sterile glucose is not available. During the brief recovery that the latter should provide, sugar should be given by mouth.

If there is any doubt about the cause of loss of consciousness in a diabetic, insulin must *never* be given. It can be lethal to a patient in hypoglycaemic coma.

Circulatory collapse in patients on corticosteroid treatment

The response of patients on long-term corticosteroid treatment to surgery is unpredictable, but near-fatal circulatory collapse can follow minor dental extractions under anaesthesia in a patient taking as little as 5 mg of prednisone a day. All patients who are having systemic corticosteroids, and even those who have had these drugs in the past, are at risk. Adrenocortical function may possibly take up to 2 years to recover. Corticosteroid skin preparations used lavishly, particularly for widespread eczema, also have systemic effects and have been known to cause severe reactions.

Since large doses of corticosteroids given for a short period are safe and can be life-saving, management should lean towards being overprotective. Prevention is all important (Ch. 10). When overstressed, patients on systemic corticosteroids have died of circulatory collapse, despite all supportive efforts.

Causes of collapse

General anaesthesia, surgical or other trauma, infections or other stress are the main causes.

Signs and symptoms

1. Pallor
2. Rapid, weak or impalpable pulse
3. Loss of consciousness
4. Rapidly falling blood pressure.

Management

1. Lay the patient flat and raise the legs
2. Give at least 200 mg hydrocortisone sodium

succinate intravenously (the intramuscular route can be used if a vein cannot be found but absorption is slower)
3. Call an ambulance for immediate transfer to hospital
4. Give oxygen and, if necessary, artificial ventilation
5. Consider other possible reasons for loss of consciousness.

Anaphylactic reactions

Penicillin is the most common cause of acute anaphylactic reactions. Similar reactions due to histamine release by intravenous barbiturate anaesthetics or sedatives are rare. Anaphylactic reactions can also be precipitated by insect stings, foods (nuts or shellfish particularly), and exceptionally rarely by aspirin or latex gloves.

In general, the quicker the onset the more severe the reaction. A severe reaction to penicillin may start within a minute of an injection, but immediate loss of consciousness is more likely to be due to fainting. A reaction starting 30 min after an injection is unlikely to be dangerous. Acute reactions to oral penicillins are exceptionally rare but can develop after half an hour or more because of slower absorption from the gut.

Collapse is due to widespread vasodilatation and increased capillary permeability causing potentially fatal hypotension.

Signs and symptoms

The clinical picture is variable. Typical features include:

1. Initial facial flushing, itching, paraesthesiae or cold extremities
2. Bronchospasm (wheezing) is sometimes a prominent feature
3. Loss of consciousness
4. Pallor going on to cyanosis
5. Cold clammy skin
6. Rapid weak or impalpable pulse
7. Facial oedema or sometimes urticaria
8. Deep fall in blood pressure.

Death can quickly follow if treatment is delayed or inappropriate.

Management

1. Lay the patient flat, with the legs raised, to improve cerebral blood flow
2. Give adrenaline (0.5–1 ml of 1:1000) by intramuscular injection
3. Give 10–20 mg chlorpheniramine diluted in the syringe with 10 ml of blood or saline slowly intravenously
4. Give 200 mg of hydrocortisone sodium succinate intravenously
5. Give oxygen and, if necessary, assisted ventilation
6. Call an ambulance.

Adrenaline acts rapidly. It raises cardiac output, combats excessive capillary permeability and bronchospasm, and also inhibits release of mediators from mast cells. The action of adrenaline is relatively short lived and administration can be repeated every 10 min if necessary until the patient responds. Circulatory collapse is probably largely due to histamine release which is combatted by the parenteral chlorpheniramine. However, there should be no delay in giving hydrocortisone in the hope that adrenaline alone may be effective. Hydrocortisone takes an hour or so to take effect, but maintains the blood pressure for some hours and combats the continued effect of the antigen–antibody reaction.

The patient should be transferred to hospital as soon as possible where the circulation can be supported by intravenous fluids and any other necessary measure can be provided. The patient must also be given a card warning against the use of penicillin in the future.

Myocardial infarction

A patient may suddenly lose consciousness as a result of myocardial infarction, but typically has severe chest pain as described below.

Cardiac arrest

Cardiac arrest can follow myocardial infarction or the acute hypotension of an anaphylactic reaction or corticosteroid insufficiency. Alternatively, it may be the result of an anaesthetic accident and due to hypoxia, anaesthetic overdose or severe hypotension.

Dentists should be aware of and alert to the possibility of cardiac arrest and be able to recognise it when it happens. The dental team should know what to do in such an emergency and also the extent of their limitations.

Speed of response is essential. The dental team should have practised and, once the emergency is recognised, be able to institute cardiopulmonary resuscitation immediately.

Signs and symptoms

1. Loss of consciousness
2. Absence of arterial pulses (the carotid artery, anterior to sternomastoid should be felt).

It is essential to start resuscitation before respiratory arrest and eventual cyanosis, pupil dilatation and loss of reaction to light, and absence of measurable blood pressure become apparent.

Management

1. Summon help and get another assistant to telephone for an ambulance and state that there has been a cardiac arrest.

2. Put the patient on a firm flat surface, such as the floor, if possible. If the patient is too heavy to lift out of a dental chair and can be laid supine there, resuscitation can be carried out by the operator and assistant standing beside the chair, An operator's stool can be placed under the headrest to stabilise the chair.

3. Clear the airway and keep it clear by extending the neck and holding the jaw forward.

4. Start external cardiac compression immediately. Kneel (or stand) beside the patient and put one hand over the other on the patient's lower sternum. Depress the sternum about 1.5–2 in. (4–5 cm) at about 80 times a minute. Compression must be forceful and the danger of cracking a rib must be disregarded. The optimal pressure is about 40 or 50 kg (allow the weight of the upper part of the body to be applied through stiffly extended arms). External cardiac compression is tiring and, if possible, another person should take over as soon as the first operator shows signs of fatigue.

5. The assistant should inflate the lungs between each five compressions of the sternum, either using a mouth-to-mouth procedure or with a self-inflating bag with oxygen supplementation, as described below.

6. Persist until expert help arrives or there are signs of restoration of blood pressure with disappearance of facial pallor, and a good spontaneous pulse. Other signs of success are contraction of the pupils, return of reflex activity such as the blink reflex and reaction of the pupils to light, lightening of unconsciousness and purposeful spontaneous movements – not twitching or convulsions.

7. Transfer the patient to hospital for advanced life support.

If no signs of life appear within 15 min (timed by the clock) recovery is unlikely.

Unless the operator is skilled in its use, time should not be wasted in trying to pass an endotracheal tube. However, a self-inflating bag with an oxygen supply should be available to provide positive-pressure ventilation. A plastic airway should be put in the patient's mouth and the mask applied firmly over the nose and mouth with the resuscitation bag attached. The patient's lungs should be inflated with oxygen by squeezing the bag, so that the chest is visibly expanded at each respiration. Passive recoil of the chest wall causes spontaneous expiration as soon as the pressure is removed.

If a self-inflating bag is not available, mouth-to-mouth ventilation can be given preferably with an intervening Laerdal pocket mask.

During artificial ventilation the patient's nose must be closed. Deep inflations are given by the operator and time allowed for passive recoil of the chest. If there is no airway adjunct available, direct mouth-to-mouth resuscitation with the nose occluded must be given.

Causes of failure

The most common mistakes are:

1. Giving external cardiac compression without artificial ventilation.

2. Giving artificial ventilation without external cardiac compression.

3. Failing to clear the airway or to make sure that it remains open by failing to hyperextend the head adequately.

4. Failing to close the nose during mouth-to-mouth ventilation.

5. Failing to make a close fit with the mask on the patient's face when using an inflating bag.

6. Failing to make sure that ventilation is adequate, as shown by the movement of the chest.

7. Timidity in applying external cardiac compression, and as a result using insufficient force to compress the heart.

8. Failing to release pressure on the chest completely between compressions and preventing cardiac filling as a consequence.

9. Compressing the chest too rapidly to allow enough time for the heart to fill between compressions.

10. Putting the hands in the incorrect position.

11. Failing to act sufficiently quickly and fretting about details rather than getting on with the essentials of external cardiac compression and artificial ventilation.

Stroke

Patients are usually hypertensive and middle-aged or elderly.

Signs and symptoms

1. Loss of consciousness
2. Weakness of an arm and leg on one side
3. Drooping of the side of the face.

However, the picture varies with the size and site of brain damage. Subarachnoid haemorrhage as a result of rupture of a berry aneurysm on the circle of Willis is the only cause of stroke in a younger person. There is typically intense headache followed by coma without localising signs.

Management

1. Maintain the airway
2. Call an ambulance and transfer the patient to hospital.

CHEST PAIN OR DIFFICULTY IN BREATHING

Angina

A patient with coronary atheroma could conceivably have a first anginal attack as a consequence of an emotional response to dental treatment. However, more patients will already have had attacks and carry medication.

Signs and symptoms

Acute chest pain.

Management

1. Give the patient his antianginal drug (usually 0.5 mg of glyceryl trinitrate sublingually)
2. If there is no relief within 3 min the patient has probably had a myocardial infarction.

Myocardial infarction

Myocardial infarction is a common cause of death and must be recognised, as the patient's fate may be decided by treatment given in the first few minutes. Several aspects of dentistry, particularly apprehension, pain or the effect of drugs could contribute to make this accident more likely in a susceptible patient.

Some patients die within a few minutes after the start of the attack and it is rash to try over-ambitious management. Drugs, apart from those described below, should not be used as, without continuous monitoring, they can sometimes do more harm than good.

Signs and symptoms

1. Severe crushing retrosternal pain
2. Vomiting
3. Weak or irregular pulse.

Pain can radiate to the left shoulder or down the left arm and is occasionally felt only in the left jaw. Vomiting is common and there is sometimes shock or loss of consciousness.

Management

1. Place the patient in a comfortable position that allows easy breathing (do not lay flat if there is left ventricular failure and pulmonary oedema).

2. Send an assistant to telephone for an intensive-care ambulance.

3. Give 50/50 nitrous oxide and oxygen from a

general anaesthetic or relative analgesia machine, to relieve pain and anxiety.

4. Constantly reassure the patient.
5. Give oxygen if necessary.

Aspirin is a valuable antiplatelet drug but it is only feasible to give a fibrinolytic drug such as streptokinase in hospital where lignocaine or other antidysrhythmic drugs can be given as appropriate.

Asthma and status asthmaticus

Causes

Loss of or forgetting to bring a salbutamol inhaler. Anxiety, infection or exposure to a specific allergen can contribute.

Signs and symptoms

1. Breathlessness
2. Expiratory wheezing (this may be disguised by shallow breathing)
3. Rapid pulse (usually over 110 per minute)
4. Accessory muscles of respiration may start to come in action.

Management

1. Reassure the patient
2. Do not lay the patient flat
3. Give the antiasthmatic drugs normally used (such as salbutamol inhaler)
4. Give hydrocortisone sodium succinate (200 mg) intravenously
5. Give oxygen
6. Ideally, if there is no response within 2–3 min salbutamol (500 μg/ml) should be given by IM or SC injection (***Note:* amino-phylline has no advantages, is more dangerous and is no longer recommended for acute asthma)**
7. Call an ambulance for transfer to hospital.

CONVULSIONS

Epilepsy

Hunger, menstruation and some drugs such as methohexitone, tricyclic antidepressants or alcohol may sometimes precipitate a fit.

Signs and symptoms of a tonic–clonic attack

1. Sometimes there is a brief warning cry as the chest muscles contract and air is forced through a closed larynx
2. Consciousness is lost immediately
3. The patient's body becomes rigid (tonic phase) and becomes cyanotic
4. Widespread jerking movements start (clonic phase)
5. There is sometimes incontinence or frothing of the mouth
6. The patient usually becomes flaccid after a few minutes
7. Consciousness is regained after a variable period, but the patient may remain confused.

Management

1. Put the patient prone in the coma ('recovery') position as soon as fits have stopped
2. Make sure the airway is clear after convulsions have subsided
3. Prevent the patient from damaging himself but do not try to put anything in the mouth in an attempt to prevent the patient biting the tongue
4. Do not give any medication but await recovery
5. Reassure the patient as soon as consciousness returns
6. Only allow the patient to return home when fully recovered and preferably accompanied by a responsible adult.

Status epilepticus

If convulsions do not stop within 15 min or are rapidly repeated the patient is in status epilepticus and can die from anoxia.

Management

1. Give 10 mg intravenous diazepam to an adult patient
2. If venous access cannot be obtained give 5 mg of intramuscular midazolam (absorption of intramuscular diazepam is too slow and erratic)
3. Repeat diazepam or midazolam if there is no recovery within 5 min
4. Maintain the airway and give oxygen

5. Call an ambulance and transfer the patient to hospital.

Fainting

As described earlier, transient convulsions can result from fainting.

OTHER EMERGENCIES

Haemorrhage

Causes

1. Prolonged bleeding is usually due to traumatic extractions. A major vessel is unlikely to be opened during dental surgery and patients are unlikely to lose a dangerous quantity of blood if promptly managed. Postextraction bleeding is only an emergency in the sense that the dentist may be woken up at 3 o'clock in the morning by a frightened patient.
2. Occasionally bleeding is due to unsuspected haemophilia or other causes such as anticoagulant treatment.

Management

1. Reassure the patient.
2. Usher excited relatives out of the surgery.
3. Clean the mouth with swabs and locate the source of bleeding.
4. Give a local anaesthetic, remove ragged tissue, squeeze up the socket mouth, and put a suture over it.
5. When bleeding has been controlled, ask about the history and especially any family history of prolonged bleeding.
6. If bleeding is uncontrollable despite suturing or if the patient is obviously anaemic or debilitated, then transfer to hospital for investigation and management of any haemorrhagic defect.
7. In the interim limit bleeding as much as possible with a pressure pad over the socket and by supporting the patient's jaw with a firm barrel bandage.
8. Tranexamic acid (500 mg in 5 ml, by slow intravenous injection) may be effective in a mild haemophiliac and may be given in the hospital.

Drug reactions and interactions

Apart from the anaphylactic reactions discussed earlier, very few other drug reactions or interactions endangering life are likely to be seen in the dental surgery.

1. *Noradrenaline*, when used as a vasoconstrictor in high concentration (1:20 000), has caused deaths from acute hypertension, some from cerebral haemorrhage. Quite apart from its dangers, noradrenaline has no advantages and should not be used in local anaesthetic solutions. The treatment is to give an α blocker such as phentolamine.

   There is no clinical evidence of hypertensive reactions to *adrenaline* used in normal concentration and quantity.
2. *Monoamine oxidase inhibitors* can cause severe reactions with opioids, particularly pethidine. The reaction can be very sudden in onset. Monoamine oxidase inhibitors also interact with indirectly acting sympathomimetic agents (drugs such as ephedrine used as a nasal decongestant) to cause acute severe hypertension. The treatment is to give an α blocker such as phentolamine. Adrenaline or noradrenaline do not cause hypertensive reactions with monoamine oxidase inhibitors (MAOIs).
3. *General anaesthetics*, particularly intravenous barbiturates, are the main cause of fatalities in the dental surgery (Ch. 18).
4. As already described, patients on long-term *corticosteroid* treatment, when exposed to stress, can suffer circulatory collapse as a result of adrenal suppression.

Appendix: Antibiotic prophylaxis of infective endocarditis and related problems

The Endocarditis Working Party of the British Society for Antimicrobial Chemotherapy made the following recommendations (1993) for patients with congenital or acquired heart defects, or with prosthetic heart valves or a history of infective endocarditis. For these patients antibiotic prophylaxis should be given when ***extractions, scaling*** or ***periodontal surgery*** are to be carried out.

For the purposes of general practice only the recommendations for patients in group A are relevant. Apart from the fact that general anaesthesia in general practice is discouraged, ***few of the recommended regimens for patients in groups B and C could reasonably be administered in general practice***.

A. Patients not requiring a general anaesthetic *and with no special risks*

i. Patients who are not allergic to the penicillins and who have not received penicillin more than once in the previous month:

Amoxycillin

Adults: a single dose of 3 g orally 1 h before the operation, taken in the presence of the dentist or dental surgery assistant.

Children under 10 years: half the adult dose.

Children under 5 years: a quarter of the adult dose.

ii. Patients allergic to the penicillins or who have received penicillin more than once in the previous month:

Clindamycin

Adults: 600 mg single oral dose taken under supervision 1 h before the dental procedure.

Children age 5–10 years: half the adult dose.

Children under 5 years: a quarter of the adult dose.

B. Patients requiring a general anaesthetic but not allergic to the penicillins

Amoxycillin parenterally

Adults: intravenously 1 g, or intramuscularly 1 g in 2.5 ml of 1% lignocaine at the time of induction, followed by 500 mg of amoxycillin orally 6 h later.

OR (if agreed by the anaesthetist)

Oral amoxycillin

Adults: 3 g, 4 h before induction and repeated as soon as possible after the operation.

OR

Amoxycillin and probenecid orally

Adults: 3 g amoxycillin plus oral probenecid 1 g, 4 h before induction.

C. Special problem patients who should always be referred to hospital

a. Those who have had a previous attack of infective endocarditis (thus indicating susceptibility to the disease), *irrespective of whether or not a general anaesthetic is to be given.*

b. Patients who are to have a general anaesthetic, but who have a prosthetic heart valve.*

c. Patients who are allergic to the penicillins or have received a penicillin more than once in the

* It is controversial as to whether these patients are at special risk, but since it is a possibility, general anaesthesia allows a more potent antimicrobial mixture to be given.

previous month, and are to have a general anaesthetic.

i. Patients not allergic to the penicillins and who have not received a penicillin more than once in the previous month:

Amoxycillin plus gentamicin

Adults: amoxycillin 1 g intravenously or 1 g intramuscularly in 2.5 ml of 1% lignocaine plus gentamicin 120 mg intravenously or intramuscularly at the time of induction. A further 0.5 mg of amoxycillin should be given orally 6 h later.

Children 5–10 years: amoxycillin, half the adult dose; gentamicin 2 mg/kg.

Children under 5 years: amoxycillin a quarter of the adult dose; gentamicin 2 mg/kg.

ii. Patients allergic to the penicillins or who have received a penicillin more than once in the previous month, and are to have a general anaesthetic:

Vancomycin plus gentamicin

Adults: vancomycin 1 g by slow intravenous infusion over at least 100 min followed by 120 mg of gentamicin intravenously at the time of induction or 15 min before the surgical procedure.

Children under 10 years: vancomycin by slow intravenous infusion 20 mg/kg followed by gentamicin 2 mg/kg intravenously.

OR

Teicoplanin plus gentamicin

Adults: teicoplanin 400 mg intravenously plus gentamicin 120 mg at the time of induction or 15 min before the surgical procedure.

Children under 14 years: teicoplanin 6 mg/kg intravenously plus gentamicin 2 mg/kg intravenously.

OR

Clindamycin

Adults: clindamycin 300 mg by intravenous infusion over at least 10 min at the time of induction or 15 min before the surgical procedure, followed by 150 mg orally or by intravenous infusion over at least 10 min 6 h later.

Children 5–10 years: half the adult dose.

Children under 5 years: a quarter of the adult dose.

Additional measures (all patients)

1. Irrigation of the gingival margins or pockets with an antiseptic such as 0.5% chlorhexidine before the dental procedure will reduce the severity of any resulting bacteraemia and may usefully supplement antibiotic prophylaxis in those at risk.

2. Regular dental care for the maintenance of optimal dental health in those at risk should reduce the frequency and severity of any bacteraemias and also reduce the need for extractions.

3. More important still is that, even when antibiotic cover has been given, *patients at risk should be instructed to report any unexplained illness*. Infective endocarditis is often exceedingly insidious in origin and may develop 2 or more months after an operation. Late diagnosis considerably increases both the mortality or disability among survivors.

4. Patients at risk should carry a warning card to be shown to their dentist at each visit to indicate the danger of infective endocarditis and the need for antibiotic prophylaxis. These cards are available free of charge from the British Heart Foundation, 14 Fitzhardinge Street, London W1H 4DH, UK.

PATIENTS WITH PROSTHETIC HIP REPLACEMENTS

Antibiotic prophylaxis for dental procedures on these patients is not recommended. These procedures have been carried out on an enormous scale in recent decades, but there is considerable doubt whether any of these prosthetic joints have ever been infected as a result of a dental procedure.

PATIENTS WITH IMMUNODEFICIENCY DISEASES

Though these patients can develop septicaemias or metastatic infections by oral microbes, there is little evidence of such infections as a consequence of dental procedures. Remarkably, there appears to be little or no evidence of patients with AIDS being at greater risk of infective endocarditis than other patients. In any case, it would be impossible to devise a practical regimen as the range of bacteria that cause opportunistic infections is so wide.

There appears therefore to be no special case for antimicrobial prophylaxis for dental treatment on immunodeficient patients unless they have heart defects.

Index